# Dictionary of Nutrition
and Food Technology

*Should this book become sufficiently familiar through usage to earn the title 'Bender's Dictionary', it would probably be more correct to call it 'Benders' Dictionary', in view of the invaluable assistance of D., D.A. and B.G., guided, if not driven, by A.E.*

# Dictionary of Nutrition and Food Technology

Sixth Edition

## Arnold E. Bender
DSc(hc), PhD, HonMAPHA, HonFRSH, FIFST

*Formerly Professor of Nutrition and Dietetics, Queen Elizabeth College, University of London*

Butterworths

London   Boston   Singapore   Sydney   Toronto   Wellington

⬤ PART OF REED INTERNATIONAL P.L.C.

First published 1960
Second edition 1965
Third edition 1968
Fourth edition by Newnes–Butterworth 1975
Fifth edition by Butterworth Scientific 1982
Reprinted 1984
Sixth edition 1990

© **Butterworth & Co (Publishers) Ltd, 1990**

**British Library Cataloguing in Publication Data**

Bender, Arnold E. (Arnold Eric), *1918*–
  Dictionary of nutrition and food technology.—6th ed.
  1. Man. Nutrition   2. Food. Processing
  I. Title
  613.2

ISBN 0-408-03753-9

**Library of Congress Cataloging in Publication Data**

Bender, Arnold E. (Arnold Eric)
  Dictionary of nutrition and food technology/
Arnold E. Bender.—6th ed.
    p.   cm.
  Includes bibliographical references.
  ISBN 0-408-03753-9 :
  1. Nutrition—Dictionaries. 2. Food—Dictionaries. I. Title.
  [DNLM: 1. Food-Processing Industry—dictionaries.
  2. Nutrition—dictionaries.   QU 13 B458d]
TX349.B4   1990
641'.03—dc20
DNLM/DLC                                          90-1936

Composition by Genesis Typesetting, Laser Quay, Rochester, Kent
Printed and bound by Hartnolls Ltd, Bodmin, Cornwall

# Preface

The study of food and nutrition starts with genetic selection then proceeds to food production (farming, animal production, fishing, etc.) via food science to the technology of food processing, packaging and distribution, its preparation and consumption and then, logically, to its fate in the body and medical aspects of good or poor diets. Along the way are the complex sociological and physiological aspects of food choice.

All this involves many disciplines and basic sciences – chemistry, physics, biochemistry, biophysics, microbiology, physiology, and the social sciences, along with legal and medical aspects. It is clearly difficult for any one person to be familiar with all the technical terms used. So many readers and practitioners involved in food and nutrition may need to seek the meaning of, at least, some of them.

At the same time individuals – laymen, journalists, managers in the food industry and policy makers in nutrition and public health areas – are reading literature dealing with food and nutrition; they may need to look up explanations which might be commonplace to the specialists.

Changes are continuous in this area with 'new' foods, new processes, new safety hazards (or old ones that have become more important), rapid developments in methods of food analysis and quality control, and particularly in our understanding of the relations between diet and health. All this gives rise to a need for a dictionary.

At the same time some terms become obsolete and disappear from current textbooks so that readers of the earlier literature may be at a loss.

All these items, so far as the author is aware, are included so that the reader of food literature need not be left wondering.

If it is true to say that it is difficult for any one person to be familiar with all the terms used, then this must apply equally to the author, who apologises for errors of omission and commission in the hope of assistance from readers and reviewers.

Arnold E. Bender

# Note on food composition

Any specified food will differ in composition from sample to sample, quite apart from variations due to experimental error and methods of analysis, which partly explains why foods of the same type show compositional differences between data published in different countries. For this reason all compositional data presented here must be regarded as an approximation to the average for that type of food and not with precision – as, indeed, must all composition tables.

Since vitamin A can be present in foods as preformed retinol and as its precursor carotene, it is usual to quote figures in terms of 'retinol equivalents'. Vitamin E is present in foods in several forms of different biological potencies and figures are quoted as alpha-tocopherol equivalents.

Niacin is present in foods as the preformed vitamin and can also be formed in the body from the amino acid, tryptophan. Tables of food composition usually state niacin figures in terms of niacin equivalents (preformed niacin plus 1/60 of the tryptophan): the figures of niacin content of foods shown here are for the preformed vitamin only.

# Contents

# A

$a_w$   Available water. See *water activity*.

**abalone**   A snail-like shellfish (gastropod mollusc) of the genus *Haliotis*, found particularly in waters around Australia, and also Japan, California, Channel Islands and France. The meat is canned and frozen. Also called ormer. Analysis per 100 g: 19 g protein, 3 g carbohydrate, 100 kcal (400 kJ).

**Abbé refractometer**   See *refractometer*.

**Abernethy biscuit**   Scottish biscuit made from flour, sugar, butter, eggs, milk and caraway seeds; named after Dr John Abernethy (1764–1831) of St Bartholomew's Hospital, London.

**abomasum**   See *rumen*.

**absinthe**   Green liqueur prepared from oils of wormwood, angelica, anise and marjoram. It is toxic and the manufacture has been banned in many countries. The toxic principle is oil of thujol, which is a cerebral convulsant and is cumulative.

**absorptiometer**   Instrument used to measure the absorption of light, and therefore used as a quantitative measure of coloured solutions. Frequently (incorrectly) called colorimeter. Many substances, minerals, vitamins, amino acids, will react with a particular reagent to form a coloured complex. The colour developed is proportional to the amount present and is measured in an absorptiometer or a true colorimeter.

**acarbose**   Generic name for a group of complex oligosaccharides isolated from culture broth of *Actinomycetes*, which inhibit the enzymes glucoamylase, sucrase, maltase and dextrinase; used experimentally to restrict digestive hydrolysis of dietary carbohydrates and so reduce postprandial hyperglycaemia and hyperinsulinaemia.

   The core structure, acarviosine, is made up of a substituted cyclohexene ring and 4,6-dideoxy-4-amino-D-glucose.

**acaridicides**   Chemicals used to kill mites and ticks.

**acarviosine**   See *acarbose*.

**accelase**   Mixture of proteolytic enzymes including an exopeptidase from the dairy starter bacterium, *Streptococcus lactis*; used to shorten maturation time of cheese and intensify the flavour of processed cheese.

1

**Ac'cent** Trade name (International Mineral & Chemical Corpn, USA) for monosodium glutamate. See *glutamic acid*.

**acerola** West Indian cherry; see *cherry, West Indian*.

**acesulfames** Also acesulphames. Class of artificial, non-nutritive sweeteners from oxathiazinone. The potassium salt, called acesulfame-K, is 200 times as sweet as sucrose; not metabolised and excreted unchanged; good shelf life.

**acetate, active** The form in which the acetyl radical, $CH_3CO-$, is transferred from one compound to another, as the acetyl–coenzyme A complex (see *coenzyme A*). The metabolism both of glucose and of fats involves the formation of active acetate.

**acetate replacement factor** See *lipoic acid*.

**acetic acid** One of the simplest organic acids – $CH_3COOH$. Formed by fermentation of ethyl alcohol (secondary fermentation) and formed in some fermented foods together with lactic acid, both of which serve to preserve such foods – i.e. the process of pickling. May also be added to foods and sauces to preserve them.

*Acetobacter* Genus of bacteria of family Bacteriaceae, which oxidises alcohol to acetic acid. *Acetobacter pasteurianus* (also known as *Mycoderma aceti* and *Bacterium aceti* or *pasteurianum*) is one of this type and is used in the manufacture of vinegar. Also grow in film on beer wort, pickle brine and fruit juices. See also *vinegar*.

**acetoglycerides** Differ from the triglycerides in that either one or two of the long-chain fatty acids attached to the glycerol molecule are replaced by acetic acid. There are three types: diacetotriglycerides (e.g.diacetomonostearin); monoacetotriglycerides (e.g. monoacetodistearin); and monoacetodiglycerides (e.g. monoacetomonostearin), in which one hydroxyl group of the glycerol is free. Also known as partial glyceride esters.

They are non-greasy and have lower melting points than the corresponding triglycerides, and are used in shortenings and spreads, as films for coating foods, and as plasticisers for hard fats.

**acetoin** Acetyl methyl carbinol, $CH_3COCHOHCH_3$, precursor of diacetyl, butter flavour. Produced by bacteria during butter ripening and by yeast during fermentation.

**acetone bodies** See *ketone bodies*.

**acetylcholine** Acetyl derivative of choline (which see) which is liberated at certain nerve endings (cholinergic nerves) to stimulate the muscle.

**ACH index** Arm, chest, hip index. The arm girth, chest diameter and hip width used as a method of assessing the state of nutrition.

**achlorhydria**   Deficiency of hydrochloric acid in the gastric secretion.

**achromotrichia**   Loss of hair pigment. See *pantothenic acid*; *para-amino benzoic acid*.

**achroodextrin**   Product formed during the enzymic breakdown of starch to maltose; it is a dextrin that gives no colour with iodine (hence achro).

**acid–base balance**   Body fluids are maintained just on the alkaline side of neutrality, pH 7.3–7.45, by buffers in the blood and tissues. Buffers include proteins, and sodium and potassium phosphate and bicarbonate.

Acidic products of the body's metabolism are excreted in the urine in combination with bases such as sodium and potassium. These bases are thereby lost to the body and the acid–base balance is maintained by replacing them from the diet.

Buffer materials in the blood and tissues are termed the alkaline reserve.

**acid calcium phosphate**   See *calcium acid phosphate*.

**acid foods and basic foods**   Refers to the residue of the metabolism of the food – the minerals sodium, potassium, magnesium and calcium are base-forming, and phosphorus, sulphur and chlorine are acid-forming, and which of these predominates determines whether the food leaves an acid or basic residue. Meat, fish, eggs, cheese and cereals leave an acid residue; milk, vegetables and some fruits leave an alkaline residue; fats and sugar contain no minerals and so are neutral foods.

Fruit juices contain acids and their sodium salts and have an acid taste, but the organic portion is completely oxidised and the residual sodium leaves an alkaline residue.

See also *acid–base balance*.

**acid number**   With reference to fats, a measure of hydrolytic rancidity. Defined as milligrams of caustic potash required to neutralise the free fatty acids in 1 g of the fat.

The acid number, also known as the acid value, is an index of the efficiency of refining, during which process the free fatty acids are removed and the acid number falls to very low values; it is also an index of the deterioration in storage.

**acidophilus therapy**   Consumption of milk containing a high concentration of viable *Lactobacillus acidophilus* (the milk itself being unfermented) as a treatment for constipation. The effect is said to be due to the implantation of these organisms in the intestine.

**acidosis**   Increase in the ratio between acid and base in the blood plasma, or a reduction in its buffering power. Causes may be alteration in carbon dioxide excretion, metabolic overproduction of acid or excessive loss of base. See also *acid–base balance*.

**acid rebound** Term used in reference to the secretion of gastric acid to signify the increase in acidity of the stomach that results from the administration of alkalies. There is conflicting evidence as to whether this really occurs.

**acid value** See *acid number*.

**ackee** Fruit of *Blighia sapida* common in West Indies. Unripe fruits contain hypoglycin (α-amino-β-methylene cyclopropanyl-propionic acid – hypoglycin A, and its peptide – hypoglycin B) in quantities sufficient to reduce blood glucose levels and cause 'vomiting sickness', coma and death.

**aconitine** Toxic alkaloid of monkshood (*Aconitum*); slows the pulse and reduces blood pressure; fatal in small doses.

**acorn sugar** Quercitol, extracted from acorns; pentahydroxy-cyclohexane.

**ACP** Acid calcium phosphate. See *calcium acid phosphate*.

**acraldehyde** See *acrolein*.

**acrodynia** Specific type of dermatitis seen in animals fed on diet deficient in vitamin $B_6$.

**acrolein** Acraldehyde, $CH_2=CHCHO$. Formed when glycerol is heated to a high temperature, and responsible for the acrid odour and lachrymatory vapour produced when fats are over-heated.

**Acronize** Trade name (Cyanamide Co., USA) for the antibiotic chlortetracycline (used, for example, as 'acronized ice').

**ACTH** Abbreviation for adrenocorticotropic hormone, which see.

**actin** See *actomysin*.

**activators** With reference to enzymes, substances that increase the activity of the enzyme in a non-specific manner. Those substances that are part of the activating system, and are required before the enzyme can activate its substrate, are activators. Substances that are part of the reaction system but play no part in the activation of the substrate are coenzymes. Many inorganic radicals are activators; thus, salivary amylase requires the presence of chloride; others are potassium, calcium, magnesium, phosphate.

**active oxygen method** A method of measuring the stability of fats and oils by bubbling air through the heated material and following the formation of peroxides. Also known as the Swift stability test.

**actomyosin** The two principal proteins of muscle, actin (about 13% of muscle protein) and myosin (about two-fifths of muscle protein), form actomyosin during muscle contraction with the simultaneous hydrolysis of ATP to ADP.

**Addison's disease**   Destruction of the cortex of the suprarenal glands; symptoms are low blood pressure, anaemia, muscular weakness, fall in metabolic rate. Treatment partly successful by taking sodium chloride, or by implantation of pellets of deoxycorticosterone acetate.

**additives**   Include all materials deliberately added to food to help manufacture and preserve food, improve palatability and eye-appeal; for example, emulsifiers, flavours, thickeners, curing agents, humectants, colours, vitamins, minerals, and mould, yeast and bacterial inhibitors. Most of these are controlled by law in all countries.

**additives, baking**   See *baking additives*.

**adenine**   See *nucleic acids*; *purines*.

**adenosine**   Combination of the base adenine with the sugar ribose. See *adenosine nucleotides*.

**adenosine diphosphate** (ADP)   See *adenosine nucleotides*.

**adenosine monophosphate**   See *adenylic acid*.

**adenosine nucleotides**   Adenosine triphosphate (ATP) has three phosphate moieties esterified to adenosine. Two of these are associated with a high free energy of hydrolysis, and are often called 'high-energy' phosphates; they are readily available for transfer to other compounds, and are a common method of energy transfer in reactions. In general, oxidative (energy-yielding) metabolism leads to the synthesis of ATP from ADP, while synthetic reactions, which require energy, involve the use of phosphate from ATP to yield ADP (adenosine diphosphate).

Cyclic AMP (cAMP) is formed from ATP by the action of adenyl cyclase; this enzyme is frequently activated in cell membranes by hormones and neurotransmitters, and acts as a second messenger for the hormone; it is a common allosteric effector of regulatory enzymes.

**adenosine triphosphate**   See *adenosine nucleotides*.

**adenylic acid**   Combination of the base adenine with the sugar ribose, and phosphoric acid. Also known as adenosine monophosphate, or AMP; of importance in muscle metabolism.

**adenyl pyrophosphate**   See *adenosine nucleotides*.

**adermin**   See *vitamin $B_6$*.

**adipose tissue**   Groups of cells that store and mobilise fat; constitutes one-fifth to one-quarter of the total body mass – more in fat people. Composed of 82–88% fat, 2–2.6% protein and 10–14% water and contains 8–9 kcal (34–38 kJ) per gram or 3600–4000 (15.1–16.8 MJ) per pound.

**Adirondack bread**   Baked product made from ground maize, butter, wheat flour, eggs and sugar (USA speciality).

**adlay**   A tall grass, *Coix lachryma-jobi*, Job's tears, which grows wild in parts of Africa and Asia and is used as a cereal to eke out rice supplies in countries in S.E. Pacific area. Same tribe as maize – Tripsaceae.

Analysis per 100 g: 14 g protein, 4 g fat, 4 mg Fe, 0.3 mg vitamin $B_1$, 0.2 mg vitamin $B_2$, 3 mg niacin, 360 kcal (1.5 MJ).

**ADI**   Acceptable daily intake: refers to chemical additives used in food processing.

**ADP**   See *adenosine nucleotides*.

**adrenal glands**   Also called suprarenal glands; situated just above each kidney. Comprise the inner part, or medulla, which secretes adrenaline and noradrenaline (which see), and the outer cortex, which secretes steroid hormones.

Steroid hormones include steroid sex hormones, corticosterone (affects carbohydrate metabolism and is anti-inflammatory) and aldosterone (controls excretion of salt and water through the kidneys).

**adrenaline**   Hormone secreted by the medulla of the adrenal glands; the first hormone to be discovered. It is secreted under conditions of emotional stress, and causes an increase in blood pressure, blood sugar levels and metabolic rate, thus mobilising the body's reserves of energy.

Also known as epinephrine, chemically hydroxy, dihydroxy-phenyl-ethylmethylamine.

**adrenocorticotropic hormone**   Hormone extracted from the anterior part of the pituitary gland of animals and used in the treatment of rheumatoid arthritis. Acts by stimulating the adrenal gland to secrete corticosteroids.

**adverse reactions (to food)**   (1) Food aversion – an unpleasant reaction caused by emotions associated with the food rather than the food itself; it does not occur in a blind trial.

(2) Food intolerance – a reproducible unpleasant reaction to food which is not psychologically based, subdivided into: (a) allergy – the body's immune system reacts to traces of a substance (to which the individual has been previously exposed); (b) irritants (e.g. highly spiced foods); (c) pharmacological effects caused by substances in the food, e.g. natural toxicants, caffeine; (d) inability to metabolise the substance because of enzyme defects.

**aequum**   Amount of food necessary to maintain body weight under normal or specified conditions of activity (rarely used).

**aerobes**   Micro-organisms that need oxygen for growth. Obligate aerobes cannot survive in the absence of oxygen.

**aesculin**   (esculin)   Dihydroxycoumarin glucoside found in the leaves and the bark of the horse chestnut tree, *Aesculus hippocastanum*. Has effect on capillary fragility, which see.

**AFD** Accelerated freeze-drying. See *freeze-drying*.

**aflatoxins** Group of complex difurano-coumarins (about 15 are known) formed by some strains of the mould, *Aspergillus flavus*, which can grow on groundnuts and cereals when stored under damp and warm conditions. Originally identified as turkey X disease in UK in 1960.

Aflatoxin B1 is a most potent liver carcinogen in experimental animals and thought to be the cause of primary carcinoma of the liver of human beings in parts of Africa.

If cows consume feed infected with *A. flavus* the aflatoxin B1 is secreted in the milk as aflatoxin M1, so the aflatoxin content of animal feed is strictly limited.

**agar** Dried, purified stems of a seaweed, *Gelidium algae, Gracilaria* and other genera. Partly soluble, and swells with water to form a gel. It has a wide temperature range between gelling and melting points.

Used in soups, jellies, ice-cream, meat and fish pastes, in bacteriological media, for sizing silk, as adhesive and as a stabiliser for emulsions. Also called agar-agar, Macassar gum and vegetable gelatine.

Agar is a galactan, i.e. a complex of galactose units, but it is not digested by man.

**agene** Nitrogen trichloride, once used as bleaching and 'improving' agent for wheat flour in bread making but found to combine with methionine to form methionine sulphoximine, which caused 'canine hysteria' and so was abandoned.

**ageusia** Lack or impairment of sensitivity to taste stimuli.

**agglomeration** Production of a free-flowing, dust-free powder from substances such as dried milk powder and wheat flour. The process consists of moistening with droplets of water and drying in a stream of air; the agglomerates are readily wettable.

**agglutinins** See *lectins*.

**aging** (1) Term applied to chemicals used to oxidise (age) wheat flour for bread making. Freshly milled flour produces a weaker and less resilient dough and less 'bold' loaf than flour which has been stored for some weeks or 'aged' chemically. Substances such as ammonium persulphate, ascorbic acid, chlorine, sulphur dioxide, potassium bromate and cysteine are used as oxidising agents; nitrogen peroxide and benzoyl peroxide, to bleach the flour; chlorine dioxide (and at one time nitrogen trichloride – agene), to bleach the flour and 'improve' the dough. Regulations in many countries control which of these may be used and the amounts.

(2) In reference to wine aging, refers to the development of a 'bouquet' and smooth, mellow flavour and the disappearance of harsh yeasty flavours by slow oxidation and the formation of esters.

(3) With reference to meat, see *rigor mortis*.

**aginomoto**  See *glutamic acid.*

**aglycone**  The non-sugar part of a glycoside.

**agnelloto**  Envelope of pasta stuffed with minced meat or vegetables; cut in half-moon shape, so differing from ravioli, which is cut in squares.

**A/G ratio**  See *albumin/globulin ratio.*

**air classification**  Separation of fractions of powdered material in a current of air by size and composition of the particles on the basis of weight and density. Particularly applied to fractionation of the endosperm of milled wheat flour; the smaller particles are richer on protein – fractions range from 3% to 25% protein.

**aitchbone**  Cut of meat (UK) = rumpbone (USA) = loin or haunch.

**Ajinomoto**  Trade name (Hercules Powder Co.) for range of flavour enhancers – Ajinomoto IMP, disodium inosinate; Ajinomoto GMP, disodium guanylate; Ajinomoto, monosodium glutamate.

**akutok**  Dried strips of caribou meat prepared by Eskimos; outer crust, inside only partly dry.

**alactasia**  Reduction or absence of the digestive enzyme, lactase, resulting in impaired tolerance to milk products.

**alanine**  A non-essential amino acid, amino propionic acid. The alpha amino acid is found in all proteins; there is also beta-alanine (the amino group attached to the second carbon atom), which is part of the molecule of pantothenic acid, of carnosine and of anserine.

**albacore**  Long-finned species of tunny fish, *Thynnus germo*, usually canned as tuna fish.

**albedo**  White pith of the inner peel of citrus fruits, also known as the mesocarp; 20–60% of the whole fruit. Consists of sugars, cellulose and pectins; used as a source of pectin for commercial manufacture.

**albumen**  Variant spelling of albumin (which see), used generally to mean white of egg. See also *egg-white.*

**albumin**  Often used as a non-specific term for protein (e.g. albuminuria means protein present in urine), but strictly refers to simple proteins soluble in water and coagulated by heat, such as ovalbumin in egg, serum albumin in blood, lactalbumin in milk.

**albumin/globulin ratio**   Ratio between the blood albumin and the globulins; in normal human serum, 1.82. Change in the A/G ratio is of diagnostic value.

**albumin index**   A measure of the quality of an egg; the ratio between the height of the albumin and the width when broken on to a flat surface. As the egg deteriorates, the albumin index decreases, i.e. the egg white spreads.

**albumin milk**   See *protein milk*.

**albuminoids** (scleroproteins)   Fibrous proteins that have supporting or protective function in animals (in plants cellulose fulfils this function). Three types: (1) collagens in skin, tendons and bones, resistant to pepsin and trypsin, converted to water-soluble gelatin by boiling with water; (2) elastins in tendons and arteries, not converted to gelatin; (3) keratins, proteins insoluble in dilute acids and alkalies, not attacked by any animal digestive enzymes, comprise horns, hoofs, feathers, scales, nails.

**albumoses**   Old name for proteoses, which see.

**alcaptonuria**   A rare inborn error of metabolism of the two amino acids phenylalanine and tyrosine. Their metabolism ceases at homogentisic acid, which is excreted in the urine. Homogentisic acid oxidises to black melanoid pigments; hence, the urine of alcaptonurics slowly turns black. The defect appears to be harmless.

**alcohol**   Generally refers to ethyl alcohol or ethanol, $C_2H_5OH$, although it is the second member of the series of alcohols of the general formula $C_nH_{2n+1}OH$. Produced by yeast fermentation of sugars, and the basis of a large number of alcoholic beverages ranging from low alcohol beers containing 2% ethanol to spirits with 40%. See also *alcoholic beverages*.

**alcohol, denatured**   Alcohol to which unpleasant materials have been added to prevent it being drunk – e.g. methylated spirits contains 10% methyl alcohol, a blue dye and unpleasant-smelling pyridine. Denatured alcohol is used for industrial purposes and not subject to Excise Duty.

**alcoholic beverages**   Yeast can convert sugar into ethanol until the concentration reaches about 12–14% w/v, at which the yeast dies off. Consequently, this is the maximum alcohol content of wines, depending on the amount of sugar in the grapes. If fermentation is stopped before all the sugar has been fermented, the wine will be relatively sweet.

In some countries wines are labelled 'dry' when they contain less than 8 g carbohydrate per litre; less than 4 g/l is labelled 'suitable for diabetics'; 25–45 g/l is medium; and sweet wines contain more than 45 g/l.

Fortified wines have extra alcohol added as 'spirit' or as brandy.

See also *beer*; *spirits*; *wine*.

**aldehydes** A large class of organic substances derived from primary alcohols by oxidation, and containing the grouping $-CHO$. For example, acetaldehyde, benzaldehyde.

**alderman's walk** Name given in London to longest and finest cut from haunch of venison or lamb.

**aldosterone** Hormone secreted by the adrenal cortex which controls the excretion of salt and water through the kidneys.

**ale** See *beer*.

**alecost** Aromatic herbaceous perennial, *Tanecetum balsamita*; formerly used to flavour ale, and in salads, and as medicinal herb.

**aleurone layer** Single layer of large cells under the bran coat and outside the endosperm of cereal grains; about 3% by weight of the grain, rich in protein. Botanically part of the endosperm but during milling remains attached to the inner layer of bran.

Contains about 20% of the thiamin, 30% of the riboflavin and 50% of the nicotinic acid of the grain.

**alewives** River herrings, *Pomolobus pseudoharengus*, mostly used for canning after salting.

**algae** Sub-group of the division of plants termed Thallophyta which show no differentiation into root, stem and leaf. They are mainly aquatic, and include seaweeds such as dulse and Irish moss, which have long been eaten by man.

Unicellular varieties have been grown experimentally as novel sources of foods; these include *Chlorella, Scenedesmus* and *Spirulina*. Protein content, 50–60% of dry weight.

**alginates** Salts of alginic acid found as the free acid and calcium salt in many seaweeds. Alginic acid is a polysaccharide complex built from mannuronic acid units.

Salts such as iron, magnesium and ammonium alginates form viscous solutions. They hold large amounts of water and are useful as thickeners, stabilisers, and gelling, binding and emulsifying agents in ice-cream, synthetic cream. The propylene glycol ester is used under the trade name of 'manucol ester'.

**alginic acid** See *alginates*.

**alimentary canal** The digestive tract, comprising, in man, mouth, oesophagus, stomach, duodenum, and small and large intestines.

**alimentary pastes** Shaped dried doughs made from semolina or wheat flour with water, and sometimes egg and milk. The dough is partly dried in hot air, then more slowly.

Macaroni – tubular-shaped, about ¼ inch diameter; at ¾ inch it is called fovantini or maccaroncelli; at ½ inch, zitoni.

Spaghetti is solid rod about 3/32 inch diameter; vermicelli is a third of this thickness.

Noodles are shaped into sheets or ribbons.

Farfals are ground, granulated or shredded.

**aliment de sevrage**   Protein-rich baby food, 20% protein. Algerian version made from wheat, chick peas, lentils, skim milk powder and sugar, with added vitamin D. Senegal version made from millet flour, peanut flour, skim milk powder and sugar, with vitamins A and D and calcium.

**aliphatic**   Name given to those organic chemicals that have open-chain structure, in distinction from the cyclic compounds, which contain rings of carbon compounds.

**alkali formers**   See *acid foods and basic foods*.

**alkaline reserve**   See *acid–base balance*.

**alkaloids**   Unspecific term originally applied (Meissner, 1819) to basic nitrogen-containing compounds of plant origin. In fact some substances classed as alkaloids are not basic (e.g. colchicine) and are synthesised in animal tissues (phenylalkylamines and indoles). A pharmacological definition includes naturally occurring organic bases which possess marked pharmacological effects in animals (about 200 such compounds are known). Many are found in plant foods such as potato, tomato (*Solanum* alkaloids), ergot, animal foods (tetrodotoxin in puffer fish, tetramine in shellfish), decarboxylated amino acids (tryptamine, tyramine, histamine); a number are used in drug treatment, such as morphine, colchicine, quinine, atropine.

**alkalosis**   Decrease in the acid–base ratio in the blood plasma, or an increase in its buffering power. Causes may be excessive loss of carbon dioxide; excessive intake of base, as in antacid drugs; loss of gastric juice by vomiting; high intake of sodium or potassium salts of weak organic acids. See also *acid–base balance*.

**alkannet** (alkanet, alkannin, alkanna)   Colouring obtained from root of *Anchusa tinctoria* (*Alkanna tinctoria*); legally permitted in food in most countries; colouring principle is alkannin. Insoluble in water but soluble in alcohol and ether. Blue in alkalies, blue with lead, crimson with tin, violet with iron. Used for colouring fats, cheese, essences (and inferior port wine). Also known as orcanella.

**allantoin**   Oxidation product of uric acid; end-product of purine metabolism in most mammals except man and the anthropoid apes (where end-product is uric acid).

**All-Bran**   Trade name (Kellogg Co.) for a breakfast cereal prepared from wheat bran.

Analysis per 100 g: 13 g protein, 2.5 g fat, 46 g available carbohydrate, 250 kcal (1 MJ), 28 g dietary fibre, 1.7 g Na, 9 mg Fe, 1 mg thiamin, 1.5 mg riboflavin, 16 mg niacin, 1.8 mg vitamin $B_6$, 2.8 µg vitamin D.

**allergen**   See *adverse reactions (to food)*.

**allergy**   See *adverse reactions (to food)*.

**allicin**   Sulphur compound responsible for the flavour of garlic.

**alligator pears**   See *avocado*.

**Allinson bread**   A whole-wheat bread named after Allinson, who advocated its use in England at the end of the nineteenth century, as did Graham in the United States (thus, Graham bread).

**allolactose**   A sugar, which may be a modification of lactose, which, together with gynolactose, has been claimed to be found in human milk.

**allotriophagy**   Unnatural desire for foods; alternative words, cissa, cittosis and pica.

**alloxan**   Pyrimidine derivative that can induce diabetes when given orally or by injection, by damaging the islets of Langerhans (that part of the pancreas which secretes insulin).

**alloxan diabetes**   Experimental diabetes caused by alloxan.

**alloxazine**   Three-ring structure, the central part of riboflavin. The latter is dimethyl-ribityl-isoalloxazine.

**allspice**   Dried fruits of the evergreen *Pimenta officinalis*, also known as pimento or Jamaican pepper (differs from pimiento). The name 'allspice' derives from the volatile oil, which has an aroma similar to a mixture of cloves, cinnamon and nutmeg. Used to flavour meat products.

**allysine**   Semi-aldehyde of amino-adipic acid, formed in connective tissue by oxidative deamination of peptide-bound lysine.

**almond, sweet**   Ripe seeds of *Prunus amygdalus* var. *dulcis*; yields sweet almond oil.

**almond oil, bitter**   Essential oil from seeds of almond tree (*Prunus amygdalus*) or apricot tree (*Prunus armeniaca*); mostly manufactured from the apricot. Contains 95% benzaldehyde, with hydrocyanic acid and benzaldehyde cyanhydrin. When freed from hydrocyanic acid, is used as flavour, in perfumes and in cosmetics.

**aloe**   Dried juice of leaves of *Aloe perryi*; used in medicine. Contains a glycoside, aloe-emodin or rhabarberone, aloe oil, and aloin or barbaloin.

**Alpha-Laval centrifuge**   Continuous bowl centrifuge for separating liquids of different densities for clarifying. Widely used for cream separation.

**aluminium**  One of the most abundant elements in Nature, as it occurs in rocks and clay. It is found in animal and plant tissues in traces but has not been shown to be essential to either.

There is a popular misconception that aluminium cooking vessels are in some way harmful, but the fact that relatively large doses of aluminium hydroxide are often consumed as an antidote to gastric hyperacidity demonstrates the harmlessness of aluminium.

'Alum' baking powders, in which sodium aluminium sulphate was the acid constituent, used to be used.

'Silver' beads used to decorate confectionery may be coated with either silver foil or an aluminium copper alloy.

**ALV**  Available lysine value. See *available lysine*.

**alveographe**  Measures stretching quality of dough as index of protein quality for baking. A standard disc of dough is blown into a bubble and the pressure curve and bursting pressure measured; gives the stability, extensibility and strength.

**Amama**  Trade name (Glaxo Laboratories) for a protein-rich baby food based on casein (1 part) and groundnut flour (10 parts) – obsolete.

**amaranth**  Burgundy-red colour, fast to light; trisodium salt of 1-(4-sulpho-1-naphthylazo)-2-naphthol-3,6-disulphonic acid.

**Amaranthus**  Genus of plants of which some varieties are cultivated for their leaves and seeds (*A. paniculatus*) and others for leaves (*A. polygamus* and *A. gracilis*).

Composition of seeds per 100 g: protein 11–23 g, oil 5–20 g, carbohydrate 34–65 g. Leaves are promoted in S.E. Asian countries as a dietary source of carotene.

**ambergris**  Morbid concretion obtained from the intestine of the sperm whale. Contains cholesterol, ambrein, benzoic acid. Appears as a mottled or striped grey-brown or black wax. Used in drugs and perfume.

**amberlite**  Group of polystyrene resins used to absorb specific radicals from solutions. The sulphonic acid derivative, strongly acidic (IR120), and the carboxylic acid, weakly acidic (IRC150), are used for cation exchange; basic types used for anion exchange (IR4B, IR45, IRA400). Used for water softening, metal recovery, purification of chemicals, chemical analysis, particularly amino acids. See also *ion-exchange resins*.

**Ames test**  *In vitro* screening test for mutagenic potential of substances (including food additives). Bacteria already mutant at an easily detected locus treated with test material for reversal of the mutation; e.g. strain of bacteria that cannot multiply unless histidine is present in the growth medium reverts to form that can do so.

**amino acid** Characterised by an amino group and an acid group attached to the same carbon atom. Proteins are made of combinations of large numbers of amino acids of twenty different kinds.

Eight of these amino acids must be provided in the diet – i.e. the essential amino acids: lysine, methionine, valine, tryptophan, threonine, leucine, isoleucine and phenylalanine. Possibly arginine and histidine are essential for infants.

The remaining twelve can be synthesised in the body so long as a source of nitrogen is available in the diet. These are the non-essential amino acids: histidine, glycine, arginine, alanine, aspartic acid, glutamic acid, proline, hydroxyproline, serine, cystine, cysteine and tyrosine.

**amino acid, limiting** That essential amino acid present in the protein in question in least amount (relative to the dietary needs). The ratio beween the amount of the limiting amino acid and the requirements serves as a chemical estimation of the nutritive value of the protein. See *chemical score*.

Most cereal proteins are limited by lysine, and most animal and vegetable proteins by the sulphur amino acids (methionine plus cystine).

In complete diets it is the sulphur amino acids that are usually limiting.

See also *lysine*; *methionine*.

**amino acid oxidase** See *flavoproteins*.

**amino acid profile** Amino acid composition of a protein.

**amino acids, antiketogenic** Those which are metabolised to glucose. They are glycine, alanine, serine, cystine, aspartic acid, glutamic acid, arginine, proline and hydroxyproline.

**amino acid score** See *protein quality*.

**amino acids, ketogenic** Those which are metabolised to acetoacetic acid (ketone bodies). They are leucine, isoleucine, phenylalanine and tyrosine.

**amino acids, non-protein** Occur in higher plants; some are toxic to animals and so potentially to man, e.g. mimosine (in *Leucaena*), djenkolic acid (Djenkola bean), *S*-methyl cysteine sulphoxide (kale and garlic), hypoglycin A (Ackee fruit) oxalylaminoalanine (*Lathyrus* pea).

**aminogram** Diagrammatic representation of the amino acid composition of a protein.

**aminopeptidase** Enzyme of the pancreatic juice which splits polypeptides to dipeptides. Removes the terminal unit of the polypeptide chain at the end at which the amino radical is free; hence, is an exopeptidase.

**aminopterin** Aminopteroylglutamic acid, specific antagonist to folic acid.

**amla** Indian gooseberry, *Emblica officinalis Gaertn*; important in Ayurvedic medicine. Contains 600 mg vitamin C/100 g pulp; reported to reduce hypercholesterolaemia.

**ammonotelic** Descriptive of animals that excrete their waste nitrogen as ammonia – e.g. various worms, leeches, molluscs, sea urchins, fish.

**amomum** Group of tropical plants including cardamom and grains of paradise whose seeds have pungent and aromatic properties.

**AMP** See *adenosine nucleotides*.

**amphetamine** See *anorectic drugs*.

**amphoteric** See *isoelectric point*.

**amydon** Starchy material made by steeping wheat flour in water and drying the starch sediment in the sun; used for many centuries for thickening broths.

**amygdalin** Glucoside in almonds, apricot and cherry stones, hydrolysed by the enzyme emulsin to glucose, hydrocyanic acid and benzaldehyde. The benzaldehyde gives the characteristic odour.

**amylases** Enzymes that hydrolyse starch and glycogen to maltose.

Alpha-amylase, or dextrinogenic amylase, breaks starch down to small dextrin-like molecules and does not proceed to maltose.

Beta-amylase, or maltogenic amylase, is specific for the 1,4-alpha-glucosidic linkages of starch and liberates maltose. Complete degradation of starch requires attack by both these enzymes.

Salivary amylase and pancreatic amylase in animals behave like the alpha-amylase. Also known as diastase.

See also *Z-enzyme*.

**amyloamylose** Old name for amylose, as distinct from erythroamylose, old name for amylopectin.

**amylodyspepsia** Inability to digest starch.

**amylograph** Measures the viscosity of flour paste as it is heated from 25 °C to 90 °C (the same temperature rise as in baking) and serves as a measure of the diastatic activity of the flour.

**amyloins** Carbohydrates that are complexes of dextrins with varying proportions of maltose.

**amylolytic** General adjective applied to enzymes that can split starch into soluble products.

**amylopectin** Starch consists of 20–25% amylose and the remainder is amylopectin.

Amylose consists of long straight chains of glucose ($\alpha$-D-glucopyranosyl) units linked 1,4: blue colour with iodine.

Amylopectin is a larger molecule also linked 1,4 but with 4–5% of the glucose units linked α-1,6 at branch points (purplish colour with iodine) See also *amylases*.

**amylopsin** Pancreatic amylase.

**amylose** See *amylopectin*.

**anabiosis** Suspended animation (with stoppage of respiration and the heart-beat), caused by freezing or freezing and drying, as achieved, for example, by Alaskan and Siberian insects during cold spells.

**anabolism** The process of building up or synthesising. See *metabolism*.

**anaemia** A shortage of red blood cells (see *blood, red cells*). May be caused by dietary shortage of iron (nutritional iron-deficiency anaemia), by deficiency of the various vitamins involved in the formation of red blood cells, by lack of intrinsic factor (see *pernicious anaemia*) leading to failure to absorb vitamin $B_{12}$ (pernicious anaemia); primary cause is often chronic loss of blood due to intestinal damage caused by parasites.

**anaerobes** Micro-organisms that grow in the absence of oxygen. Obligate anaerobes cannot survive in the presence of oxygen. Facultative anaerobes normally grow in oxygen but can also grow in its absence.

**analysis, gastric** See *fractional test meal*.

**analysis, proximate** An analysis for the major ingredients, usually nitrogen (as a measure of the protein), and fat and ash (as a measure of the mineral salts); these are added together and subtracted from 100 to give what is called 'carbohydrate by difference'. The latter may be corrected for crude fibre. See *carbohydrate by difference*.

**ananas** Pineapple.

**anatto** See *annatto*.

**anchovy** A fish, *Engraulis encrasicholus*. Usually prepared semi-preserved with 10–12% salt and sometimes benzoic acid.

**aneurine** Obsolete name for vitamin $B_1$.

**angelica** Bright green crystallised sticks used for decorating and flavouring confectionery goods, prepared from the young stalks of *Angelica archangelica*. This is a tall umbelliferous herb (not to be confused with wild English angelica, *Angelica sylvestris*), and the crystallised material is imported from S. France.

The roots are used with juniper berries for flavouring gin and the seeds are used in vermouth and Chartreuse. Essential oils are distilled from the roots, stem and leaves.

**angostura** Essential oil distilled from the bark of *Galipea cusparia*. Contains galipol, cadinene, galipene and pinene; used in preparation of bitters and liqueurs.

**Ångström unit**  One ten-millionth part of a millimetre, or one ten-thousandth part of a micrometre; symbol, Å.

**angular stomatitis**  An affection of the skin at the angles of the mouth, characterised by heaping up of epithelium into ridges, giving the appearance of fissures; a symptom of riboflavin deficiency but also a symptom of other diseases.

**anhydrovitamin A**  Form of retinol in which the OH group has been removed by treatment with HCl, with a corresponding shift in the double bonds. Once incorrectly called cyclised or spurious vitamin A. Has very slight biological activity. When fed in large doses to rats, a more active material called rehydro-vitamin A is obtained.

**animal protein factor**  Name given to certain growth factor or factors which were found to be present in animal but not vegetable proteins. Vitamin $B_{12}$ was identified as one of these.

**anion**  See *ionisation*.

**anise**  See *aniseed*.

**aniseed** (anise)  The dried fruit of *Pimpinella anisum* (parsley family). Chief component of the volatile oil is anethole (methoxypropenyl benzene). The seed is used to flavour baked goods, meat products and drinks.

**anisette**  Liqueur based on aniseed.

**annatto**  Also known as bixin, butter colour, orlean and rocou; colour extracted from pericarp of the fruit of tropical shrub *Bixa orellana*. Major ingredient is the carotenoid, bixin, insoluble in water; also, of minor importance, orellan, water-soluble. Used to dye cotton and silk, in wood stains – and cheese. Seeds are sometimes used for flavouring, especially in Caribbean food.

**anomers**  A pair of stereoisomers related to each other in the same way as alpha and beta glucose are related, are termed anomers.

**anorectic drugs** (anorexigenic drugs)  Drugs that depress the appetite and are used an an aid to weight reduction – e.g. amphetamine (or dextro-amphetamine or dexedrine), preludin (phenmetrazine hydrochloride), Tenuate (diethylpropion).

**anorexia**  Lack of appetite.

**anorexia nervosa**  Psychological disturbance resulting in a refusal to eat; sensations of hunger usually not felt. There may be a restriction of the diet to particular foods. The result is great weight loss, atrophy of tissue and fall in basal metabolic rate.

**anosmia**  Lack or impairment of sensitivity to odour stimuli.

**anserine**  Beta-alanyl methylhistidine; a dipeptide originally isolated from goose muscle; found in muscle of mammals, fishes and birds; function unknown.

**Antabuse** Tetra-ethyl thiuramdisulphide, drug used in the treatment of alcoholism. The drug alone has no effect, but if alcohol is subsequently taken, it gives rise to headache, palpitation, nausea and vomiting.

**antacids** Bases or buffers that neutralise acid; used generally in relation to the partial neutralisation of stomach acidity. Substances such as magnesium carbonate, sodium bicarbonate, magnesium hydroxide, glycine, etc., are used.

**anthocyanins** Violet, red and blue water-soluble colouring matter of many fruits, flowers and leaves. Consist of glucose plus anthocyanidins (these consist of two 6-membered carbon rings containing one oxygen atom). Examples are delphinidin, pelargonidin, cyanidin. Can attack iron and tin and cause trouble in canned foods.

**anthoxanthins** Alternative name for flavonoids, which see.

**antibiotics** Substances produced by living organisms which inhibit the growth of other organisms. Classic example is penicillin, produced by the mould *Penicillium notatum*, which inhibits bacteria and is used to control infections by susceptible bacteria.

When added to the diet of animals in small quantities (a few grams per tonne of food), many antibiotics stimulate growth, possibly by increasing the efficiency of food absorption or by controlling mild infections. To prevent the development of antibiotic-resistant strains of bacteria, the use as feed additives is limited to varieties not used therapeutically, such as nisin. The latter is also used as a food preservative. See also *nisin*; *oleandomycin*; *penicillin*; *tetracyclines*.

**antibodies** Proteins formed in the blood in response to 'foreign' proteins – antigens. These proteins are immunoglobulins of which there are five types, IgM, G, A, D and E.

Immunity to infection is due to the presence in the blood of antitoxins (specific antibodies) formed in response to the initial infection with bacterial antigens.

**anti-caking agents** Added to powder foodstuffs to prevent caking – e.g. small amounts of anhydrous disodium hydrogen phosphate added to salt or sugar; aluminium calcium silicate or calcium or magnesium carbonate in table salt; calcium silicate in baking powder.

**anticoagulants** With reference to blood, substances that prevent clotting by interfering with the mechanism. Oxalate and citrate are anticoagulants, as they combine with the calcium which is needed; dicoumarin and heparin inhibit the formation of prothrombin, needed to release fibrin from fibrinogen; hirudin inactivates the thrombin.

**antidiuretics** Drugs that reduce the rate of formation of urine, i.e. reduce water loss from the body.

**antienzymes** Substances that specifically inhibit the action of digestive enzymes – produced by the lining of the digestive tract, secreted by intestinal parasites, found in raw legumes (antitrypsin, antiamylase); destroyed by heat.

**antifoaming agents** Octanol (capryl alcohol), sulphonated oils, silicones; reduce foaming often caused by the presence of dissolved protein or other stabiliser.

**antigalactics** Substances that suppress the secretion of milk.

**antigen** Protein material (bacteria, food, pollen) which, when introduced into the blood or tissues, stimulates the formation of a specific antibody (immunoglobulin).

**anti-grey hair factor** Absence of either para-aminobenzoic acid or pantothenic acid can cause the loss of hair colour in rats; not related to loss of hair pigment in human beings.

**anti-mould agents** See *antimycotics*.

**antimycotics** Substances that inhibit mould growth, such as sodium and calcium propionate, methyl hydroxybenzoate, quaternary ammonium chloride, sodium benzoate, sorbic acid.

**antioxidants** Substances that retard the oxidative rancidity of fats – e.g. propyl gallate, octyl gallate, dodecyl gallate, butylated hydroxyanisole (BHA) and butylated hydroxytoluene (BHT). Many fats, particularly vegetable oils, contain naturally occurring antioxidants, such as tocopherol, which protect the oils from rancidity for a limited period. See *induction period*.

**antisialagogues** Substances that arrest the flow of saliva.

**anti-spattering agents** Added to fats used in frying – e.g. lecithin, sucrose esters (laurates and stearates), and sodium sulphoacetate derivates of mono-and diglycerides. They function by preventing the coalescence of water droplets.

**anti-staling agents** Substances that retard the staling of baked products, and also soften the crumb – e.g. sucrose stearate, polyoxyethylene monostearate, glyceryl monostearate, stearoyl tartrate.

**antivitamins** Substances that interfere with the function of vitamins or destroy them. Dicoumarol in spoiled sweet clover inhibits function of vitamin K; thiaminase in raw fish destroys thiamin; the drug methotrexate inhibits folate.

**AOM** See *active oxygen method*.

**apastia** Refusal to take food as an expression of mental disorder.

**APF** Animal protein factor.

**aphagosis** Inability to eat.

**apo-carotenal** See *carotenal*.

**apoenzyme** See *enzyme*.

**apoerythein**  Name suggested for intrinsic factor. See *pernicious anaemia*.

**apoferritin**  The protein part of ferritin, the iron storage complex in the intestinal mucosal cells.

**Apollinaris water**  An alkaline, highly aerated water, containing sodium chloride and calcium, sodium and magnesium carbonates; obtained from a spring in the valley of the Ahr (Prussia).

**aporinosis**  Term for any disease due to deficiency of an element in diet. (Greek *aporos*, scarce.)

**aporrhegma**  Ptomaine or other toxic substance split off from an amino acid during the bacterial decomposition of a protein.

**aposia**  Absence of feeling of thirst.

**apositia**  Aversion for food.

**apparent digestibility**  See *digestibility*.

**appertisation**  Term applied by the French to the process of destroying all the micro-organisms of significance in food, i.e. 'commercial sterility'; a few organisms remain alive but are quiescent. (Named after Nicholas Appert, a confectioner of Paris, 1752–1841, who invented the process of canning.)

**apple**  Fruit of many species of *Malus sylvestris* (origin of name of malic acid).

Analysis per 100 g: 84 g water, 2 g dietary fibre (3.7 in 100 g skin), 46 kcal (0.2 MJ); only 3 mg vitamin C in eating apples, 15–20 mg in cooking apples.

**apple butter**  Apple that has been boiled in an open kettle to a thick consistency. Similar to apple sauce but darker in colour, owing to the prolonged boiling.

**apple jack**  American name for apple brandy; distilled cider, also known as Calvados.

**apple, liquid**  American preparation of apple juice plus pulverised apple pulp in suspension.

**apple nuggets**  Crisp granules of apple of low moisture content. Dehydrated apples of 24% moisture content are cut into small cubes and dried down to 2% moisture; used to make apple sauce.

**apricot**  Fruit of *Prunus armeniaca*.

Analysis per 100 g (without stones): 87 g water, 7 g sugar, 2 g dietary fibre, 1000–2500 µg carotene, 7 mg vitamin C, 30 kcal (0.1 MJ). Dried apricots, per 100 g: 15 g water, 43 g sugar, 24 g dietary fibre, 4 mg iron, 3000–4000 µg carotene, trace of vitamin C.

**arachidonic acid**  Fatty acid with 20 carbon atoms and four double bonds, 20:4ω6, (see *linoleic acid* for nomenclature). Three times as potent as linoleic acid in curing symptoms of essential fatty acid deficiency; found in animal tissues – fish, eggs, liver, brain – formed from linoleic acid so not strictly an EFA although so potent (see *essential fatty acids*).

**arachin** One of the globulin proteins from the peanut. Precipitated by 40% saturated ammonium sulphate from a salt extract of peanut. Conarachin can be precipitated from the residue by 85% saturated ammonium sulphate.

**arachis oil** Peanut or groundnut oil; extracted from *Arachis hypogea* – earthnut, groundnut, monkey nut, peanut. About 50% oleic acid, 30% linoleic acid, less than 1% linolenic acid.

**arctons** See *refrigerants*.

**argentation** Addition of silver ions to the support or mobile phase in chromatography of fats to facilitate separation of fats of differing degrees of unsaturation.

**arginase** Enzyme that hydrolyses arginine to urea and ornithine, the last stage of urea synthesis from the amino groups of the amino acids. Present in most animal cells.

**arginine** Chemically, aminoguanido valeric acid. Dibasic amino acid that is non-essential to adult man. Since it is partly essential to growing rats (growth only 80% of optimum in its absence), it may similarly be partly essential to children. It is essential to the chick.

**argol** Crust of crude cream of tartar (potassium acid tartrate) which forms on the sides of wine vats (also called wine stone). White argol from white grapes, red argol from red. 50–85% potassium hydrogen tartrate and 6–12% calcium tartrate. Used in vinegar fermentation, as mordant in dyeing, and in the manufacture of tartaric acid.

**ariboflavinosis** Deficiency of riboflavin (vitamin $B_2$) characterised by swollen, cracked, bright red lips (cheilosis), enlarged, tender, magenta-red tongue (glossitis), cracking at the corners of the mouth (angular stomatitis) and congestion of the blood vessels of the conjunctiva.

**Arlac** Protein-rich baby food (42% protein) made in Nigeria by Cow & Gate Ltd, from peanut flour and skim milk powder with added vitamins $B_1$, $B_2$, $B_{12}$ and D and minerals.

**Armenian bole** (ferric oxide) Occurs naturally as hematite or prepared by heating ferrous sulphate, etc. Used in metallurgy, polishing compounds, paint pigment and as a food colour.

**Arogel** Trade name, Arogel 909 P (Morningstar-Paisley, USA), for a potato starch preparation used as thickener in gravies, sauces and canned foods; it is stable to heat.

**arrowroot** Tuber of the West Indian plant *Maranta arundinacea*, mainly used to prepare arrowroot starch, the most refined of all feculas. The starch contains only a trace of protein (0.2%) and is free from vitamins. It is used in bland, low-salt and protein-restricted diets and, unfortunately, as an infant food in some West Indian islands.

**arsanilic acid**   Used to stimulate growth in poultry.

**arsenic**   Toxic chemical believed to react with cellular sulphydryl groups. FAO/WHO (1976) suggested a maximum acceptable total daily load of 50 µg/kg body weight (although organic and inorganic forms can have different potential toxicities). It can accumulate in fish and shellfish and in crops treated with arsenical pesticides.

**artichoke, globe**   Young flower heads of *Cynara scolymus* (edible part is fleshy base). Analysis per 100 g (boiled): water 84 g, carbohydrate 1.2 g, protein and fat traces, only traces of vitamins, 7 kcal (28 kJ).

**artichoke, Jerusalem**   Underground tubers of *Helianthus tuberosus* (of the Compositae family). Analysis per 100 g: protein 1.5 g, carbohydrate 3 g, only traces of vitamins, 18 kcal (80 kJ). Also known as girasole, and sunflower artichoke – source of the indigestible polysaccharide, inulin.

**ascorbic acid**   Vitamin C, also called L-xyloascorbic acid, in distinction from D-araboascorbic acid (isoascorbic acid or erythorbic acid), which has only slight vitamin C activity.

Erythorbic acid has strong reducing properties, and is used as an antioxidant in foods and to preserve the red colour of fresh or preserved meats.

Physiological properties of ascorbic acid are described under vitamin C.

**ascorbic acid, mono dehydro**   Intermediate stage in the route from ascorbic acid to dehydroascorbic acid; it is a free radical formed in very small concentrations and with a short life.

**ascorbic acid oxidase**   Plant enzyme that oxidises ascorbic acid to the dehydro form. In the living tissue it appears to be separated from the vitamin, but in the wilting leaf or, for example, in shredded cabbage, the enzyme comes into contact with its substrate and there is a rapid destruction of the vitamin. For preservation of the vitamin in greens on cooking, it is recommended that the vegetables be plunged into boiling water, when the enzyme is destroyed.

**ascorbin stearate**   Ester of ascorbic acid (vitamin C) and stearic acid; a fat-soluble form of the vitamin which is used as an antioxidant at concentrations around 0.1%.

**ascorbyl palmitate**   Ester of ascorbic acid and palmitic acid used an an anti-staling agent in bakery products. Amounts of 0.1–0.4% by weight of the flour retard staling for 2–4 days.

**aseptic filling**   Refers to filling containers (cans) with food that has already been sterilised and so must be maintained under aseptic conditions. Continuous sterilisation as the food passes along narrow pipes allows more rapid heating, with less effect on the quality of the food.

**ash** Residue left behind after all the organic matter has been burned off. Serves as a measure of the inorganic salts that were present in the original material.

**asparagine** Amide of the amino acid aspartic acid; serves in plants as a store of ammonia. During the growth of seedlings ketonic acids are formed during photosynthesis, and these are aminated to amino acids at the expense of the ammonia in asparagine.

**asparagus** Young shoot of *Asparagus officinalis*.

Analysis per 100 g: protein 1.4 g, fat 0.1 g, Ca 14 mg, Fe 0.6 mg, kcal 14 (60 kJ), vitamin A 220 μg, vitamin $B_1$ 0.11 mg, vitamin $B_2$ 0.13 mg, nicotinic acid 0.9 mg, vitamin C 22 mg.

**aspartame** Artificial sweetener, *N*-L-aspartyl-L-phenylalanine methyl ester; 200 times as sweet as 4% solution of sucrose. Stable for only a limited time in solution (some months) when it breaks down to diketopiperazine derivative. Discovered 1965; used in soft drinks, dessert mixes, as 'table-top sweetener' etc.

**aspartic acid** A non-essential amino acid; amino succinic acid (dibasic). Its amide is asparagine.

**aspartyl-phenylalanine methyl ester** Dipeptide ester. See *aspartame*.

*Aspergillus* See *moulds*; *takadiastase*.

**aspic jelly** A clear jelly made from fish, chicken or meat stock, sometimes with added gelatin, flavoured with lemon, tarragon vinegar, sherry, peppercorns and vegetables, and used to glaze meat or game, among other foods. Name derived from the herb espic or spikenard.

**astaxanthin** A carotenoid pigment; the pink colour of salmon muscle.

**astringency** Literally, a 'drawing together'; property of foods, especially unripe fruits and cider apples, thought to be due to the destruction of the lubricant properties of the saliva and contraction of epithelial tissues of the tongue by precipitation by tannins, which see.

**atherosclerosis** Degenerative disease of the arteries in which there is an accumulation on the inner wall of a complex of lipids, complex carbohydrates, blood products and fibrous tissue – called atheroma – which leads to narrowing of the lumen of the arteries. When it occurs in the coronary artery, it can lead to failure of the blood supply to the heart muscle (ischaemia).

**Atmungsferment** Name given by Warburg to the respiratory enzyme, later called cytochrome oxidase

**ATP** (adenosine triphosphate)   See *adenosine nucleotides*.

**Atwater factors**   Factors used to calculate the energy available from foodstuffs after allowing for the losses of digestion and the incomplete combustion of the nitrogen part of proteins. The complete heat of combustion of proteins is 5.7, of fats 9.4 and of carbohydrates 4.1 kcal/g; Atwater factors are, respectively, 4, 9 and 4 kcal/g. See also *energy*; *Rubner factors*.

**AT-10**   See *tachysterol*.

**aubergine**   Also known as egg plant, *Solanum melongena*, native of S.E. Asia; 3–5 inches in diameter and up to 12 inches long, purple in colour. Composition per 100 g: carbohydrate 6 g, protein 1.4 g, vitamin $B_1$ 0.06 mg, $B_2$ 0.05 mg, nicotinic acid 0.8 mg, vitamin C 5 mg.

**aurantiamarin**   Glucoside present in the albedo of the bitter orange; partly responsible for the flavour.

**aureomycin**   See *tetracyclines*.

**autoclave**   A vessel in which high temperatures can be reached by using high pressure. The domestic pressure cooker is an example.

  At atmospheric pressure water boils at 100 °C; at 10 lb extra pressure the boiling point is 115 °C; at 15 lb, 121 °C and at 20 lb, 126 °C.

  Autoclaves have two major purposes. As in the domestic pressure cooker, the higher temperature permits cooking in a shorter time. The second major use is in sterilisation. Bacteria are destroyed more readily at these elevated temperatures, and autoclaves are used to sterilise food, for example in cans, and for sterilising instruments and dressings in surgery.

**autolysis**   Process of self-digestion effected by the enzymes naturally present in the tissue. For example, tenderising of game while hanging is autolytic breakdown of connective tissue.

**autotrophes**   Organisms that can synthesise their own tissues from simple inorganic salts, as distinct from heterotrophes, which must be supplied with complex ready-made foods. Thus, plants are autotrophes, animals are heterotrophes. Bacteria can be of either type. Autotrophes are not involved in food spoilage; heterotrophic bacteria include pathogens and food-spoilage organisms.

**auxins**   Plant hormones produced in the growing buds, embryos and young leaves of plants, as well as many fungi and bacteria. They are organic acids – e.g. indolyl acetic acid, indolyl butyric acid and naphthalene acetic acid. Used to stimulate root formation and control growth.

**available carbon dioxide**   See *baking powder*; *flour, self-raising*.

**available lysine**   Refers to protein-bound lysine in which the end-amino group is free, so that after enzymic hydrolysis – digestion – the lysine is available for absorption. In contrast, when the end-amino group of the lysine is bound to a reducing sugar (Maillard reaction) or by another linkage that cannot be hydrolysed during digestion, the lysine is unavailable. Such linkages are hydrolysed by acid digestion *in vitro*, so giving rise to a discrepancy between chemical and biological determination of protein quality.

**available nutrients**  In some foodstuffs nutrients shown to be present by chemical tests may not be available, or be only partly available, to the animal. For example, the calcium combined in phytin, and the lysine that is combined with sugar in the Maillard complex, are not available, since they cannot be liberated by the digestive enzymes. Also termed *bioavailable*.

**avenalin**  The globulin protein present in oats.

**avenin**  The glutelin protein present in oats.

**aversion, food**  See *adverse reactions (to food)*.

**Avicel**  Trade name (American Viscose Co.) for microcrystalline alpha-cellulose – natural cellulose partly hydrolysed with acid and reduced to a fine powder. Disperses in water and has the properties of a gum; used to make oily foods such as cheese, peanut butter, as well as syrups and honey, into dry granular powders; also used in sauces and dressings.

**avidin**  Protein in white of egg which combines with vitamin H (biotin) and renders it unavailable to the body. It is inactivated in cooked eggs. See *biotin*.

**avitaminosis**  Absence of a vitamin; may be used specifically, as avitaminosis A.

**avocado** (alligator pear)  Fruit of *Persea americana*. Unusual among fruits in its high fat content, 17–27%.

Analysis per 100g: 69g water, 4g protein, 22g fat, 1.8g carbohydrate, 5–30mg vitamin C, 220kcal (920kJ). 7–14% of the fat is linoleic acid.

**axerol, axerophthol**  Suggested names for vitamin A but not used.

**azaserine**  Diazoacetyl derivative of the non-essential amino acid serine. Appears to interfere with the metabolism of serine and acts as an anti-cancer agent.

**azeotrope**  A mixture of water and organic solvent that distils at a temperature below the boiling point of either. Use is made of this property in azeotropic drying, when the addition of the solvent allows the water to be distilled off at a reduced temperature.

**azlon**  Name given to textile fibres produced from proteins, such as casein, zein.

**azo dyes**  A group of compounds formed by combining a diazonium salt with an aromatic amino- or hydroxy-compound; they contain two nitrogen atoms combined together and are all strongly coloured.

*Azotobacter*  Genus of bacteria of family Bacteriaceae which can use atmospheric nitrogen and synthesise nitrogenous tissue from it.

**azorubin**  Red colour, carmoisine.

# B

**baba**  French cake invented by King Stanislas I of Poland and named after Ali Baba. 'Rum baba' flavoured with rum; French modification using 'secret' syrup was called brillat-savarin or savarin.

**babaco**  Seedless fruit, *Carica pentagona* of same family as paw paw (*Carica papaya*); discovered in 1920s in Ecuador and introduced into New Zealand in 1973.

Analysis per 100 g; 0.7 g protein, 8.5 g sugars, trace of fat and starch, 30 mg vitamin C.

**babassu oil**  Edible oil from the Brazilian palm nut; similar to coconut oil, and used in food, soap and cosmetics.

**Babcock test**  Test for fat in milk. The sample is mixed with sulphuric acid in a Babcock bottle, centrifuged, diluted and recentrifuged. The level of the fat in the neck of the bottle is read off.

**bacalao**  South American name for klipfish, which see.

**bacitracin**  Antibiotic isolated from an organism of the *Bacillus subtilis* group; a polypeptide.

**bacon**  The smoked and cured meat made from pig – back, sides and belly (old French for pig).

Gammon (usually top of hind leg), analysis per 100 g: 25 g protein, 19 g fat, 270 kcal (1.1 MJ).

Rasher (single slice) can contain up to 40% fat. Pig meat is exceptionally rich in thiamin, containing about 0.5 mg per 100 g (up to 1 mg in lean meat), about ten times as much as beef; riboflavin (0.2–0.3 mg) and niacin (3–7 mg) are similar in amounts to those of other meats.

**bacteria**  Microscopic, unicellular plants which do not contain chlorophyll; mostly 0.5–3 μm in size. They are responsible for much food spoilage and for disease; but are also made use of, as in biological oxidation, and fermentation, such as the pickling process and the souring of milk.

Some bacteria, the so-called pathogens, produce toxins which cause disease. Some are spore-formers and in this form they are more resistant to heat and sterilising agents. Bacteria contain

45–85% dry matter as protein and are grown on petroleum residues, methane or methanol for animal feed.

**bacterial count** See *plate count*.

**bacteriophage** Group of viruses that attack bacteria; composed of nucleoprotein and capable of multiplying in host cells. They are smaller than bacteria and can pass through ordinary bacterial filters. Cause of considerable trouble in culture suspensions – e.g. in milk starter cultures, since these readily become infected with phages.

*Bacterium aceti* See *Acetobacter*.

**bactofugation** Belgian process for removing bacteria from milk by high-speed centrifuging.

**bactometer** Device for rapid (few hours) estimation of bacterial contamination by measuring early stages of nutrient breakdown by the bacteria through electrical impedance (capacitance and inductance).

**badminton** Drink of claret, sugar and soda water.

**bagasse** Mill residues from sugar-cane, consisting of the crushed stalks from which the juice has been expressed; 50% cellulose, 25% hemicelluloses, 25% lignin. Sometimes also applied to residues from other plants, such as beet.

Used as fuel and as cattle feed, in preparation of paper and fibre board, and in manufacture of furfural.

**bagel** Circular bread roll with hole in the middle made from fermented wheat flour dough (recipe includes egg) boiled before baking; Jewish speciality.

**baguette** A French bread, long and thin, about 60 cm and weighing 250 g.

**bain marie** Double saucepan (French for water-bath).

**baker's cheese** See *cheese, cottage*.

**baking additives** Materials added to flour products for a variety of purposes, including bleaching of the flour, aging (which see), slowing rate of staling, improving texture.

**baking powder** Mixture that liberates carbon dioxide when moistened and heated. Sodium bicarbonate is the source of $CO_2$, and an acid substance is required, such as cream of tartar, calcium acid phosphate, sodium pyrophosphate or sodium aluminium sulphate. Quick-acting powders contain tartrate and liberate $CO_2$ in the dough before heating; slow-acting powders contain phosphate and liberate most of the $CO_2$ during heating.

Legally must contain not less than 8% available, and not more than 1.5% residual, $CO_2$. Golden raising powder (similar but coloured yellow; formerly called egg-substitute) must contain not less than 6% available, and not more than 1.5% residual, $CO_2$.

**bal-ahar**  Protein-rich baby food (22–26% protein) made in India from wheat flour, oil-seed flour and vegetables, with added vitamins and calcium.

**balance**  With reference to diet, means net gain (positive balance) or loss (negative balance); used in reference to nitrogen, mineral salts, etc. When intake equals excretion, the body is in equilibrium with respect to the nutrient in question. Balanced diet is one containing all nutrients.

**Balling**  A table of specific gravity published by von Balling in 1843, giving the weight of cane sugar in 100g of solution corresponding with s.g. determined at 17.5°C.

It is used in calculating the percentage extract in beer worts. It was corrected for slight inaccuracies by Plato, 1900. Extracts are referred to as per cent Plato.

For s.g. greater than unity, s.g. = 200 divided by (200 minus scale reading); for s.g. less than unity, s.g. = 200 divided by (200 plus scale reading).

**ball mill**  Vessel in which material is ground by rolling heavy balls; used for hard materials.

**Balmain bug**  A variety of lobster found in Australia.

**Bambarra groundnut**  *Voandzeia subterranea* (Madagascar peanut, earth pea): resembles true groundnut but seeds are low in oil content. Seeds are hard and need soaking or pounding before cooking.

Analysis per 100g: 18g protein, 6g fat, 60g carbohydrate, 370kcal (1.5MJ), 65mg Ca, 6mg Fe, 0.3mg vitamin $B_1$, 0.1mg vitamin $B_2$, 2mg nicotinic acid.

**bamboo shoots**  Thick, pointed shoots of *Bambusa vulgaris* and *Phyllostachys pubescens* eaten in eastern Asia.

Analysis per 100g: 2.3g protein, 0.2g fat, 6g carbohydrate, 35kcal (0.15MJ), 0.15mg vitamin $B_1$, 0.07mg vitamin $B_2$, 0.6mg nicotinic acid, 4mg vitamin C.

**bamies**  See *okra*.

**banana**  Fruit of genus *Musa*; but since the cultivated kinds are sterile hybrid forms, they cannot be given exact species names.

Dessert bananas have a high sugar content (17–19%) and are eaten raw (see also *plantain*).

Analysis per 100g: 1g protein, 0.3g fat, 27g carbohydrate, 116kcal (0.49MJ), 0.5mg Fe, 30μg vitamin A, 0.05mg vitamin $B_1$, 0.05mg vitamin $B_2$, 0.7mg nicotinic acid, 10mg vitamin C. Sodium content is low, 1.2mg per 100g, so used in low-sodium diets.

**banana, false**  *Ensete ventricosum*, closely related to the banana; fruits are small and contain seeds (bananas are sterile and have no seeds); the rhizome and inner tissues of the stem are eaten after cooking (major food in S. Ethiopia).

Analysis of rhizome per 100g: 1.5g protein, 45g carbohydrate, 190kcal (0.8MJ), 5mg Fe, 0.02mg vitamin $B_1$, 0.05mg vitamin $B_2$, 0.2mg nicotinic acid, 0.5mg vitamin C.

**banana figs**  Bananas are split longitudinally and sun-dried without treating with sulphur dioxide. The product is dark in colour and sticky.

**banian days**  Days on which no meat was served; named after Banian (Hindu) merchants who abstained from eating flesh. Obsolete term for 'days of short commons'.

**bannock**  Flat round cake made of oat, rye or barley meal; baked on a hearth or griddle.

Pitcaithly bannock is a type of almond shortbread containing caraway seeds and chopped peel.

**bap**  A soft, white, flat, floury-coated Scottish breakfast roll.

**Barbados cherry**  See *cherry, West Indian*.

**Barbados sugar**  See *sugar*.

**barding**  See *larding*.

**Barfoed's test**  For all monosaccharides. Barfoed's solution is copper acetate in acetic acid, which gives a red precipitate of cuprous oxide with monosaccharides.

**barium meal**  A meal containing barium sulphate, which is opaque to X-rays, and allows examination of the shape and movements of the stomach for diagnostic purposes.

**barley**  Grain of *Hordeum vulgare*, of considerable importance as human and animal food and in brewing; one of the hardiest of cereals.

The whole grain with only the outer husk removed is called pot, scotch or hulled barley (this requires several hours' cooking).

Pearl barley – most of the bran and germ removed, ash reduced from 2.5 to 1%, vitamin $B_1$ to one-tenth.

Analysis per 100g: protein 9g, fat 1.4g, Ca 20mg, Fe 0.7mg, vitamin $B_1$ 0.15mg, vitamin $B_2$ 0.08mg, nicotinic acid 2.5mg.

Barley meal is ground hulled barley; barley flour is ground pearl barley; barley flakes are the flattened grain.

**barleycorn**  (1) Single grain of barley.

(2) Measure of length – ⅓ inch (0.85cm).

**barley, malted**  See *malt*.

**barley sugar**  Sugar confectionery made by melting and cooling sugar; originally by boiling with decoction of barley.

**barley water**  Drink made by boiling pearl barley with water.

**Barlow's disease**  Infantile scurvy; also Moeller's disease and Cheadle's disease.

**barm**  Another name for yeast or leaven, or the froth on fermenting malt liquor.

Spon or virgin barm (short for spontaneous) is made by allowing wild yeast to fall into a sugar medium and multiply there.

**Barmene** Trade name (English Grains Ltd) for yeast extract – prepared from autolysed brewer's yeast – plus vegetable juices, used for flavouring.

Analysis per 100g: 38g protein, 13g carbohydrate, 6mg thiamin, 6mg riboflavin, 60mg nicotinic acid, 3mg pantothenic acid, 1.5mg pyridoxine, 1mg folic acid.

**barrel** UK – 36 imperial gallons (163.6 litres); USA 25 imperial gallons (113.7 litres).

**basal metabolic rate** (BMR) When the body is at complete rest, free from draughts, at moderate room temperature and 12–14 hours after a meal, energy is being used at the basal rate – the basal metabolism. This energy is needed to maintain the heart beat, respiration, etc., but largely to maintain body temperature and the tension of the muscles. BMR is therefore related to muscle mass and the surface area of the body. It may be calculated from surface area; the output per square metre varies with age and sex.

For male infants BMR is 50–70kcal per square metre per hour, falling steadily with age to 30–40kcal at the age of 70, about 10% less for women.

Average BMR, about 1500kcal (6MJ) per day. It is under control of the thyroid gland, increased in fever and hyperthyroidism, and by administration of thyroxine or dried thyroid, and reduced when the thyroid is underactive.

See also *energy*; *surface area*.

**Basedow's disease** Exophthalmic goitre, hyperthyroidism.

**base formers** See *acid foods and basic foods*.

**basic foods** See *acid foods and basic foods*.

**basic 7 foods plan** Division of foods into seven groups, with the recommendation that some food from each group should be eaten every day, so ensuring a well-mixed diet.

Group 1, green and yellow vegetables. Group 2, oranges, tomato, grapefruit and raw salads. Group 3, potatoes and other vegetables and fruits. Group 4, milk and cheese. Group 5, meat, poultry, fish and eggs. Group 6, bread, flour, cereals. Group 7, butter, margarine.

**basil** May be one of four different types of herb, but the main one is the European sweet basil, *Ocimum basilicum*. Used in seasoning.

**batata** See *potato, sweet*.

**Bath bun** Small English cake made with yeast (Dr W. Oliver of Bath, 1750).

**Bath chap**   Cheek and jawbones of the pig, salted and smoked. Originated at Bath.

**Bath cheese**   Small English cheese made from cow's milk with subsequent addition of cream.

**Bath Oliver**   Biscuit made with yeast (Dr W. Oliver of Bath, 1750).

**Baudouin test**   Colour test for sesame oil used to detect traces of sesame in other oils. In some countries sesame oil is added to all oils except olive oil to facilitate detection of adulteration of the olive oil (similarly for adulteration of ghee).

**Baumé**   Scale used to measure density of liquids. Specific gravity at 60°F (15.5°C) corresponds to degrees Baumé for all liquids heavier than water.

**Baycovin**   Trade name (Bayer Co.) for diethyl pyrocarbonate.

**bdelygmia**   Extreme loathing for food.

**Bé**   Abbreviation for degrees Baumé.

**beans**   See *legumes, food*.

**beans, baked**   Usually mature haricot beans, *Phaseolus vulgaris*, (see *legumes, food*), cooked by autoclaving.

**beans, broad**   *Vicia faba*. See *legumes, food*.

Analysis after cooking, whole beans without pod, per 100 g: water 84 g, protein 4 g, carbohydrate 7 g, kcal 43 (176 kJ), Fe 1 mg, nicotinic acid 3 mg, vitamin C 15 mg. Also known as horse bean.

**beans, butter**   Several varieties of *Phaseolus vulgaris*. See also *legumes, food*.

Analysis after cooking, per 100 g: water 70.5 g, fat trace, protein 7 g, carbohydrate 17 g, kcal 93 (390 kJ), Fe 1.7 mg.

Also known as Lima bean (USA), curry bean, madagascar bean and sugar bean.

**beans, French**   *Phaseolus vulgaris*, eaten unripe in the pod.

Analysis of cooked pod and beans per 100 g: water 95.5 g, fat trace, protein 0.8 g, carbohydrate 1.1 g, kcal 7 (30 kJ), Fe 0.6 mg, carotene 600 µg, vitamin C 5 mg.

Mature bean is the haricot bean. See also *legumes, food*.

**beans, haricot**   Ripe seeds of *Phaseolus vulgaris* (unripe seed is the French bean).

Analysis of cooked bean per 100 g: water 70 g, fat trace, protein 6.6 g, carbohydrate 16.6 g, kcal 89 (370 kJ), Ca 65 mg, Fe 2.5 mg.

Also known as Navy, string, pinto or snap beans (USA).

**beans, runner**   *Phaseolus multiflorus*, eaten unripe with pod.

Analysis after cooking, per 100 g: water 93.6%, protein 0.8%, carbohydrate 0.9 g, kcal 7 (30 kJ), Fe 0.6 mg, carotene 300 µg, nicotinic acid 0.5 mg, vitamin C 5 mg.

**beans, string** Usually runner beans, *Phaseolus multiflorus* but can also be haricot beans, *P. vulgaris*.

**béarnaise sauce** Thick French sauce made with egg yolk, butter, wine vinegar or white wine, and chopped shallots; named after the chef who invented it in about 1835.

**béchamel sauce** One of the basic French sauces made with milk, butter, flour. Named after Louis de Béchamel, court of Louis XIV, often called white sauce.

**bêche-de-mer** Sea slug, *Stichopus japonicus*, also called trepang; an occasional food in most parts of the world.

Analysis per 100 g: protein 22 g, carbohydrate 1 g, fat trace, Ca 120 mg, Fe 1.4 g, kcal 95 (400 kJ).

**beechwood sugar** Xylose.

**beef** Flesh of ox; composition varies with amount of fat present and the particular cut – e.g. brisket, forerib, rump, silverside, etc.

Dressed carcass, analysis per 100 g raw: 280 kcal (1.17 MJ), 16 g protein, 24 g fat, 59 g water, 1.9 mg Fe, 3.3 mg Zn, 0.05 mg thiamin, 0.2 mg riboflavin, 4 mg niacin, 0.2 mg vitamin E, 0.2 mg vitamin $B_6$, 1 µg vitamin $B_{12}$, 4 µg free folate, 0.5 mg pantothenate.

Rump steak, fried, analysis per 100 g: 250 kcal (1.0 MJ), 29 g protein, 15 g fat, 56 g water, 0.08 mg thiamin, 0.35 mg riboflavin, 5.5 mg niacin, 0.33 mg vitamin E, 0.3 mg vitamin $B_6$, 2 µg vitamin $B_{12}$, 4 µg free folate, 0.8 mg pantothenate; traces of other vitamins.

**beefalo** Cross between bull and buffalo which can be fattened on range grass rather than requiring cereal and protein supplement.

**beef tea** An extract of stewing beef prepared by simmering for 2–3 hours. Used to be used for invalids, as the meat extractives stimulate the appetite. See also *Bovril*; *meat extract*.

**beer** Alcoholic beverage produced by fermentation of cereals. The first step in manufacture is malting of the barley. It is allowed to sprout, when the enzyme amylase develops and hydrolyses the starch to dextrins and maltose. The sprouted barley is dried and extracted with hot water (the process is called mashing) to produce wort. After the addition of hops for flavour the wort is allowed to ferment.

Ale is a light-coloured beer made by top fermentation and containing more alcohol and hops.

Porter is made from partly charred malt and is darker in colour; it is also a top fermentation.

Stout is similar to porter, but contains more extract and a higher alcohol content.

Lager is made by bottom fermentation, is low in alcohol content, is rich in extract and is aged after fermentation.

Most beers, ale and stout contain 3–7% alcohol and 30–60 kcal per 100 ml.

**beestings**   The first milk given by the cow after calving.

**beet, common red**   Root of *Beta vulgaris*.

Analysis per 100 g, boiled: water 83 g, protein 1.8 g, fat trace, carbohydrate 10 g, kcal 44 (185 kJ), Fe 0.7 mg, Ca 30 mg, carotene trace, vitamin $B_1$ 0.02 mg, vitamin $B_2$ 0.04 mg, nicotinic acid 0.06 mg, vitamin C 5 mg.

**beet, leaf, silver, spinach**   Swiss chard.

**beet sugar**   Sucrose extracted from the sugar beet. It is identical with sucrose extracted from any other source.

**beeturia**   Production of red-pigmented urine after eating beet-root; occurs in only one person in eight and not consistently. The colour is due to the pigment betanin.

**bee wine**   Wine produced by the usual alcoholic fermentation of sugar, but using yeast in the form of a clump of yeast and lactic bacteria. The clump rises and falls with bubbles of carbon dioxide produced; hence the 'bee'.

**Bemax**   Trade name (Vitamins Ltd) of a wheat germ preparation.

Analysis per 100 g: protein 27.8 g, fat 9.3 g, carbohydrate 44.7 g, Ca 54 mg, Fe 7.7 mg, kcal 368 (1.55 MJ), vitamin $B_1$ 1.6 mg, vitamin $B_2$ 0.7 mg, nicotinic acid 7 mg.

**Benedictine**   French liqueur invented and manufactured by Benedictine monks at the Abbey of Fécamp; approximately 30% alcohol, 30% sugar, 300 kcal (1.3 MJ) per 100 ml.

**Benedict–Roth spirometer**   Apparatus for determining metabolic rate by measuring the amount of oxygen consumed.

**Benedict's test**   For reducing sugars; solution of copper sulphate, sodium citrate and sodium carbonate which gives a green, yellow or red precipitate on heating with a reducing agent, depending on the amount present. Benedict's quantitative re-agent also includes potassium thiocyanate and potassium ferro-cyanide.

**benniseed**   See *sesame*.

**bentonite**   See *Fuller's earth*.

**benzidine test**   Very sensitive test for blood. The substance under test is added to a saturated solution of benzidine in glacial acetic acid, followed by hydrogen peroxide. A blue or green colour is positive. See also *peroxidase*.

**benzoate**   See *benzoic acid*.

**benzoic acid**   $C_6H_5COOH$. Preservative normally used as sodium, potassium or calcium salt in acid foods such as pickles and sauces. Occurs naturally in cranberries, prunes, greengages, cinnamon and in very high concentrations in cloudberries. Excreted from the body in the urine conjugated with glycine (hippuric acid).

**bergamot** (1) Pear-shaped orange, *Citrus bergamia*, grown almost exclusively in Calabria, Italy, for its peel oil.

(2) An ornamental herb, *Monarda didyma*, dried leaves of which were used to make Oswego tea.

(3) Type of pear, *Pyrus persica*.

**beriberi** Result of a severe vitamin $B_1$ deficiency; common in the Far East, where white (polished) rice forms the bulk of the diet and vitamin $B_1$ is poorly supplied.

There are two forms of beriberi: the wet form, where oedema is present, and dry beriberi, where there is extreme emaciation. In both forms there is a degeneration of the nerves affecting the lower limbs first, gastrointestinal disorders, mental symptoms, an enlarged heart with an increased rate of beat; death ultimately results from cardiac failure.

**berries** Botanical name for fruits in which seeds are embedded in pulpy tissue – e.g. strawberry, currant, tomato.

**betaine** Trimethylglycine. Occurs in beetroot and cottonseed; also known as lycine and oxyneurine (obsolete names). Related to choline; possesses labile methyl groups.

**betanin** Violet-red pigment in beetroot, related to anthocyanins.

**beta-oxidation** One of the routes of fatty acid metabolism. Oxidation at the carbon atom beta to the carboxyl group of the fatty acid (i.e. next but one), with the formation of the beta-ketonic acid. Acetic acid then splits off, leaving a fatty acid two carbon atoms shorter than the original.

**betel** Leaf of the creeper *Piper betel* or *betle*, which is chewed in some parts of the world for its stimulating effect (due to presence of the alkaloids arecoline and guvacoline). The leaves are chewed with nuts of the areca palm, *Areca catechu*, which is therefore often called the betel palm, and the nut is called the betel nut.

**bezoar** A hard ball of undigested food which forms in the stomach and can cause intestinal obstruction. Foods with a high content of indigestible pectin such as orange pith can form bezoars if swallowed without chewing.

**BHA** Butylated hydroxyanisole.

**BHT** Butylated hydroxytoluene.

**BIBRA** British Industrial Biological Research Association.

**Bicarnesine** Trade name for synthetic carnitine.

**bifidus factor** A N-containing carbohydrate in human milk that stimulates growth of *Lactobacillus bifidus* in the intestine which lowers pH and suppresses *E.coli* and other pathogens. See also *lactulose*.

**biffins** Apples that have been peeled, partly baked, then pressed and dried.

**bigarade** French term for the bitter orange; see *orange, bitter*.

**bilberry** Berry of shrub of species *Vaccinium*. Variously named whortleberry, blaeberry (Iceland), windberry, huckleberry. Not cultivated but grows wild.

Analysis per 100 g: water 76.6–87 g, protein 0.7 g, free acid 1.1–1.7 g, sugar 3.8–6.8 g, pentosans, etc., 0.6–1.4 g, fibre 3.7–12.0 g, ash 0.3–1.0 g.

**bile** Liquid produced by the liver and stored in the gall bladder which is embedded in the liver. It consists of bile salts (sodium glycocholate and sodium taurocholate), bile pigments (bilirubin and biliverdin) and cholesterol. The bile salts play a part in the digestion of fats, as they lower the surface tension and aid the formation of a fine emulsion of fat. The bile pigments are waste products formed from the breakdown of haemoglobin and they are excreted in the faeces.

The bile travels from the gall bladder to the duodenum via the bile duct.

**bile salts** See *bile*.

**bilirubin** One of the bile pigments; formed by the degradation of haemoglobin; a reduction product of biliverdin.

**biliverdin** One of the bile pigments; formed by the degradation of haemoglobin.

**biltong** Dried meat strips (South Africa). The meat is cut in 2 inch strips, 2–3 feet long, along the muscle fibres, salted, spiced and dried in air for 10–14 days.

Analysis per 100 g: 11.5 g water, 1.9 g fat, 12.5 g ash, 65 g protein, 300 kcal (1.3 MJ).

**binge–purge syndrome** A feature of the psychiatric illness, bulimia (which see) characterised by ingestion of excessive amounts of food and the excessive use of laxatives.

**biocides** Chemicals used to destroy unwanted organisms – herbicides, insecticides, fungicides.

**biocytin** One of the bound forms of biotin which occurs naturally, the lysine derivative; not fully usable by all organisms until it has been hydrolysed to free biotin.

**bioflavonoids** Alternative name for flavonoids. See *vitamin P*.

**biological oxygen demand** (BOD) Micro-organisms consume oxygen for their respiration and the uptake of oxygen by a contaminated material, e.g. sewage, water, milk, etc., is a measure of microbial activity. Also termed biochemical oxygen demand.

**biological value** A quantitative measure of the nutritive value of a protein food carried out under conditions where quality of the protein is the limiting factor. Defined as the amount of absorbed protein retained in the body (expressed as a ratio) – i.e. digestibility is not taken into account. If digestibility is included (i.e. the amount retained is expressed as a fraction of the amount in the diet), the measure is net protein utilisation. NPU = BV × digestibility.

Previously expressed as a percentage scale, now as a ratio; thus, the perfect protein has BV = 1.0 (100% retained). Examples are egg and human milk protein, 0.9–1.0; meat, fish and cow's milk, 0.75–0.8; wheat bread, 0.5; peanut, 0.4–0.45; gelatin, zero. When fed as mixtures, these proteins complement one another. See *complementation*.

**bios** Name given in 1901 by Wildiers to factor in cell-free extract of yeast necessary for growth of yeast. Later the precipitate was shown to be bios I (identified 1920 as inositol); and the filtrate, bios IIa, beta-alanine, and IIb biotin (isolated 1936).

**Biostat** Trade name (Pfizer Ltd, USA) for ice containing the antibiotic oxytetracycline.

**biosterol** Obsolete name for vitamin A.

**biotin** Also known as vitamin H, identical with bios IIb and with coenzyme R (growth factor and respiratory stimulant for the organism *Rhizobium*, present in the root nodules of legumes).

Molecule has three asymmetric C atoms and eight stereoisomers: only D-biotin is biologically active.

Essential to a wide variety of animals, including man, but synthesised in the intestines. Is inactivated by combination with avidin, a protein in raw egg-white, and deficiency symptoms can be produced by feeding raw egg-white (not cooked). Deficiency causes dermatitis, loss of fur and disturbances of the nervous system in experimental animals.

Present in liver, kidney, egg yolk, yeast, vegetables, grains, nuts.

**biotoprotein** A soluble biotin protein complex that occurs naturally.

**biphenyl** Diphenyl, which see.

**birch beer** Non-alcoholic carbonated beverage flavoured with oil of wintergreen or oil of sweet birch and oil of sassafras.

**Birs dryer** Tower 60–70 m high, up which air at ambient temperature is blown while the product is sprayed from the top and so dried without heat.

**biscuit** Essentially a bakery confectionery dried down to low moisture content; name derived from Latin for twice-cooked. Made from soft flour; mostly rich in fat and sugar and consequently of high energy content, 420–510 kcal (1.7–2.1 MJ) per 100 g.

Termed cookie in the USA, where the word biscuit means a small cake-like bun.

**biscuit check**  The development of splitting and cracks in biscuits immediately after baking.

**Biskoids**  Trade name (Andomia Products) for saccharin.

**Bitot's spots**  Foam-like irregular plaques on the conjunctiva of the eye, often seen in vitamin A deficiency but not considered to be a characteristic deficiency sign.

**bitters**  Gentian, quassia and calumba, and, in small doses, quinine and strychnine. Used to stimulate gustatory nerves in the mouth and thus stimulate appetite.

**biuret test**  For proteins (actually for peptide bonds). Violet colour is developed when a drop of copper sulphate is added to a solution of protein in caustic soda.

**bixin**  Carotenoid pigment found in the seeds of the tropical plant *Bixa orellana*; the crude extract is the colouring agent annatto, which see.

**blackberry**  Berry of bramble, *Rubus fruticosus*.

Analysis per 100 g: protein 1.2 g, fat 1.0 g, 57 kcal (0.24 MJ), Fe 1.0 mg, vitamin A 50 µg, vitamin $B_1$ 0.03 mg, vitamin $B_2$ 0.05 mg, nicotinic acid 0.4 mg, vitamin C 24 mg.

**blackcurrant**  Fruit of the bush *Ribes nigra*. Of special interest because of its high vitamin C content.

Analysis per 100 g: protein 0.9 g, fat trace, carbohydrate 6.6 g, water 77 g, 30 kcal (0.12 MJ), Fe 1.3 mg, vitamin A 90 µg, vitamin $B_1$ 0.03 mg, vitamin $B_2$ 0.06 mg, nicotinic acid 0.25 mg, vitamin C 200 mg.

**black jack**  See *caramel*.

**black PN**  Food colour, tetra sodium salt of 8-acetamido-2-(7-sulpho-4-*p*-sulphophenyl-azo-1-naphthylazo)-1-naphthol-3,5-disulphonic acid. Also called Brilliant black BN. Not very stable.

**black tongue**  A symptom of nicotinic acid deficiency in dogs, historically useful in the isolation of the vitamin.

**blaeberry**  See *bilberry*.

**blanching**  A partial pre-cooking. Fruits and vegetables are blanched before canning, dehydrating or freezing, for a variety of reasons: softening of texture, shrinkage, removal of air, destruction of enzymes, removal of undesirable flavours. Consists of dipping in hot water, 82–93°C, for one-half to five minutes. Also done to remove excess salt from preserved meat and to aid removal of skin, e.g. from almonds. Can result in losses of 10–20% of sugars, salts and protein, some of the vitamins $B_1$, $B_2$ and nicotinic acid, and up to one-third of the vitamin C.

**blancmange powders**  Usually a cornflour base with added flavour and colour.

**bland diet**   One that contains the minimum of crude fibre or roughage and is therefore non-irritating and soothing to the intestine.

**bleach figure (for flours)**   Measure of extent of bleaching from relative paleness of extracted (yellow) pigments.

**bleaching**   In the context of food, usually refers to the bleaching of flour. (See *aging*.) Also refers to the bleaching of oils, a stage in the purification by which colloidally dispersed impurities and natural colouring matters are removed by activated earth or fuller's earth.

**bleaching agents**   See *aging*.

**bleeding bread**   A bacterial infection with *Bacillus prodigiosus* which stains the bread bright red. Under optimal conditions of warmth and damp the infection can appear overnight, and contamination of shewbread with this organism in churches has led to accusations and riots against religious minorities over the centuries.

**bloaters**   See *red herrings*.

**blood cells, white**   See *leucocytes*.

**blood, citrated**   Blood that has been prevented from clotting by the addition of citrate, which combines with the calcium. (See *coagulation, blood*.) 600 mg sodium citrate will prevent coagulation of 100 ml blood.

**blood, defibrinated**   Blood clots rapidly after it has been shed, when the soluble protein fibrinogen is converted into insoluble fibrin. If the blood is stirred with a rod, the fibrin can be removed as it forms and the blood, still containing the cells, will remain fluid. This is defibrinated blood.

**blood, oxalated**   Blood that has been prevented from clotting by the addition of oxalate, which combines with the calcium. (See *coagulation, blood*.) 160 mg sodium oxalate will prevent the clotting of 100 ml blood.

**blood, red cells**   Carry the red colouring matter, haemoglobin, which is the means of transporting oxygen and carbon dioxide in the blood stream. The cell, or erythrocyte, is 8.8 μm in diameter, 1.9 μm at its greatest thickness; 5 million per cubic millimetre of blood; exists for 120 days, then destroyed in the body, the iron being re-used.

**blood sugar**   The blood sugar is glucose, normally present (before breakfast) at 5 mmol/l (80–100 mg per 100 ml). The level rises after a meal (to around 7.5 mmol/l (150 mg per 100 ml)) but rapidly returns to normal as glucose is taken up by the tissues (except in cases of diabetes mellitus, which see).

Glucose provides the energy for muscular activity and it is stored in the liver and muscles after conversion to glycogen.

**blood sugar test**  See *glucose tolerance*.

**blood volume**  Average: males, 5.3 litres, females 3.8 litres; 78 and 66 ml per kg body weight, respectively. Can be calculated from Wilson's formula: volume (ml) = 43 × weight (kg) + 131 × height (inches) − 6250. Determined by injecting known amount of a dye, such as Evans Blue, and determining the degree of dilution in a sample of the blood.

**blood, white cells**  See *leucocytes*.

**bloom**  Fat bloom is the whitish appearance on the surface of chocolate which sometimes occurs on storage. It is due to a change in the form of the fat at the surface or to fat diffusing outward and being deposited on the surface.

**Bloom gelometer**  Instrument used for measuring the strength of jellies, and also for any test of firmness, e.g. staleness of bread.

For jelly strength the jelly is prepared at 6.66% concentration and chilled at 10°C for 16–18 hours. The instrument measures the load in grams needed to produce a 4 mm depression in the gel with a ½-inch diameter plunger.

Gelatin at 250 Bloom grams is used in jellied meat, at 200 in marshmallows.

**blueberry**  High-bush blueberry (*Vaccinium corymbosum*) and low-bush (*V. augustifolium*) grown in North America.

**blue cheese**  See *cheese, blue*.

**blue value**  (1) Of vitamin A, refers to the transient blue colour produced by reaction with antimony trichloride, the depth of colour being proportional to the amount of the vitamin present.

(2) Referring to starch, it is an index of the free soluble starch, i.e. the amylose, in a food, e.g. potatoes.

**blue VRS**  Sodium salt of 4,4'-di(diethylamino)-4",6"-disulphotriphenylmethanolanhydride.

**BMI**  See *body mass index*.

**BMR**  See *basal metabolic rate*.

**bobby veal**  From calves younger than 3 months.

**BOD**  See *biological oxygen demand*.

**body-building food**  Term indiscriminately used, usually refers to proteins. The Code of Practice suggests that no claim should be made for the body-building properties of a food unless a reasonable amount of protein (not specified) is present in a normal portion.

**body fluid**  See *water balance*.

**body mass index**  Weight (kg) divided by height (m) squared; used as index of obesity. Same as Quetelet's index, which see.

**body surface**  See *surface area*.

**bog butter**  Norsemen, Finns, Scots and Irish used to bury firkins of butter in bogs to ripen it for the strong flavour that developed.

**boheic acid**  Substance isolated from China tea (*Thea bohea*) by Rochelder, 1847, considered to be 'tannin'.

**boiled sweets**  Sugar and water boiled at such a high temperature, 149–166°C, that practically no water remains and a vitreous mass is formed on cooling. Actually a supersaturated solution of sugar.

**bole**  See *Armenian bole*.

**Bombay duck**  Fish found in Indian waters; eaten fresh or after salting and curing. *Harpodon nehereus* or *Saurus ophiodon*; the name is a corruption of bombil, local name of the fish.

**bomb calorimeter**  See *calorimeter*.

**bone**  Organic matrix of collagen, osseoalbumoid and osseomucoid, with an inorganic mixture of 85% calcium phosphate, 10% calcium carbonate and 1.5% magnesium phosphate. The inorganic mixture has the crystal structure of the mineral hydroxyapatite, which is composed of one molecule of calcium hydroxide to three of calcium phosphate. Fluoride and sulphate are also present in bone.

**bone broth**  Prepared by prolonged boiling of chopped bones. Of little nutritive value, consisting of 2–4% gelatin, with very little calcium.

**bone charcoal**  Bones degreased, broken to required size and heated in closed retorts. The organic matter is carbonised, leaving about 10% carbon deposited on a framework of calcium phosphate. Used to purify solutions by virtue of its properties of absorbing colouring matter and impurities.

**bone meal**  Prepared from degreased animal bones and used as a supplement to both animal feed and human food as a source of both calcium and phosphate; also used as plant fertiliser as a source of phosphate.

**Bontrae**  Trade name (General Mills, Inc., USA) for textured vegetable protein preparation made by spinning or extrusion.

**borage**  A herb, *Borage officinalis*, not grown on a commercial scale. The flowers and leaves are sometimes used to flavour beverages and have a flavour resembling that of cucumber.

**borax**  Sodium salt of boric acid.

**boric acid**  Derived from boron; has, in the past, been used as a food preservative (in bacon and margarine), but accumulates in the body.

**Boston brown bread**  In the United States, a spiced pudding steamed in the can.

**bottle house**  Old UK term for manufacturer of glass containers, i.e. bottles and jars as distinct from tableware.

**bottles**  The customary wine bottle holds 700 to 750 ml. In Great Britain this is one sixth of a gallon or a 'reputed quart' – 26 fluid oz. (A true quart is a quarter of a gallon or 2 pints.)

The two-bottle size is a magnum; four-bottle container is a Jeroboam; six is a Methusaleh; 12 is a Salamanzer; and 20 is a Nebuchadnezzar.

**botulinum cook** Degree of heat required to ensure (virtual) destruction of all spores of *Clostridium botulinum*, which are the most resistant of bacterial spores.

Botulinum cook is the number of minutes required at 121.1°C to achieve a 12D reduction (12 decimal reductions) in spore numbers, i.e. reduced by a factor of $10^{12}$. See also *decimal reduction time*.

**botulism** Rare form of food poisoning caused by extremely potent neurotoxins of *Clostridium botulinum* (seven types of antigenically distinct toxins have been identified). Derived from *botulus*, a sausage, because the illness was originally associated with sausages in Germany.

Botulism is rare but often fatal unless antitoxin is administered, and arises from consumption of food that has been incorrectly preserved or treated and in which many of the competing micro-organisms have been destroyed. A wide range of foods have been involved, including meat, fish, milk, fruits and vegetables, and the toxin may be formed without any apparent spoilage of the food.

The toxin can be destroyed by heating at 80°C for ten minutes, but is more resistant in foodstuffs.

**boucanning** Process by which meat was preserved by sun-drying and smoking while resting on a wooden grid – boucan (West Indies).

**bouillabaisse** Fish stew common in S. France, made from several kinds of fish and shellfish, cooked with oil, spices and herbs. So named since it is repeatedly boiled.

**bouillon** Plain, unclarified beef or veal broth.

**bouquet garni** See *faggot*.

**bourbonal** Ethylvanillin; see *vanilla*.

**Bournvita** Trade name (Cadbury-Schweppes Ltd) for a preparation of malt, milk, sugar, cocoa, eggs and flavouring, for consumption as a beverage when added to milk.

Analysis per 100g: protein 11.4g, fat 7.5g, carbohydrate 67.6g, Ca 89mg, Fe 3mg, kcal 370 (1.6MJ).

**Bovril** Trade name (Bovril Ltd) for a preparation of meat extract, hydrolysed beef, beef powder and yeast extract used as a beverage, breadspread and flavouring agent.

Analysis per 100g: protein 28g, vitamin $B_2$ 3.5mg, nicotinic acid 24mg, Fe 12mg.

**Bowman–Birk inhibitors** A group of protease inhibitors found, together with Kunitz inhibitors, in soya beans.

**boysenberry**   Similar to loganberry.

**brachyose**   See *isomaltose*.

**bradycardia**   An unusually slow heart-beat; a symptom, among other causes, of certain vitamin deficiencies.

**bradyphagia**   Eating very slowly.

**brain sugar**   One-time name for galactose.

**braise**   Cook in a closed container with little liquid, usually in the oven.

**bran**   The outer layers of cereal grain which are largely removed when the grain is milled – i.e. in preparation of white flour or white rice. The germ is discarded at the same time, and there is a considerable loss of iron and other minerals, and particularly of the B vitamins as well as of dietary fibre.

Analysis of wheat bran per 100g: 8g water, 4g sugars, 23g starch, 44g dietary fibre (mostly cellulose and hemicelluloses), 2.2g N (14g crude protein), 1.1g K, 1.2g P, 13mg Fe, 16mg Zn, 0.9mg thiamin, 0.4mg riboflavin, 30mg niacin, 1.6mg vitamin E, 1.4mg vitamin $B_6$, 130µg free folate, 2.4mg pantothenate, 14µg biotin.

See also *wheatfeed*.

**Bran Plus**   Trade name (Allinson's Ltd) for untreated wheat bran with germ.

Analysis per 100g: 13.7g protein, 57.4g carbohydrate, 13g water, 3.6g fat, 4.5g ash, 7.8g fibre.

**brandy**   Spirit distilled from wine; name derived from German, brandtwein (burnt wine), corrupted to brandywine; 40% alcohol.

Age generally designated as Three Star (3–5 years old before bottling); VSOP – Very Special Old Pale, aged 4–10 or more years, the name indicating that it has not been heavily coloured with caramel; Napoleon, premium blend aged 6–20 years; XO, Extraordinary Old (Extra or Grand Reserve) possibly 50 years old.

All cognacs are brandies but legally cognac comes only from the Charente region of N.W. France (where the town of Cognac is).

**brawn**   Made from meat, ears and tongue of the pig; boiled with peppercorns and herbs, minced and pressed into a mould. Mock brawn differs in that other meat by-products are used.

**bread**   Usually refers to a loaf made from wheat or rye flour, but mixtures of many cereals may be used. Wheat flour makes a softer loaf than other cereals, because the gluten is extensible and holds pockets of air. White bread is usually made from flour of 72% extraction rate; the composition depends on the type of flour used.

Analysis per 100 g wholemeal bread (white bread in brackets); water 38 g (37 g), protein 9 g (8 g), fat 2.5 g (2 g), carbohydrate 42 g (49 g), dietary fibre 7 g (4 g), 220 kcal – 0.9 MJ (235 kcal – 1 MJ), Fe 3 mg (1.6 mg), Ca 50 mg (100 mg), vitamin $B_1$ 0.3 mg (0.2 mg), vitamin $B_2$ 0.1 mg (0.06 mg), niacin 4 mg (1.7 mg).

Brown breads are made from flours of varying extraction rates between wholemeal and white flours. Added nutrients are present in, for example, protein bread, wheat germ bread, gluten bread and milk bread.

**bread, aerated**  The dough is made with water saturated with carbon dioxide under pressure. The object is to produce an aerated loaf without the loss of carbohydrate involved in a yeast fermentation (7% of the total ingredients). The result was insipid in flavour and the method went out of use, but see *glucono-delta-lactone*.

**bread, Allinson's**  Trade name for a wholemeal loaf.

Analysis per 100 g: protein 8.2 g, fat 2 g, carbohydrate 47.1 g, Ca 26 mg, Fe 3 mg, kcal 230 (1.0 MJ).

**Bread, Bank holiday**  Bread with extra fat to soften the crumb so that it will last over a long (Bank holiday) weekend.

**bread, batch**  The moulded pieces of dough touch one another and when baked and separated only the top and bottom of the loaves have crusts.

**bread, black**  Coarse wholemeal wheat or rye bread leavened with 'sauerteig' – i.e. a mixture of fermenting micro-organisms. These include: (1) peptonising bacteria that turn the dough to a more plastic state, (2) yeast, (3) lactic or acetic bacteria that produce the sour flavour.

**bread, brown**  A loaf may not legally be described as brown (or wholemeal) unless it contains not less than 0.6% fibre (on dry weight) – i.e. a high rate of extraction.

**bread, Cornell**  Loaf of increased nutritional value by addition of 6% soya flour and 8% skim milk solids. So-called because of participation of staff of Cornell University in its development.

**breadfruit**  The starchy fruit of the tree *Artocarpus communis* or *A. incisa*. Staple though seasonal food of the West Indies; eaten roasted whole when ripe or boiled in pieces when green.

Analysis per 100 g: water 70 g, carbohydrate 26 g, protein 1.5 g, fat 0.4 g, kcal 110 (0.47 MJ), Fe 1 mg, vitamin $B_1$ 0.1 mg, vitamin $B_2$ 0.06 mg, nicotinic acid 1.2 mg, vitamin C 20 mg.

**bread, lactein**  Loaf with added milk, usually about 6% milk solids, although 3–4% milk solids are often added to the ordinary loaf in the United States.

**bread, soda**  Bread leavened with sodium bicarbonate and an acidic substance instead of yeast, although legally it may contain yeast as well.

**breads, quick**  See *quick breads*.

**bread, starch-reduced**  Bread is normally 9–10% protein and about 50% starch; if the starch is reduced either by washing some part of it out of the dough or by adding extra protein, the bread is referred to as starch-reduced, and is often claimed of value in slimming and diabetic diets.

Legally the term 'starch-reduced bread' may be applied only to bread containing less than 50% carbohydrate and the wording claiming its value as a slimming aid is legally controlled.

**breakfast food, cereal**  Legally defined as any food obtained by the swelling, roasting, grinding, rolling or flaking of any cereal. Described under individual names (e.g. *All-Bran; Bemax; Cornflakes; Wheat, puffed; Wheat, shredded; Force*).

**break rolls**  See *milling*.

**Bredsoy**  Trade name (British Soya Products Ltd) for unheated (enzyme-active) full-fat soya flour.

**brewers' grains**  Cereal residue from brewing, containing about 25% protein; used as animal feed, and also a source of unidentified growth factors.

**brewers' pounds**  Before specific gravity was used in breweries, the strength of wort was expressed as the difference between the weight of a barrel of wort and that of a barrel of water (360lb). The excess weight over 360lb is denoted by brewers' pounds.

**brewing**  See *beer*.

**Brillat-Savarin**  French gourmet, 1755–1826, name given to several dishes and a consomme; also see *baba*.

**brine**  Salt solution of varying concentrations used in pickling. 'Fresh' brine may have added nitrite; 'live' brine contains micro-organisms that convert nitrate to nitrite (pickling salts).

**brislings**  Young sprats, *Clupea sprattus*. Canned brislings contain 300μg vitamin A and 25–50μg vitamin D per 100g.

**British Industrial Biological Research Association**  Joint Government–industry sponsored body that investigates food additives.

**Brix**  A table of specific gravity based on the Balling tables (which see), calculated in grams of cane sugar in 100g solution at 20°C, i.e. degree Brix = percentage sugar. Used to refer to concentration of sugar syrups used in canned fruits.

**broasting**  Cooking method in which the food is deep fried under pressure, which is quicker than without pressure and the food absorbs less fat.

**broil**  US term for grill.

**broiler chicken**  See *chicken*.

**bromatology** Science of foods (from the Greek *broma*, food).

**bromelains** Proteolytic enzymes in pineapple (*Ananas comosus*) and related members of Bromelidaceae; available as by-products from commercial pineapple production, usually from the stems; similar in activity to ficin (from the fig) and papain (from pawpaw), and used to tenderise meat, to treat sausage casings and to chill-proof beer.

**brominated oils** Brominated olive, peach, apricot kernel, soya oils, etc., used to help to stabilise emulsions of flavouring substances in soft drinks; also described as weighting oils.

**brose** Scottish dish made by pouring boiling water on oatmeal or barley meal; fish, meat or vegetables may be added.

**broth** Soup made from meat or bone extractives, with vegetables, meat, farinaceous material, spices and herbs. Legally, in the case of canned soups, the 'meat nitrogen' content must be equivalent to not less than 1% protein.

**brown colours** *Brown FK.* A mixture of the disodium salt of 1,3-diamino-4,6-di(*p*-sulphophenylazo) benzene and the sodium salt of 2,4-diamino-5-(*p*-sulphophenylazo)toluene – 'kipper brown'.

*Chocolate-brown FB.* The product of coupling diazotised naphthionic acid with a mixture of morin and maclurin (see *fustic*).

*Chocolate-brown HT.* Disodium salt of 2,4-dihydroxy-3,5-di(4-sulpho-1-naphthylazo) benzyl alcohol. Both these colours are 'baking browns'.

**brownie** American cake made with chocolate.

**browning reaction** See *Maillard reaction*; *phenol oxidases*.

**Brussels sprouts** Leaf buds of *Brassica oleracea gemmifera*.
Analysis per 100 g: protein 3.6 g, fat 0.4 g, Ca 26 mg, Fe 1.0 mg, kcal 36 (0.15 MJ), vitamin A 90 μg, vitamin $B_1$ 0.06 mg, vitamin $B_2$ 0.12 mg, nicotinic acid 0.5 mg, vitamin C 70 mg.

**bubble-and-squeak** Old English dish originally made from cold salt beef fried with cooked cabbage (name arose from the noise of frying vegetables). More commonly a mixture of cabbage and potato fried together.

**buckling** Hot-smoked herring. (The kipper is cold-smoked.)

**buckwheat** A cereal, *Fagopyrum esculentum* and other species, also known as Saracen corn and, when cooked, as kasha (Russian). Unsuitable for bread-making, eaten as the cooked grain, porridge or pancakes.
Analysis per 100 g: protein 11 g, fat 2 g, carbohydrate 70 g; kcal 350 (1.5 MJ), Fe 3 mg, vitamin $B_1$ 0.3 mg, vitamin $B_2$ 0.3 mg, nicotinic acid 3 mg.

**Budde's process** For preserving milk; see *milk, Buddeised*.

**buffers**  Substances that resist change in acidity or alkalinity. Salts of weak acids and weak bases are buffers, also proteins and amino acids by virtue of their content of both acidic and basic groups. See also *acid–base balance*.

**buffy layer**  Nutritional assessment of vitamin C status is best carried out on the leucocytes. However, when these are sedimented from blood they are contaminated with blood platelets, the mixture being termed the buffy layer or buffy coat preparation.

**bulgur**  Prepared, precooked wheat originating in the Near East. Wheat is soaked, cooked and dried; it is lightly milled to remove the outer bran and cracked. Eaten with soups, cooked with meat, etc.

Bulgur is the oldest processed food known; also called ala and American rice; cooked with meat it is called kibbe.

**bulimia nervosa**  A psychiatric illness characterised by powerful and intractable urges to overeat, followed by self-induced vomiting and excessive use of purgatives. Mostly affects women between 15 and 30; considered to be a variant of anorexia nervosa, which see.

**bullace**  Wild damson.

**bullock's heart**  See *custard apple*.

**bully beef**  Name given by troops in First World War to corned beef (canned salted beef).

**buni**  Coffee beans left in the field to dry; generally hard and of poor quality.

**bunt**  See *smut*.

**burghul**  Alternative name for bulgur.

**burning feet syndrome**  Aching and throbbing in the feet, later spreading upwards to the knees; results from long periods on a diet poor in protein and B vitamins.

Claimed to be cured by pantothenic acid but not confirmed, and the whole vitamin B complex appears to be necessary.

**busa**  See *milks, fermented*.

**bushel**  Dry measure of capacity, equivalent to 80 lb of distilled water at 17 °C with barometer reading 30 inches, i.e. 8 gallons or 4 pecks. Used as a measure of corn, potatoes, etc.

The weight of a bushel varies with the product – e.g. wheat 60 lb; maize 56 lb; rye 56 lb; barley 48 lb; oats 32 lb; paddy rice 45 lb.

The American measure is the Winchester bushel, which is 3% greater.

**butane diol** (butylene glycol)  $CH_3CHOHCHOHCH_3$. Colourless liquid soluble in both water and ether, with an energy content of 6 kcal (24 kJ) per g.

**butt**  Cask for beer or wine containing 108 imperial gallons.

**butter**  Prepared from milk fat by souring the cream either naturally or with a bacterial culture (starter) followed by churning. Usually not less than 80% fat, the remainder being water; 2% salt sometimes added; contains trace of protein and lactose; 740 kcal (3 MJ) per 100 g; may be coloured with annatto. Vitamin A about 1000 µg per 100 g, partly as carotene, higher in summer than winter; vitamin D 0.6–1.0 µg, vitamin E 2 µg.

**butter, black**  Butter that has been browned by heating, vinegar, salt, pepper or other seasoning then being added, and used as a sauce.

**butterine**  See *margarine*.

**buttermilk**  Residue left after churning butter, 0.1–2.0% fat with the other milk constituents proportionately increased. Has a slightly acid flavour together with a distinctive flavour due to diacetyl and related substances.

**buttermilk, cultured**  The modern equivalent of sour buttermilk, produced by acid-producing streptococci in skim milk.

**butter, Mowrah**  See *vegetable butters*.

**butter, process or renovated**  Butter that has been melted and rechurned with the addition of milk, cream or water.

**butter, vegetable**  See *vegetable butters*.

**butter, whey** (serum butter)  Made from the small amount of fat left in whey. It has a fatty acid composition slightly different from that of ordinary butter.

**butylated hydroxyanisole** (BHA)  Antioxidant used for fats and fatty foods, derived chemically from phenol, not destroyed by heat and therefore useful in baked products; active at concentration of 0.01–0.1%.

**butylated hydroxytoluene** (BHT)  Antioxidant used for fats and fatty foods.

**butyric acid**  Short-chain fatty acid, with the formula $CH_3CH_2CH_2COOH$. Occurs as the triglyceride as 5–6% of butter fat; small amounts in other fats.

**butyrine**  Alternative name for alpha-amino-*n*-butyric acid; found in the blood stream, derived from threonine and not present in the diet.

**BV**  Biological value.

**bynin**  Name given (by Osborne and Campbell, 1896) to an alcohol-soluble protein of malt; later shown to be identical with the alcohol-soluble protein of barley, and the name was abandoned.

# C

**CA**  See *gas storage, controlled*.

**cabbage**  Leaves of *Brassica oleracea capitata*.

Analysis per 100g: protein 1.1g, fat 0.1g, Ca 35mg, Fe 0.3mg, kcal 17 (0.07MJ), vitamin A 20µg, vitamin $B_1$ 0.04mg, vitamin $B_2$ 0.03mg, nicotinic acid 0.2mg, vitamin C 35mg.

**cacao butter**  Cocoa butter.

**cachexia**  An extreme state of general ill-health, with malnutrition, wasting, anaemia, and circulatory and muscular weakness.

**cadaverine**  1,5-pentanediamine, formed by decarboxylation of lysine, and found in decomposing meat and fish; toxic.

**cadmium**  This mineral accumulates in the body throughout life, reaching 20–30mg (200–300µmol), but does not appear to be a dietary essential. Cadmium poisoning is a recognised industrial hazard. In Japan it has been incriminated in itai-itai disease, a severe and sometimes fatal loss of calcium from bone tissue – the disease occurred in an area where rice was grown on land irrigated with contaminated waste waters. Experimentally, the toxic effects of small doses of cadmium can be reversed with zinc (possibly owing to competition).

**caecum**  First part of the large intestine, separated from the small intestine by the ileo-colic sphincter. It is small in carnivorous animals, very large in herbivores as it is involved in cellulose digestion, of intermediate size in man.

**caffeine**  Alkaloid drug (trimethylxanthine) found in coffee and tea. Raises blood pressure, stimulates kidneys and averts fatigue temporarily.

Coffee beans contain 1% caffeine; hence, the beverage contains about 18mg per oz or 100mg per cup. Tea contains 1.5–2.5% caffeine, about 12–15mg per oz of beverage. Cola drinks contain 3–4.5mg per oz.

Also called theine.

**caffeol**  Volatile oil giving characteristic flavour and aroma to coffee.

**calabash**  See *gourds*.

**calamondin**  Citrus fruit resembling a small tangerine, with a delicate pulp and a lime-like flavour.

**calcifediol**  25-hydroxy derivative of vitamin D.

**calciferol**  Old name for ergocalciferol or vitamin $D_2$, made by irradiation of ergosterol. See *vitamin D*.

**calcitriol**  1,25-dihydroxy derivative of vitamin D.

**calcium**  The major inorganic ingredient of bones and teeth, totalling about 1–1.5kg in the adult body. The small amounts in blood (2.1–2.6mmol/l, 9–11 mg/100ml) and in the soft tissues play a vital role in metabolic reactions, and control the heart beat and the excitability of muscle and nerve.

Recommended daily intake about 0.5 g/day; higher in growing children and during lactation.

Absorption requires vitamin D. Richest sources are milk and cheese; added to flour in some countries.

See also *hypercalcaemia*; *parathyroid glands*; *phytic acid*.

**calcium acid phosphate**  Also known as monocalcium phosphate, and acid calcium phosphate or ACP, $Ca(H_2PO_4)_2$.

Used as the acid ingredient of baking powder and self-raising flour since it reacts with bicarbonate to liberate carbon dioxide.

Chemically similar to 'superphosphate' fertiliser but purer.

**calcium gluconate**  Water-soluble salt of calcium and gluconic acid useful for intravenous administration (e.g. in the relief of tetany).

**calcium–phosphate ratio**  Rickets can be caused in the rat by feeding a diet with a high ratio of calcium to phosphate, and it was thought at one time that the ratio for man should lie between $1:2$ and $2:1$, but within the range normally ingested phosphate does not appear to have any effect on the absorption of calcium, except possibly in young infants.

**calculus**  Stone formed in tissues such as kidney and gall bladder. Kidney stones consist of uric acid, urates, and calcium oxalate, carbonate and phosphate. Possibly of dietary causation.

Renal calculus – stones in kidney or ureter.

Vesical calculus – prostatic gland obstruction.

Biliary calculus – gallstone, which see.

**Calfos**  Trade name (Croda Food Ingredients Ltd) for a prepared bone meal, i.e. calcium phosphate used as a source of calcium and of phosphate in foods. Similarly Calphos is a trade name (Joseph Crosfield and Sons Ltd).

**calorie**  The unit of heat used in nutrition is the kilocalorie, amount of heat required to raise the temperature of 1 kg of water from 15 °C to 16 °C, abbreviated to kcal or written with a capital C to distinguish it from the small calorie.

**calorie conversion factors**  See *Atwater factors*; *energy conversion factors*; *Rubner factors*.

**calories, empty**  Refers to foods that supply only energy with little, if any, of the nutrients.

**calorie values**  See *energy*.

**calorimeter** (bomb calorimeter)  Instrument for measuring the amount of oxidisable energy present in a substance by burning it in oxygen and measuring the heat released. The heat liberated by burning a food in this way will coincide with the metabolisable energy in that food only if it can be completely metabolised. For example, proteins liberate 5.65 kcal/g in the bomb calorimeter in which the nitrogen is oxidised to the dioxide, but only 4.4 kcal/g in the body where the nitrogen is excreted as urea and uric acid, etc. (containing 1.25 kcal/g).

**calorimetry, direct** Direct measurement of heat production. It is measured in man in a respiration calorimeter (Atwater–Benedict type); the subject is placed inside the calorimeter, which is a small room with insulated walls. The heat produced is measured by the rise in temperature of water flowing round the walls. This type of apparatus was used in the early days of research into energy metabolism.

**calorimetry, indirect** Measurement of energy output by calculation from the oxygen consumption and carbon dioxide output. See *spirometer*.

**caltrops** See *chestnut, water*

**calvados** See *apple jack*.

**Calvin cycle** Carbon fixation in plants. See *photosynthesis*.

**cAMP** See *adenosine nucleotides*.

**Campbell's process** A method of drying milk by first concentrating by blowing hot air through, followed by drum-drying; patented in England 1901.

**Campden process** The preservation of food by the addition of sodium bisulphite, which liberates sulphur dioxide. Also known as cold preservation, since it replaces heat sterilisation.

**Campden tablets** Tablets of sodium bisulphite.

**camu-camu** A Peruvian fruit from the bush *Myrciaria paraensis*; burgundy red in colour, 6–14 g weight, 3 cm diameter: 3000 mg vitamin C per 100 g pulp.

**canapés** Small open sandwiches.

**canbra oil** Oil extracted from genetically selected variety of rapeseed with not more than 2% erucic acid. See *erucic acid*.

**Canderel** Trade name (originally G. D. Searle) for tablets of aspartame.

**Candida** See *yeasts*.

**candied peel** Used in confectionery; prepared by softening the peel, often of citrus fruits, and boiling for prolonged period with sugar syrup.

**candy** (1) Crystallised sugar made by repeated boiling and slow evaporation.

(2) United States term for sugar confectionery.

**candy doctor** See *sugar doctor*.

**cane sugar** Sucrose extracted from the sugar cane; identical with sucrose prepared from any other source, such as sugar beet.

**canihua** Seeds of *Chenopodium pallidicaule*, grown in Andes, Peru, for food. 14% protein, 4% fat, 52% starch.

**canner's alkali**  Mixture of sodium hydroxide and sodium carbonate used to remove skin from fruit before canning (sodium hydroxide alone more frequently used).

**canning, aseptic**  Foods are pre-sterilised at very high temperatures, 150–175 °C, for a few seconds and then sealed into cans under aseptic conditions. The flavour, colour and vitamin retention are superior with this short time–high temperature process compared with conventional canning.

The rate of bacterial spore destruction is approximately multiplied tenfold for every 10 °C rise in temperature, while the rates of chemical reactions responsible for loss of quality are doubled for every 10°C rise in temperature.

**canola**  Variety of rape low in glucosinolate. See *rape*.

**canthaxanthin**  A red carotenoid pigment, chemically related to beta-carotene but without any vitamin A activity. Suggested use as addition to the diet of broiler chickens to impart a pigmented skin and shanks, and to the diet of trout to produce the bright colours of wild trout; these colours are normally derived from natural foodstuffs, which may be variable or in short supply.

Similarly, beta-apo-8′-carotenal, which is four-fifths of the beta-carotene molecule, can be used in chick diets to increase the colour of the egg yolks.

**capers**  Buds of unopened flowers of *Capparis spinosa* (Europe and North Africa): flavour for pickles and sauces.

**capillary fragility**  Refers to the resistance to rupture of the walls of a blood vessel, which would result in the leakage of red blood cells into the tissue spaces. There is some evidence that the flavonoids (see *vitamin P*) increase the resistance to rupture, and this has given rise to unverified suggestions that this group of compounds will protect against the common cold by increasing the resistance of the capillaries to infection.

**capon**  Castrated cockerel; slightly increased growth with more tender flesh than the cockerel. Surgery mostly replaced by 'chemical caponisation', i.e. implantation of pellets of female sex hormone.

**capric acid**  One of the fatty acids, $C_9H_{19}COOH$. Occurs as triglyceride in coconut, in goat and cow butter and in the fat of the spice bush.

**caproic acid**  One of the fatty acids, $C_5H_{11}COOH$. Found as triglyceride in goat and cow butter and coconut fat.

**caprylic acid**  One of the fatty acids, $C_7H_{15}COOH$. Occurs as triglyceride in goat and cow butter, coconut oil and human fat.

**capsicum**  See *pepper*.

**caramel**  Amorphous brown material formed by heating carbohydrates in the presence of acid or alkali. Also known as burnt sugar. Manufactured from various sugars, starches or starch hydrolysates, and used for both colour and flavour in a wide variety of foods – soft drinks, alcoholic beverages, baked goods, sauces, canned meats and stews.

**caramels** See *toffee*.

**caraway** Dried ripe fruit of *Carum carvi*. Main component of the volatile oil is carvone, with smaller amounts of limonene. Used for the liqueur kümmel, and on bread and rolls.

**carbohydrate by difference** In the analysis of foods it is difficult to determine the various carbohydrates and they are usually approximated by subtracting the measured protein plus ash plus fat from total. The figure can be corrected by subtracting dietary fibre which is non-available carbohydrate.

Carbohydrate by difference is the sum of: (a) unavailable carbohydrate – pentosans, pectins, hemicelluloses and celluloses; (b) available carbohydrate – dextrins, starch and sugars; (c) non-carbohydrates, such as organic acids and lignin.

**carbohydrate metabolism** See *glucose metabolism*.

**carbohydrates** Substances composed of carbon, hydrogen and oxygen with two atoms of hydrogen for every oxygen. They include polysaccharides such as starch, dextrins and glycogen which are digested to glucose, and sugars such as lactose, fructose and glucose, as well as undigestible materials (see *carbohydrates, unavailable*).

They form the major part of the diet of man in the form of starch and sucrose in particular, and provide energy at the rate of 4 kcal or 16 kJ per g. The loss of water in the formation of disaccharides and polysaccharides from the monosaccharides results in slight differences in energy content – monosaccharides 3.74 kcal or 15.6 kJ, disaccharides 3.95 kcal or 16.5 kJ, starch 4.18 kcal or 17.5 kJ and glycerol 4.32 kcal or 18.0 kJ per g.

**carbohydrates, unavailable** The term includes pentosans, pectins, hemicellulose, cellulose, lignin and gums which are not digested and therefore unavailable to monogastric animals, but some are available to ruminants.

**carbon dioxide, available** See *baking powder*; *flour, self-raising*.

**carbon dioxide storage** See *gas storage*.

**carbonic anhydrase** Enzyme that converts carbon dioxide and water into carbonic acid. This is normally a slow process and its acceleration by the enzyme is an essential part of respiration (transfer of carbon dioxide from the tissues to the lungs). Present in red blood cells; plays part in gastric secretion of hydrochloric acid; contains zinc.

**carboxymethylcellulose** Prepared from the pure cellulose of cotton or wood. Absorbs up to 50 times its weight of water to form a stable colloidal mass, and used (in combination with stabilisers) as a whipping agent, in ice-cream, confectionery, jellies, etc., and as an inert food filler in slimming aids.

Methyl cellulose is another cellulose derivative but differs from the above (and other gums) since its viscosity increases with rise in temperature instead of decreasing; hence, it is soluble in cold water and gels on heating. Used as thickener, emulsifier, in foods low in gluten, etc.

Other cellulose derivatives with similar properties are ethyl methyl cellulose, and hydroxyethylcellulose.

**carboxypeptidase** Enzyme of the pancreatic juice which splits polypeptides to dipeptides. Removes the terminal unit of the chain in which the carboxyl radical is free; hence, it is an exopeptidase.

**carcinogen** Substance able to induce cancer.

**cardamom** Dried, nearly ripe, fruit, and the seed of *Elettaria cardamomum* (ginger family). The volatile oil contains cineol and terpineol. Used as flavouring in sausages, in bakery goods and in curry powder, and used in whole, mixed pickling spice.

**carenol** Name once suggested for vitamin A but not accepted.

**carmine-fibrin** Chopped blood fibrin that has been soaked in ammoniacal carmine solution. It is used as a test for proteolytic activity, since, when digestion takes place, the liberation of the carmine into the solution acts as an indicator.

**carmoisine** Red colour, also called azorubin; disodium salt of 2-(4-sulpho-1-naphthylazo)-1-naphthol-4-sulphonic acid.

**carnitine** $\beta$-hydroxy-$\gamma$-butyrobetaine. Occurs in all animal tissues, involved in intracellular fat metabolism. Not a dietary essential for vertebrates but is a growth factor for some insects, e.g. *Tenebrio molitor*, the mealworm, and so-called vitamin $B_T$.

**carnosine** $\beta$-alanyl histidine; dipeptide found in muscle of most animals.

**carob seed** Seeds and pod of *Ceratonia siliqua*, also known as locust bean and St John's bread. Contains a sweet pulp rich in sugar and gums 21% protein, 1.5% fat; used for fodder and for the preparation of carob-seed gum used for emulsifiers, cosmetics and textile sizes.

**Carophyll** Trade name (Hoffman La Roche) for apo-8-carotenal. See *carotenal*.

**carotenal** ($\beta$-apo-8'-carotenal) Red-orange carotenoid pigment which is an intermediate in the metabolism of $\beta$-carotene; used as a food colour in many countries; has vitamin A activity.

**carotene** Red pigment in plants; obvious in carrots, red palm oil and yellow maize, masked by chlorophyll in leaves.

It is converted into retinol in the body. About one-third of the vitamin A of western diets is supplied as carotene. Present to only a limited extent in animal tissues: for example, there is some carotene as well as retinol in milk.

Occurs in three forms – α-, β- and γ-carotenes – and lends name to a range of pigments of similar structure, the carotenoids, only a few of which are vitamin A-active.

Before the preparation of pure retinol β-carotene was used as the vitamin A standard – 0.6 μg of β-carotene = 1 i.u. of vitamin A. α- and γ-carotenes have only half the vitamin A potency of β-carotene.

Since carotene is poorly absorbed from foods (about 33%) and the efficiency of conversion to vitamin A in the body is one-half of the available β-carotene, the utilisation efficiency is taken as one-sixth. Thus, 1 μg of β-carotene in the diet is equivalent to 0.167 μg retinol.

Used as a colouring material in foods and as a source of vitamin A in vegetarian and kosher margarines.

**carotenoids** A group of yellow to red pigments occurring widely in plants and animals and structurally related to carotene. Some are converted into retinol in the body – the carotenes, crypto-xanthin, echinenone, torularhodin and apocarotenal; others are not – canthaxanthin, lycopene, zeaxanthin, bixin.

**carotenols** Carotenoid pigments carrying the hydroxyl group. The term 'xanthophylls' is often used collectively for these hydroxylated carotenoids, apart from the substance xanthophyll itself.

**carotin** Obsolete spelling of carotene.

**caroto-albumin** Carotene–protein complex in the blood serum, presumed to be the mode of transport of carotene in the body.

**carrageenan** Anionic polysaccharide composed of sulphated galactose units extracted from red algae, especially *Chondrus crispus* (Irish moss) and *Gigartina stellata*.

Increases viscosity, binds water to form a gel and reacts with proteins to form emulsions – used in milk drinks, processed cheese, low-energy foods, etc.

**carrot** Root of *Daucus carota*, commonly used as a vegetable; an extremely rich source of carotene – 5–15 mg per 100 g. The lower range is present in the young carrots harvested in early summer, higher values in the older carrots.

Analysis per 100 g: water 90 g, sugars 5 g, protein 0.7–0.9 g, 20 kcal (90 kJ).

**Carr–Price reaction** Test for vitamin A which gives a blue colour with a solution of antimony trichloride in chloroform (the Carr–Price reagent).

**Carter's spread** Name given to a mixture of butter (68%) with hydrogenated oil (12.4%) plus salt, preservative and lecithin, used as a breadspread.

**cartilage** Consists mainly of collagen, chondromucoid (protein plus chondroitin sulphuric acid) and chondroalbumoid (a protein similar to elastin). New bone growth consists of cartilage on which calcium salts are deposited at a later stage to form the bone.

**Cartose** Trade name (Winthrop Laboratories, USA) for a steam hydrolysate of maize starch used as a carbohydrate modifier in milk preparations for infant feeding. Consists of a mixture of dextrin, maltose and glucose.

**casein** A heterogeneous group of phosphoproteins precipitated from skim milk at pH 4.6 and 20 °C – isoelectric casein. Consists of 12–15 fractions separable by electrophoresis or differential solubilities in urea. Comprises about 75% of the total milk proteins. Also precipitated by the enzyme rennin in an insoluble form, whereas isoelectric casein can be solubilised by NaOH at pH 6.7 as the sodium salt or the hydrogen form by additional acid.

**casein, Hammarsten's** See *Hammarsten's casein*.

**casein, iodinated** (caseoiodine) Casein with about 9% iodine introduced into the molecule; has some thyroactive properties similar to those of thyroxine.

**caseinogen** Obsolete name used in Great Britain for the form in which casein is present in milk; when it had been precipitated, it was then termed casein.

**caseoiodine** Iodinated casein containing about 9% iodine.

**Casilan** Trade name (Glaxo Laboratories Ltd) for a casein preparation used as a protein concentrate – 90% protein, 1.8% fat, 3.8% mineral salts.

**cassareep** The juice of the bitter cassava or manioc. It is boiled to a thick syrup and used as a base for sauces.

**cassava** (manioc) Tuber of the plant *Manihot utilissima*. Staple article of diet in many tropical countries, although an extremely poor source of protein.

One of the most productive crops, yielding (e.g. in Nigeria) 13 million kcal per acre, compared with yam, 9 million, sorghum, 1 million, and maize, 1 million.

Analysis per 100 g: protein 0.9 g, fat 0.2 g, Ca 25 mg, Fe 0.5 mg, kcal 109 (0.46 MJ), vitamin $B_1$ 0.04 mg, vitamin $B_2$ 0.02 mg, nicotinic acid 0.4 mg, vitamin C 27 mg.

The juice from the roots is cassareep, used in sauces and fermented with molasses. The leaves are eaten as a vegetable. The tuber is a source of tapioca, which see.

**cassia** Inner bark of a tree grown in the Far East – used as a seasoning; similar in appearance and flavour to cinnamon.

**cassina** Beverage (tea substitute) made from cured leaves of a holly bush, *Ilex cassine*; contains 1–1.6% caffeine and 8% tannin.

**castor oil** From the castor oil bean, *Ricinus*. The oil itself is non-irritating, but in the small intestine is hydrolysed by lipase to liberate ricinoleic acid, which is an irritant to the gastrointestinal mucosa and therefore acts as a purgative.

**catabolism** See *metabolism*.

**catadromous (fish)** Live in fresh water and go to sea to spawn, e.g. salmon.

**catalase** Enzyme in plants and animals which splits hydrogen peroxide into water and gaseous oxygen. It is a conjugated protein containing haem (identical with the haem of haemoglobin) as its prosthetic group.

**catalyst** Substance that alters the rate of a chemical reaction; mostly of use when it accelerates the reaction. Metallic platinum is a catalyst in the manufacture of sulphuric acid; metallic nickel is a catalyst for the hardening of oils with hydrogen.

Enzymes are defined as organic catalysts produced by living cells.

**catchup** Alternative spelling of catsup or ketchup. See *ketchup*.

**cathepsins** Group of intracellular proteolytic enzymes in animal tissues. Probably function in the normal breakdown and re-synthesis of tissue proteins. Are responsible for the autolytic softening of the flesh when game is 'hung'.

There are four enzymes in the group, cathepsins I, II, III and IV, respectively similar to pepsin, trypsin, aminopeptidase and carboxypeptidase.

**cation** See *ionisation*.

**catsup** See *ketchup*.

**cauliflower** White edible flower of *Brassica oleracea botrytis*. Horticulturally, varieties that mature in summer and autumn are called cauliflowers and those that mature in winter are broccoli, but commonly both are called cauliflower.

Analysis per 100 g raw: 93 g water, 1.5 g sugars, 2.1 g dietary fibre, 1.9 g protein, 13 kcal (55 kJ), 0.1 mg thiamin, 0.1 mg riboflavin, 0.6 mg niacin, 50–90 mg vitamin C, 0.2 mg free folate, 0.6 mg pantothenate, trace carotene.

**caviar(e)** Salted hard roe of the sturgeon (Acipenseridae family).

Analysis per 100 g: 30 g protein, 20 g fat, nil carbohydrate, 340 kcal (1.42 MJ).

**Celacol** Trade name (Courtauld Ltd) for derivatives of cellulose, methyl, hydroxyethyl, etc.

**celeriac** Turnip-rooted celery, *Apium graveolens* var. *rapaceum*, of which the swollen base of the stem is the edible part; closely related to celery but the stems are small and bitter.

Analysis per 100g, boiled: 90g water, 2g carbohydrate, 4.9g dietary fibre, 1.6g protein, 14kcal (60kJ), traces of B vitamins, about 4mg vitamin C.

**celery** Edible stems of *Apium graveolens*.

Analysis per 100g, raw: 93.5g water, 1.3g carbohydrate, 1.8g dietary fibre, 0.9g protein, 8kcal (36kJ), trace of B vitamins, approximately 7mg vitamin C.

Related to celeriac, *Apium graveolens* var. *rapaceum*, which is grown for the swollen base at its stem.

**celiac disease** See *coeliac disease*.

**cellobiose** Two molecules of glucose joined together in the 1,4'-β position (as distinct from the 1,4'-α bond in maltose). Cellobiose is the basic structural unit of cellulose and does not exist in the free state in nature.

**Cellofas** Trade name (Imperial Chemical Industries Ltd) for derivatives of cellulose – e.g. Cellofas A, methyl ethyl, Cellofas B, sodium carboxymethyl.

**Cellophane** Trade name for the first of the transparent, non-porous films (1925); made from wood pulp (cellulose).

**celluflour** Powdered cellulose; used in experimental diets to provide indigestible bulk.

**cellulase** Enzyme that attacks cellulose; present in the digestive juices of various snails, wood-boring insects, and micro-organisms. The cellulase present in the intestinal micro-organisms of ruminants is responsible for the ability of these animals to obtain energy from straw, for their own digestive juices do not contain cellulase.

**cellulose** Polysaccharide that forms the supporting cell structure in plants; does not occur in animals. Consists of long chain of glucose units.

Is not digested in man or other monogastric animals, but serves a useful purpose in providing bulk for intestinal functioning. It is digested by the bacteria in the rumen of ruminating animals, which can therefore subsist on grass and hay.

Paper and wood are essentially cellulose. Commercial sources are cotton and wood pulp.

In the native state molecular weight is 600000–1.5 million; depolymerises during extraction to yield different products. Alpha-cellulose has m.wt 80000–340000. Acid hydrolysis converts this into microcrystalline cellulose, m.wt 30000–50000, used as filler in 'slimming foods'.

**cellulose derivatives** See *carboxymethylcellulose*.

**centrifuge** Machine that exerts a pull many times stronger than gravity by spinning. Used to clarify liquids by settling the heavier solid in a few minutes, a process that might take several days under gravity. Also used to separate two liquids of different densities – e.g. cream from milk.

**cephalins** Alternative spelling to kephalins, which see.

**Ceplapro** Protein-rich baby food (18–20% protein) made in granular form from degerminated maize flour, wheat, defatted soya flour and skim milk powder, with added calcium and vitamins. Made in the USA.

**cereal coffee** Prepared from roasted cereal grains.

**cereals** Any grain or edible fruit of the grass family which may be used as food. Include wheat, rice, oats, rye, barley, maize and millet.

Provide the largest single type of foodstuffs. In the Far East cereal often constitutes 90% of the diet; even in the UK bread and flour provide one-third of the calories and at the same time one-third of the protein of the average diet.

**cerebrose** One-time name for galactose.

**cerebrosides** Part of the structural matter of brain and the myelin sheath of nerves. Contain phrenosin, kerasin, fatty acid, sphingosine and galactose. This is the only structure of the body that contains the sugar galactose.

**cerelose** Commercial glucose with about 9% water.

**ceruloplasmin** Copper–protein complex which constitutes major part of circulating blood copper in man (and other mammals); involved in iron metabolism.

**cervelat** See *sausage*.

**Cetavlon** Trade name (ICI) for detergent and bacteriostat, cetyltrimethylammonium bromide.

**cetyl alcohol** Solid, waxy, straight-chain alcohol of sixteen carbon atoms, found in spermaceti (from the sperm whale) and waxes. Can be spread as a thin (monomolecular) film on the surface of water in reservoirs, where it reduces evaporation of the water.

**CF** See *citrovorum factor*.

**challah** See *cholla*.

**chalva** See *halva*.

**chamomile** Can be either of two herbs, *Anthemis nobilis* and *Matricaria recutica*. Essential oil used for flavouring liqueurs; chamomile tea, made by infusing dried flower heads, used as old-fashioned tonic; whole herb used to make herb beers.

**chapati** (chappati or chuppati) Flat, unleavened Indian bread made from wheat flour or millet.

**charcoal** See *bone charcoal*.

**charqui (or charki)** Dried meat of Brazil, chiefly from beef but also from sheep, llama and alpaca in Peru. Strips of meat cut lengthways and pressed after salting, then air-dried; finished form is in flat, thin sheets, rather flaky, so differing from the long strips of biltong. Also called jerky.

**Chartreuse**   Liqueur originally made by monks of Chartreux, using, it is said, more than 200 ingredients.

There are three varieties: green 96% of proof spirit; yellow, 74.5%; and white, 52.5%.

**Chastek paralysis**   Acute dietary disease of foxes caused by the inclusion of 10% of raw fish in the diet. It is due to a deficiency of vitamin $B_1$ caused by the presence of the enzyme thiaminase in the fish, which destroys the vitamin. It is cured by adding vitamin $B_1$ to the diet.

**CHD**   Coronary heart disease. See *ischaemic heart disease*.

**cheddaring**   In the manufacture of cheese, after coagulation of the milk, heating of the curd and draining, the curds are piled along the floor of the vat, when, in the case of Cheddar cheese, they consolidate to a rubbery sheet of curd. This stage is the cheddaring process. (Cheshire cheese is not allowed to settle so densely and has a more crumbly texture.)

**cheese**   Prepared from the curd precipitated from milk by rennin or lactic acid. Cheeses other than cottage or cream are cured by being left to mature with salt, under various conditions that produce the characteristic flavour of the particular type of cheese.

Analysis per 100 g (hard cheese): protein 25 g, fat 31 g, kcal 400 (1.7 MJ), Ca 700 mg, Fe 1 mg, vitamin A 400μg, vitamin $B_1$ 0.01 mg, vitamin $B_2$ 0.45 mg, nicotinic acid 0.1 mg.

Most of the lactose of the milk is lost with the whey.

Legally must contain not less than 40% fat on a dry weight basis, and the fat must be milk fat.

**cheese analogues**   Cheese-like products made from casein and vegetable fat.

**cheese, blue**   Cheese that contains an internal growth of the mould *Penicillium roqueforti* – e.g. Blue Vinney, Stilton and Roquefort.

**cheese, cottage**   (pot cheese, Dutch cheese, Schmierkase)   Soft, uncured white cheese made from pasteurised skim milk (or milk powder) by lactic acid starter (with or without added rennet), heated, washed and drained (salt may be added). Contains more than 80% water.

Farm cheese is as above but the curd is pressed.

Baker's cheese or hoop cheese is as cottage cheese but not washed and is drained in bags, giving a finer grain; contains more water and acid than cottage cheese.

**cheese, processed**   Natural cheese passes its peak of flavour rapidly and processing temporarily arrests the deterioration. Processed cheese is loaf cheese, melted, pasteurised, with flavouring added (pimento, caraway, etc.), plus emulsifiers, and repacked.

Nutritive value identical with that of original cheese.

**cheese, whey**   Made from whey by heat-coagulation of the proteins (lactalbumin and lactoglobulin).

**cheilosis**   See *ariboflavinosis*.

**chelating agents**   Substances that combine with metal ions and remove them from their sphere of action; hence, also called sequestrants. Used to remove traces of metals which may cause food to deteriorate, clinically to reduce absorption of a mineral, in garden soils, and in chemical operations.

**Chelsea bun**   Yeasted bun that originated in Chelsea, London, eighteenth century.

**chemical caponisation**   See *capon*.

**chemical ice**   Ice containing chemicals used as preservative – e.g. a solution of antibiotics or other chemicals frozen and used to preserve fish.

**chemical score**   Chemical method of defining the nutritional value of proteins, proposed by Block and Mitchell (1946). The limiting amino acid in the protein under consideration is expressed as the percentage of the same amino acid present in egg (taken as the standard). Chemical score numerically equals biological value.

A later modification is protein score, in which a standard amino acid reference mixture is used instead of egg protein.

**chemotherapy**   Treatment of disease by chemicals that have toxic effect on the micro-organisms.

**chenopods**   Two species, *Chenopodium quinoa* (quinoa) and *C. pallidicaule* (canihua) used for human food in Andes, Peru – see *quinoa* and *canihua*. Other chenopods considered for poultry feed – Russian thistle, Summer cypress and Garden orache.

**cherry**   Fruit of *Prunus* species.

Analysis per 100 g: protein 1.0 g, fat 0.4 g, kcal 50 (200 kJ), Fe 0.4 mg, carotene 170 µg vitamin $B_1$ 0.05 mg, vitamin $B_2$ 0.05 mg, nicotinic acid 0.4 mg, vitamin C 7 mg.

**cherry, West Indian**   Fruit of a small bushy tree native to tropical and semi-tropical regions of America – *Malpighia punicifolia*. The richest known source of vitamin C; the edible portion of the fruit contains 1000 mg of vitamin C per 100 g when ripe, and the green fruit 3000 mg.

Also known as Barbados cherry and acerola (Spanish), and Antilles cherry.

**chervil**   (1) A herb, *Anthriscus cerefolium*, with parsley-like leaves used in the fresh green state as a garnish and for flavouring salads and soups.

(2) Turnip-rooted chervil, *Chaerophyllum bulbosum*, a hardy, biennial vegetable cultivated for its roots.

**Cheshire cat**   Old English cheese measure.

**chest sweetbread**   See *pancreas*.

**chestnut, water**   *Trapa natans*, also known as caltrops and sing-haranut. Seed is eaten raw or roasted.

Analysis per 100 g: 3 g protein, 15 g carbohydrate, 75 kcal (0.32 MJ), 0.8 mg iron, 0.05 mg vitamin $B_1$, 0.06 mg nicotinic acid, 16 mg vitamin C.

Chinese water chestnut is the tuber of the sedge *Eleocharis tuberosa*, imported in cans from Hong Kong.

**chewing gum**   See *gum, chewing*.

**chick anti-pellagra factor**   Obsolete name for pantothenic acid.

**chicken**   Domestic fowl. Rock Cornish game hen (US term), 5–7 weeks old, 2 lb; poussin, up to 6 weeks old, 1–1¼ lb; double poussin, 8–10 weeks, 1¾–2 lb; spring chicken (fryer) 12 weeks, 2–3½ lb; roasting chicken, up to 8 months, 3½–5 lb; capon, castrated cockerel, up to 8 months, 6–8 lb; boiling fowl, older animal usually after laying eggs; stag (US term) tough, male chicken up to 10 months. In recent years faster-growing strains are used to produce broilers, usually 10–12 weeks old and up to 3 lb in weight.

Analysis of raw meat per 100 g: 74 g water, 20 g protein, 4 g fat, 120 kcal (0.5 MJ), 0.7 mg Fe, 1 mg Zn, 0.1 mg thiamin, 0.16 mg riboflavin, 8 mg niacin, 0.4 mg vitamin $B_6$, trace vitamin $B_{12}$, 10 µg free folate, 2 µg biotin.

**chicle**   Basis of chewing gums, the partially evaporated latex of the evergreen sapodilla tree (*Achra sapota*); contains gutta (with elastic properties, consists of polymers of isoprene) and resin (triterpenes and sterols), together with carbohydrates, waxes and tannins.

The same tree produces the sapodilla plum.

**chicory**   *Cichorium intybus*. The leaves are eaten as a salad and the root, dried and partly caramelised, is often added to coffee as a diluent to cheapen the product.

The leaves are grown in the dark to prevent the development of the bitter flavour, and so are very pale in colour. Also called succory and (in Belgium) witloof. The French call chicory 'endive belge' and endive is called 'chicorée': in the USA chicory is called endive.

Analysis per 100 g (leaf and stem): water 96 g, protein 0.8 g, fat trace, carbohydrate 1.5 g (some of which is inulin), Fe 0.7 mg.

**chili sauce**   Sauce made from tomatoes, with spices, onions, garlic, sugar, vinegar and salt – similar to tomato catsup but containing more cayenne, onions and garlic.

**chilled foods** Perishable products stored at temperatures between 0 and +7°C.

**chilli** See *pepper*.

**chillproofing** Term used in reference to beer; treatment to prevent the appearance of haze when the beer is chilled. Chillproofs include tannic acid to precipitate the proteins, materials such as bentonite to adsorb them, and proteolytic enzymes to hydrolyse them.

**chimche** Basic Korean dish (in addition to fish and rice), consisting of fermented cabbage with garlic, red peppers and pimientos. Vitamin C content – 126 mg per 100 g – led to the suggestion that the Koreans have the highest intake of vitamin C.

**Chinese eggs** Known as pidan, houeidan and dsaoudan, according to variations in the method of preparation. Prepared by covering fresh duck eggs with a mixture of caustic soda, burnt straw ash, salt and slaked line, and storing for several months (sometimes referred to as hundred-year-old eggs). The white and yolk coagulate and become discoloured, with partial decomposition of the protein and phospholipids.

**Chinese restaurant disease syndrome** Headache, sweating, nausea, weakness, thirst, flushing of face, abdominal pain, lachrymation – occurs occasionally when Chinese food rich in monosodium glutamate is eaten. Mild symptoms can result from 25 mg/kg body weight taken on an empty stomach; results follow 25–35 min after ingestion and pass off after a few hours.

**chitin** Organic base of the hard parts of insects and crustacea, and present also in small amounts in mushrooms. Similar in composition to cellulose but contains glucosamine instead of glucose; insoluble and indigestible; poly-$\beta$-(1,4)-$N$-acetyl glucosamine. Partial deacetylation yields chitosans which are used as protein-flocculating agents.

**chitterlings** Intestine of ox, calf or pig.

**chive** *Allium schoenoprasum*, a plant grown for its bulbs and its long thin leaves, both with a mild onion flavour, used in salads, soups and omelettes.

**Chlorella** See *algae*.

**chlorine** An element that is found in biological tissues as the chloride ion. The body contains about 100 g of chloride and the average diet contains 6.7 g, mainly as sodium chloride.

Free chlorine is used as a sterilising agent – e.g. in drinking water.

**chlorine dioxide** A bread 'improver'; see *aging*.

**chlorocruorin** The copper-containing protein that carries oxygen in the bloodstream of the annelid worms – analogous to haemoglobin in mammals.

**chlorophyll**  Green colouring matter of all plant materials, by the aid of which plants manufacture foodstuffs from simple salts and carbon dioxide with energy derived from sunlight, i.e. photosynthesis. This is the true distinction between plants and animals: the latter must be supplied with complex foods ready made. Bacteria are on the borderline between the plant and animal kingdoms. Chlorophyll is a mixture of chlorophyll alpha and beta and two other pigments, xanthophyll and carotene.

**chlorophyllase**  Enzyme present in all green plants, which hydrolyses chlorophyll to phytol and chlorophyllide. Reversible in action and can catalyse the synthesis of chlorophyll.

**chlorophyllide**  The green colour found in the water after cooking certain vegetables. The fat-soluble chlorophyll is converted to water-soluble chlorophyllide by removal of the phytyl side-chain by alkali or enzyme.

**chlortetracycline**  See *tetracyclines*.

**chocolate**  Made from cocoa nibs (husked, fermented and roasted cocoa beans) by refining and the addition of sugar, cocoa butter, flavouring, lecithin and, if milk chocolate, milk solids.

Analysis per 100 g: plain: 60 g sugar, 5 g starch, 0.75 g N, 29 g fat, 2 mg Fe, 530 kcal (2.2 MJ); milk chocolate: 57 g sugar, 3 g starch, 30 g fat, 1.4 g N, 1.5 g Fe, 530 kcal (2.2 MJ).

**chocolate, drinking**  Partly solubilised cocoa for preparation of the beverage, including about 75% sucrose.

Analysis per 100 g: 74 g sugars, 3.6 g starch, 1 g N, 6 g fat, 30 mg Ca, 2 mg Fe, 370 kcal (1.5 MJ).

**cholagogue**  A substance that promotes the flow of bile from the gall bladder into the duodenum.

**cholecalciferol**  See *vitamin D*.

**cholecystokinin**  Hormone secreted by the mucosa of the duodenum and jejunum and carried in the blood to the gall-bladder, which is thus stimulated to contract and secrete bile.

**cholelithiasis**  Gallstones, which see.

**choleretics**  Substances that stimulate the secretion of bile – e.g. bile salts themselves taken by mouth, or cholic acid by intravenous injection.

**cholesterol**  (cholest-5-en-3-beta-ol) Principal sterol present in tissues of higher animals, found in all body tissues, especially brain and spinal cord. Not a dietary essential, since it is synthesised in the body. Eggs contain 450 mg per 100 g, yolk, dry weight, 1.8 g, milk 14 mg, cheese 70–120 mg, brain 2.2 g, liver and kidney 300–600 mg, poultry 70–100 mg, fish 50–60 mg.

Present in plasma lipoproteins as 45% of the low-density fraction, 20% of the high-density fraction, 13% of the very low-density fraction and 5% of chylomicrons.

**choline** Essential dietary factor, trimethyl hydroxyethylammonium hydroxide, usually classed as a vitamin, although the quantities involved are far from catalytic. Functions as a source of methyl groups and in fat transport; deficiency gives rise to fatty infiltration of the liver; is part of the structure of the phospholipids of animal and plant tissues. Specific dietary deficiency does not occur; daily requirements not established but the daily intake is 0.25–0.5 g. See also *acetylcholine*.

**cholinesterase** Enzyme that hydrolyses acetylcholine (which is liberated by the nerve ending to stimulate muscle), so that the muscle can recover and become prepared for the next stimulus.

A number of substances, anticholinesterases, which inhibit the enzyme paralyse muscle. Examples are war gases of the nerve group, certain insecticides and eserine, which is used clinically in cases of excess cholinesterase (the disease myasthenia gravis).

**cholla** Loaf of white bread made in twist form (or Biblical beehive coil) from one large and one small piece of dough plaited together.

The dough is made from white flour, enriched with eggs, and a pinch of saffron, and the loaf is decorated with maw or poppy seed.

Mentioned in the Bible and translated as 'loaves'; used for benediction on the Jewish Sabbath and festivals.

**chondroitin** A polysaccharide containing galactosamine and glucuronic acid. The sulphuric acid ester, chondroitin sulphate, is found in cartilage and the organic matrix of bone. Classed as a mucopolysaccharide.

**chondrometer** Instrument used to determine specific weight of wheat (kg per hectolitre). A wet English wheat may weigh 68 kg and a dry American wheat 84 kg per hectolitre.

*Chondrus crispus* See *carrageenan*.

**Chorleywood bread process** Method of preparing dough for bread-making in which the dough is submitted to intense mechanical working (5 watt-hours or 0.4 h.p. min per pound) so that, together with the aid of oxidising agents, the need for bulk fermentation of the dough is eliminated. This is a 'no-time' dough process and saves 1½–2 hours.

Named after the British Baking Industries Research Association at Chorleywood. The process permits the use of an increased proportion (20–25% replacement) of weaker flour, and produces a softer, finer bread which stales more slowly.

**choux pastry** Light, airy pastry invented by the French chef Carême, used in éclairs and profiteroles. The batter is precooked in a saucepan, then baked. *Chou* is French for cabbage – the characteristic shape of the cream-filled puffs.

**chowder** American term for a seafood soup; often made with clams or shrimps.

**chromatography** An analytical and preparative method of separating substances by differential absorption or partition on an inert stationary phase. Carried out on columns of powders such as aluminium oxide, calcium phosphate, calcium carbonate; on columns of ion-exchange resins; on cellulose paper; on thin layers prepared on sheets of glass, plastics or foil (thin-layer chromatography – TLC). In gas–liquid chromatography (GLC) the substances pass through the column of inert material in gaseous form. HPLC, high-performance liquid chromatography, is carried out under pressure.

**chromium** Known since 1797, but shown to be a dietary essential in 1959 in animals. Later, reduced glucose tolerance was shown in poorly nourished children which responded to chromium-containing extract of yeast, termed glucose tolerance factor (GTF). GTF is a nicotinic acid derivative of chromium and its only known function is to stimulate the enzymes involved in glucose metabolism and to facilitate the interaction of insulin with cell surface receptors.

**chromoproteins** Proteins conjugated with a metal-containing prosthetic group – e.g. vertebrate haemoglobins contain iron; invertebrate haemocyanins contain copper; chlorophyll contains magnesium.

**chufa** See *tiger nut*.

**chuño** Traditional dried potato in highlands of Peru and Bolivia; tubers crushed, pressed, frozen during the night and thawed and dried in sunshine during the day (freeze-dried).

**chyle** Lymph rich in fat. See *lymph*.

**chylomicrons** Droplets of unhydrolysed fat, triglycerides, in the lymph or bloodstream. See *lymph*.

**chymase** Alternative name for rennin.

**chyme** Partly digested mass of food as it exists in the stomach.

**chymosin** Preferred name for rennin.

**chymotrypsin** Proteolytic enzyme of the pancreatic juice; attacks parts of the protein molecule different from those attacked by pepsin and by trypsin. Secreted as the inactive precursor, chymotrypsinogen, activated by trypsin.

**cibophobia** Dislike of food.

**cider, cyder** An alcoholic beverage made by fermenting apple juice; contains 5–6% alcohol (by volume) and 0.7–2.0% sugar.

　　In the USA cider or fresh cider is a name given to fresh (unfermented) apple juice, and the fermented material is called hard or fermented cider.

**cieddu** See *milks, fermented*.

**ciguatera** Poisoning from eating fish feeding in the region of coral reefs in the Caribbean Sea and the Indian and Pacific Oceans. The species of fish are normally edible, and appear to derive the toxins, ciguatoxins, from their diet. Reported in seafarers' tales in the sixteenth century.

**cinnamon** The bark of various species of the genus *Cinnamomum*; it is split off the shoots, cured and dried. During drying the bark shrinks and curls into a cylinder or 'quill'.

Ceylon or true cinnamon differs from other types (*Cinnamomum zeylanicum*) and the oil contains mostly cinnamic aldehyde, together with some eugenol. Saigon cinnamon contains also cineol; Chinese cinnamon has no eugenol. Used as flavour in meat products, bakery goods and confectionery.

**cissa** Unnatural desire for foods; alternative words, cittosis, allotriophagy and pica.

**cis–trans isomerism** Compounds with the same molecular and structural formulae but which can exist in two geometric forms exhibit *cis–trans* isomerism. When the chemical groups in the molecule are paired on the same side, the form is *cis*; on opposite sides, it is *trans*. They have different chemical and physical properties.

**citral** Important constituent of many essential oils, especially lemon. Occurs in beta and alpha forms (*cis*- and *trans*-isomers); $C_{10}H_{16}O$.

Used as the starting material for the synthesis of ionone (the synthetic perfume with the odour of violets), a stage in the synthesis of retinol.

**citrange** American citrus fruit resulting from cross between ordinary orange and the trifoliate orange, *Poncirus trifoliata*.

**citrated blood** See *blood, citrated*.

**citric acid** Tricarboxylic acid, widely distributed in plant and animal tissues. Used as flavouring and acidulant in beverages and confectionary; provides 2.47 kcal per g.

Produced on an industrial scale by fermentation of sugars with the mould *Aspergillus niger* and extracted from citrus fruits – lemon juice contains 5–8% citric acid.

**citric acid cycle** The oxidation stage in the metabolism of foodstuffs. Carbohydrates and fats are broken down to acetate (active acetate or acetyl coenzyme A), and the first step in the cycle is the combination of the acetyl with oxaloacetate to form citrate. This passes through a series of reactions in which energy is released and carbon dioxide and water produced; the end-product is oxaloacetate.

Since many of the amino acids can be converted into substances that lie on this pathway, the citric acid cycle is the common metabolic pathway for all three major foodstuffs. Also known as Krebs' cycle.

**citrin** A mixture of two flavonones found in citrus pith, namely hesperidin and eriodictin (demethylated hesperidin). See also *vitamin P*.

**citron** First of the citrus fruits to become known to Europeans; *Citrus medica*. Very sensitive to cold and can be grown only in warm regions. Very thick peel; solid, sweet and acid-free pulp with practically no juice. Used for preparing candied peel.

**citronin** Flavanone glycoside from the peel of immature Ponderosa lemons – methyoxy-dihydroxy-rhamnoglucoside.

**citrovorum factor** Name given to a growth factor for the organism *Leuconostoc citrovorum*. Now known to be tetrahydroformyl-pteroyl glutamic acid, which is believed to be the active form of the vitamin folic acid.

**citroxanthin** Also known as mutachrome. Yellow carotenoid pigment in orange peel; has vitamin A activity.

**citrulline** Amino acid formed as an intermediate in the metabolism of urea in the body. Not of nutritional importance, since it is not found in food proteins.

*Citrus* Genus including *C. limonum* (lemon), *C. aurantifolia* (lime), *C. aurantium* (sour orange), *C. sinensis* (sweet orange), *C. medica* (citron), *C. nobolis* (tangerine), *C. maxima* (grapefruit), *C. bergamia* (bergamot) and *C. grandis* (pomelo).

**clarification** The process of clearing a liquid of suspended particles; may be carried out by filtration, centrifugation, addition of particular enzymes (proteolytic or pectolytic) or addition of flocculating agents. See *isinglass*.

**clarifixation** Method of homogenising milk in which the cream is separated, homogenised and re-mixed with the milk in one machine – the clarifixator.

**Clarke degrees** See *water hardness*.

**clay** A dried mineral clay under the names of sikor, mithi, patri, khuri and khatta, sometimes used by Asians as a treatment for indigestion and as a vitamin supplement but can be toxic since it contains varying amounts of arsenic and lead.

**clementine** Citrus fruit, *Citrus nobilis* var *deliciosa*; regarded by some as a variety of tangerine and by others as a cross between tangerine and a wild North African orange.

*Clostridium* Genus of bacteria of which *C. botulinum* is responsible for rare and often fatal form of food poisoning. See *botulism*.

It is suggested that there are four groups of *C. botulinum* which grow under different conditions and have differing sensitivities to heat. Found widely distributed in soil, both virgin and cultivated. During growth in favourable food materials the organism synthesises an extremely potent neurotoxin which is released into the food when the cell dies. The spores are the most heat-resistant food poisoning organism encountered and their thermal death time is used as a minimum standard for processing foods with pH values higher than 4.5.

**clotting of blood**   See *coagulation, blood.*

**cloudberry**   Orange yellow fruit resembling raspberry in shape, *Rubus chamaemorus*; avron in Scotland, baked-apple berries in Canada. Extremely rich in benzoic acid and will not ferment and remains stable for many months.

**clove**   Dried flower buds of *Caryophyllus aromaticus*; mother of clove is the ripened fruit, inferior in flavour. Contains 10% fixed oil and a volatile oil, mostly eugenol, with small amounts of caryophyllene, vanillin and other substances. Used as flavour in meat products and bakery goods.

**CMC**   Carboxymethylcellulose.

**Co I, Co II**   Abbreviations of coenzymes I and II, officially named nicotinamide adenine dinucleotide and nicotinamide adenine dinucleotide phosphate, respectively.

**CoA**   Abbreviation for coenzyme A, which see.

**coacervation**   Heat-reversible aggregation of amylopectin – suggested as one explanation of the staling of bread.

**coagulase**   Name given to an enzyme said to be present in milk and to account for the ability of milk to clot a solution of fibrinogen.

**coagulation**   A process whereby proteins become insoluble; effected by heat, strong acids and alkalies, metals and various other chemicals.

Denaturation is the rupture of hydrogen bonds within and between the peptide chains of the protein. If the process reaches an advanced state, it becomes irreversible, there is extreme unfolding and agglomeration of the side-chains, and the aggregates of protein reach such a size that they precipitate, i.e. coagulate.

Coagulation occurs when, for example, an egg is cooked or a flour dough is baked.

**coagulation, blood**   The final stage is the precipitation of fibrils of insoluble fibrin from the soluble plasma protein fibrinogen. The mechanism is as follows: prothrombin in the plasma is converted by thromboplastin (released from blood platelets and damaged tissue) to thrombin, in the presence of calcium. The thrombin then reacts with the fibrinogen to form the fibrin clot.

Hence, the addition of oxalate or citrate, both of which combine with the calcium, will prevent clotting as effectively as heparin, hirudin and coumarin, which interfere with the prothrombin.

**cobalamin**  Vitamin $B_{12}$.

**cobalt**  Mineral believed to be a dietary essential in trace amounts, although a simple cobalt deficiency has never been observed in man. It is part of the molecule of vitamin $B_{12}$ but no other function is known.

Cobalt is not essential to plants, but 'pining disease' in cattle is due to cobalt deficiency. It is a growth factor for chicks, turkeys, pigs and rats, although large doses are toxic.

**cobamide**  Derived from vitamin $B_{12}$ (cobalamin) by removal of the cyano and dimethylbenzimidole groups.

**coca leaves**  From the S. American plant, *Erythroxylon coca*; contain cocaine, and chewed by the natives of Peru as a stimulant.

**cocarboxylase**  Coenzyme that assists the enzyme carboxylase to remove carbon dioxide from various compounds, i.e. decarboxylation.

Cocarboxylase is the diphosphate of vitamin $B_1$, alternatively known as thiamin pyrophosphate or diphosphothiamin. In deficiency of vitamin $B_1$ the body is unable to oxidise pyruvic acid, an intermediate stage in carbohydrate metabolism, which therefore accumulates in the blood.

**cochineal**  Red colour obtained from the female conchilla, *Coccus cacti*, found in Mexico, Central America and the West Indies. 70000 insects produce 1 lb of colour. Legally permitted in food in most countries. Slightly soluble in water and alcohol but not ether.

**cock-a-leekie**  Scottish soup made from leeks and chicken.

**cockles**  Marine bivalve molluscs, *Cardium edule*. Analysis per 100 g: protein 11 g, fat and carbohydrate traces, iron 30 mg, 50 kcal (200 kJ).

**cocoa**  Originally known as cacao, introduced into Europe from Mexico by the Spaniards in the early 16th century. Derived from the seed embedded in the fruit of the cocoa plant, *Theobroma cacao*.

Analysis per 100 g: 20 g fat, 20 g protein, 13 g fibril, 38 g carbohydrate, 130 mg Ca, 10 mg Fe, 1500 mg K, 950 mg sodium, 310 kcal (1.3 MJ), together with theobromine (dimethylxanthine) in amounts similar to the caffeine content of coffee; also tannins and pigments.

See also *chocolate*.

**cocoa butter**  Fat from cocoa bean used in chocolate manufacture and in pharmaceuticals; low sharp melting point, 31–35°C, melts in the mouth; mostly 2-oleopalmitostearin.

**cocoa butter equivalents**  Vegetable fats (and various mixtures) with physical and chemical properties similar to those of cocoa butter and so useful as partial or complete replacements for (expensive) cocoa butter, e.g. illipe and shea nut butter.

**cocoa, Dutch** Cocoa treated with dilute solution of alkali (carbonate or bicarbonate) to improve colour, flavour and solubility. The process is known as 'Dutching'.

**cocoa nibs** Seeds of the fruit of the cocoa plant, *Theobroma cacao*, are left to ferment, which modifies the bitterness and the colour darkens. They are then roasted and separated from the husks as two halves of the seed known as cocoa nibs. Contain about 50% fat, part of which is removed to prepare chocolate and cocoa for beverages.

**cocolait** A form of coconut 'milk' made by pressing coconut under high pressure and homogenising the oil and water emulsion plus coconut water (coconut milk) obtained. Bottled and used (e.g. in Philippines) in place of cow's milk.

**coconut** Tropical palm, *Cocos nucifera*. The dried nut is copra, which contains 60–65% coconut oil. The residue after oil extraction is used for animal feed.

The hollow unripe nut contains a watery liquid known as coconut milk – which is gradually absorbed as the nut ripens.

Composition of milk from the ripe nut: 1.4% solids, 0.2% protein, 3% carbohydrate (largely sucrose).

Analysis of mature kernel per 100g: 48–80g solids, 4g protein, 35g fat, 11g carbohydrate, 4g fibre, 375kcal (1.57MJ), 2mg Fe, traces of vitamin $B_1$, vitamin $B_2$ and nicotinic acid.

**cocoyam, new** W. African name for tannia, which see.

**cocoyam, old** W. African name for taro, which see.

**coddle** To cook slowly in water kept just below the boiling point.

**Codes of Practice** In the area of food production these refer to standards of procedure which cannot be covered by exact specifications and serve as agreed guide lines. Some are produced by government (e.g. Advertising and Labelling of Foods, Ministry of Food, 1945; Food Hygiene, 1980, Department of Health) or by trade organisations, or by the Institute of Food Science and Technology (Good Manufacturing Practice 1987) or by individual companies.

**Codex Alimentarius** Originally Codex Alimentarius Europaeus; since 1961 part of the FAO/WHO Commission on Food Standards to simplify and integrate food standards for adoption internationally.

**codfish** The composition of all non-fatty fish, such as cod, hake, haddock, flatfish, is similar. Cod = *Gadus morrhua* and other *Gadus* spp.

Cod fillet, per 100g: protein 16.4g, fat 0.5g, kcal 75 (0.31 MJ), Ca 25mg, Fe 0.7mg, vitamin A nil, vitamin $B_1$ 0.05mg, vitamin $B_2$ 0.08mg, nicotinic acid 2.2mg, vitamin C nil.

Cod, round, per 100g: protein 7.4g, fat 0.2g, 33kcal (0.13MJ), Ca 11mg, Fe 0.3mg, vitamin A nil, vitamin $B_1$ 0.02mg, vitamin $B_2$ 0.04mg, nicotinic acid 1.0mg, vitamin C nil.

**cod liver oil**  Oil from codfish liver; classic source of vitamins A and D, used for its medicinal properties long before the vitamins were discovered.

Average sample contains 120–1200μg vitamin A and 1–10μg vitamin D per gram.

British Pharmacopoeia standard: minimum 180μg vitamin A and 2μg vitamin D per gram. Ministry of Health 'Welfare' cod liver oil, 270μg vitamin A and 2.2μg vitamin D per gram.

**coeliac disease**  (idiopathic steatorrhoea, non-tropical sprue or gluten-induced enteropathy)  Inherited sensitivity to the gliadin fraction of wheat (and rye and barley) flour, in which the villi of the small intestine are severely affected and absorption of food is poor. Stools are bulky and fermenting from unabsorbed carbohydrate, and undernutrition and retarded growth result. Treatment is total exclusion of wheat, rye and barley proteins (the starches are tolerated), but rice and maize are thought to be harmless.

**coenzyme I**  (and II)  See *nicotinamide adenine dinucleotide*; *nicotinamide adenine dinucleotide phosphate*.

**coenzyme A**  Coenzyme for the transfer of acetyl groups; contains the vitamin pantothenic acid. Functions by its ability to combine with acetyl, forming acetyl CoA, and to transfer this to another compound.

Important in the oxidation of glucose at the stage between pyruvic acid and the citric acid cycle, and in fat metabolism.

**coenzyme Q**  See *ubiquinones*.

**coenzyme R**  Obsolete name for biotin.

**coenzymes**  Substances needed to assist certain enzymes. They are part of the enzyme system and differ from activators in that they play no part in the activation of the substrate.

Coenzymes react first with one enzyme, then with another, during the course of catalysis and so differ from prosthetic groups, which remain bound to the one enzyme during the course of the reaction.

Those enzymes that do require a coenzyme have an absolute specificity for that particular coenzyme, but the same coenzyme can partner a range of enzymes. Most coenzymes contain one of the B vitamins as part of the molecule; thus Coenzyme I contains nicotinic acid, Coenzyme A contains pantothenic acid, cocarboxylase is vitamin $B_1$ pyrophosphate.

**coffee**  Beverage produced from roasted beans from the berries of two principal types of shrub, *Coffea arabica* (arabica coffee) and

*Coffea canephora* (robusta coffee). Niacin is formed during the roasting process, and the coffee can contain 10–40 mg niacin per 100 g, depending on the extent of roasting. Also contains caffeine, which see.

**coffee, decaffeinated** Powdered coffee bean (or instant coffee) from which the caffeine has been extracted with solvent (e.g. methylene or ethylene chloride) carbon dioxide under pressure (supercritical $CO_2$) or water.

**coffee essence** Aqueous extract of roasted coffee; usually about 4 lb coffee per gallon of water (400 g/l).

**cognac** Brandy produced in a limited area of S. France from special varieties of grape grown on shallow soil and claimed to be distilled only in pot, not continuous, stills.

**cola drinks** Carbonated drinks containing extract of cola bean, the seed of the cola tree. The seed contains caffeine. The drinks contain 3–4.5 mg caffeine per fluid ounce.

**colchicine** Alkaloid isolated from the meadow saffron, or Autumn crocus (*Colchicum*). Old remedy for gout. Inhibits cell division, and used in experimental horticulture to produce plants with abnormal numbers of genes.

**cold preservation** See *Campden process*.

**cold-shortening (of meat)** When the temperature of muscle is reduced below 10°C while the pH remains above 6–6.2 (early in post-mortem conversion of glycogen to lactic acid) the muscle contracts in reaction to cold and, when cooked, the meat is tough.

**cold sterilisation** See *irradiation*; *sterilisation, cold*.

**'cold store' bacteria** See *psychrophilic bacteria*.

**cole** See *rape*.

**Coleman diet** High-calorie, largely liquid diet introduced by Coleman for the treatment of typhoid fever.

**coley** See *saithe*.

**coliform bacteria** Group of aerobic, lactose-fermenters, of which *Escherichia coli* is the most important member.

Many coliforms are not harmful, but since they arise from faeces, they are useful as a test of faecal contamination, particularly as a test for water pollution.

**collagen** Insoluble protein in bone, tendons, skin and connective tissue of animals and fish, converted to soluble gelatin by moist heat. See *albuminoids*; *connective tissue*.

**collagen sugar** Glycine.

**colloid** Particles (the disperse phase) suspended in a second medium (the dispersion medium); can be solid, liquid or gas suspended in solid, liquid or gas.

Examples of gas-in-liquid colloidal systems are beaten egg white, whipped cream; of liquid–liquid colloids are emulsions such as milk, salad cream.

See also *emulsifying agents*; *stabilisers*.

**colloids, lyophilic** (emulsions) Colloids in which there is a high affinity between the particles of the disperse phase and the dispersion medium. They include proteins and higher carbohydrates; very viscous; electrically charged; require large amounts of electrolytes for precipitation, which is reversible.

**colloids, lyophobic** Colloids in which there is no affinity between the particle of the disperse phase and the dispersion medium. The particles carry an electric charge and are flocculated irreversibly by electrolytes. Also called suspensoids. For example, colloids of metals and inorganic salts.

**colocasia** See *taro*.

**Colombo Plan** A co-operative effort to develop the resources and living standards of the peoples of S. and S.E. Asia, started at a meeting held in Colombo in 1950.

**colon** Last part of the intestine; consists of three parts – the ascending, the transverse and the descending colon – and finishes at the rectum.

**colorimeter** Instrument used to measure depth of colour. See also *absorptiometer*; *Lovibond comparator*.

**colostrum** The milk produced by mammals during the first few days after parturition; human colostrum contains more protein (2% compared with 1%), slightly less lactose, considerably less fat (3% compared with 5%) and overall slightly less energy than mature milk.

**colours** Those used in foods fall into three groups; natural pigments, mostly extracted from plant materials; inorganic pigments and lakes (metals complexed with organic colours); and synthetic coal-tar dyes. Most countries permit only a limited number of these to be added to foods.

**colza oil** Rapeseed oil

**COMA** Committee on Medical Aspects of Food Policy; UK Advisory Committee to Department of Health.

**comminuted** Finely divided; used with reference to minced meat products and fruit drinks made from crushed whole fruit, including the peel.

**comparator block** Method of comparing colours (often used to estimate pH). See also *Lovibond comparator*.

**comparator, Lovibond** See *Lovibond comparator*.

**Complan** Trade name (Glaxo Laboratories) for a mixture of dried skim milk, arachis oil, casein, maltodextrins, sugar, salts and vitamins. Protein 31%, fat 16%, carbohydrate 44%, Ca

825 mg, Fe 8 mg per 100 g, and vitamins A, $B_1$, $B_2$, nicotinic acid, vitamins $B_{12}$, C, D, E, K, pantothenic acid and folic acid.

**complementation**   This term is used with respect to proteins when a relative deficiency of one amino acid is compensated by a relative surplus of another consumed at the same time. The nutritive value – i.e. biological value (BV) or NPU – is then not the mean of the separate values, but higher. For example, maize, with BV 35, is limited by the amino acid lysine, but has a relative surplus of methionine; pea flour, with BV 43, is limited by methionine, but has a relative surplus of lysine; the two complement one another, so that a mixture of equal parts of the two proteins has BV 70.

**conalbumin**   One of the proteins of egg-white comprising 12% of the total solids. Has the property of binding iron in an iron–protein complex that is pink. Accounts for the pinkish colour resulting when eggs are stored in rusty containers.

**condiment**   Seasoning added to flavour foods, such as salt, mustard, ginger, curry, pepper, etc. Although some of these are relatively rich in nutrients, they are generally used in such small quantities that they make a negligible contribution to the diet.

**conditioning of meat**   After killing, the muscle glycogen is broken down to lactic acid, and this acidity gradually improves the texture and keeping qualities of the meat. When all these changes have occurred, the meat is 'conditioned'. See also *rigor mortis*.

**confectioners' glucose**   See *glucose syrups*.

**Conge machine**   Used, in the manufacture of chocolate blend, for coating, to obtain smoothness by kneading the material.

**congies**   The water from cooking rice, which contains much of the thiamin and nicotinic acid from the rice; used as a drink.

**conidendrin**   Substance isolated from a number of coniferous woods whose derivatives, norconidendrin and alpha and beta conidendrol, are antioxidants. Chemically similar to the phenolic substance nordihydroguaiaretic acid.

**connective tissue**   In fish connective tissue is found between the muscle segments (myotomes) and consists of the protein collagen. In meat it is spread through the muscle, uniting the muscle fibres into bundles and supporting the blood vessels (a kind of soft skeleton), and consists of both collagen and elastin. A higher content of connective tissue results in tougher meat. (Collagen is also present in bones and skin.)

On cooking, the insoluble collagen is converted into water-soluble gelatin, so making the material more tender, but elastin is unchanged on heating. Thus, tough meat is softened to some extent by stewing, but roasting or frying has little effect.

**consommé**   A clear soup made from meat or meat extract.

**convenience foods**   Processed foods in which a considerable amount of the preparation has already been carried out by the manufacturer – e.g. cooked meats, canned foods, baked foods, breakfast cereals, frozen foods.

**convicine**   See *favism*.

**cookie**   American term for biscuit.

**cooking**   Required to make food more palatable and more digestible. There is breakdown of the connective tissue in meat and softening of the cellulose in plant tissues.

Broiling: cooking by direct heat over flame. US term for grilling.

Pan broiling: cooking through hot dry metal over direct heat.

Sautéing: cooking with small amount of fat.

Simmering: cooking in water slightly below boiling point.

Stewing: prolonged simmering.

Fricassée: combination of sautéing and stewing.

Devilled: grilled or fried after coating with condiments or breadcrumbs.

Steaming: cooking by heat conveyed by steam either directly or through steam jacket, as in double boiler. Steaming also carried out above 100°C by means of pressure cookers.

See also *braise; connective tissue; frying; grill; roast.*

**cook-chill**   Method of catering involving cooking followed by fast chilling and storage at −1 to +5°C; shelf-life only a few days.

**cook-freeze**   Method of catering involving cooking and rapid freezing and storage between −18 and −30°C; shelf-life up to several months.

**cooking, loss of nutrients**   In general, water-soluble vitamins and minerals are lost in the cooking water, the amount depending on the surface area–volume ratio – i.e. greater losses take place from finely minced foods.

Fat-soluble vitamins are little affected except at frying temperatures. Proteins suffer reduction of available lysine if heated in the presence of reducing substances, and further losses under extreme conditions of temperature.

Dry heat, as in baking, results in some loss of thiamin and of available lysine. The most sensitive nutrient by far is vitamin C, with thiamin next.

Average losses from cereals considered in standard food tables to be: Boiling – 40% thiamin, riboflavin, nicotinic acid, vitamin $B_6$, biotin and pantothenic acid; 50% total folate. Baking – 5% nicotinic acid; 15% riboflavin; 25% thiamin, vitamin $B_6$ and pantothenic acid; 50% folate; with biotin being stable. In meat losses are approximately 20% of all the vitamins through roasting, frying and grilling and 20–60% on stewing and boiling.

**copper** Copper is part of the enzyme tyrosinase (and in plants, laccase and ascorbic acid oxidase), and is needed to assist the incorporation of iron into haemoglobin. It is therefore thought to be a dietary essential in amounts of about 2 mg per day. Traces of copper are normally present in the blood in combination with an alpha globulin as ceruloplasmin.

Deficiency in cattle gives rise to 'swayback'. Traces are also essential for plant growth.

Toxic in high concentrations, and there is a legal limit to the amount permitted in foodstuffs.

**copra** Dried coconut meat; used for production of coconut oil for margarine and soap.

**coprophagy** Eating of faeces. As B vitamins are synthesised by intestinal bacteria, animals that eat their faeces can make use of these vitamins.

**cordial, fruit** Fruit drink (UK); liqueur (USA) – original meaning in UK. See *soft drinks*.

**coriander** Dried ripe fruit of *Coriandrum sativum* (parsley family). Contains 20% fixed oil and 1% essential oil – largely linool or coriandrol (an isomer of geraniol). Used as flavour in meat products, bakery goods, tobacco, gin, and in curry powder.

**Cori cycle** The sequence of reactions through which the liver converts lactic acid back to glycogen, namely liver glycogen–blood glucose–muscle glycogen–blood lactate–liver glycogen.

**Cori ester** Name given to glucose-1-phosphate, one of the intermediates of glucose metabolism, which see.

**corm** Thickened, underground base of stem of plants, often called bulbs, as, for example, taro and onion.

**corn** In the UK a generic term for cereals. In the USA means maize.

**corn, dent** See *maize*.

**corned beef** In the USA and elsewhere this is salt beef, i.e. pickled whole meat. In the UK it is the canned product manufactured from low-quality meat after partial extraction of water-soluble materials.

Analysis of canned product per 100 g: 59 g water, 27 g protein, 12 g fat, 220 kcal (900 kJ), 1 g Na, 3 mg Fe, 2.5 mg niacin (only trace of thiamin).

**cornflakes** Breakfast cereal made from maize.

Apart from enriched proprietary preparations, analysis per 100 g: 3 g water, 7 g sugars, 74 g starch and dextrins, 3 g dietary fibre, 8 g protein, 0.5 g fat, 370 kcal (1.5 MJ).

**corn, flint** See *maize*.

**cornflour**  Purified starch from maize; in the USA called corn starch; used in custard, blancmange and baking powders.
Analysis: protein 0.5%, fat 0.3%, carbohydrate 87%, fibre 0.2%, no vitamins present.

**corn, flour**  Flour corn is a variety of maize with large, soft grains and very friable endosperm, making it easy to grind the grain to flour.

**corn grits**  See *hominy*.

**corn starch**  See *cornflour*.

**corn steep liquor**  The first stage in the preparation of starch from maize is to soak the maize in water containing sulphur dioxide for 24 h. The liquor is termed corn steep liquor. It was found to be an excellent medium for growing mould to produce penicillin; the yield was greatly enhanced beyond that obtained with synthetic media, since the liquor contained a 'biochemical precursor' of penicillin.

**corn sugar**  Glucose.

**corn syrup**  See *glucose syrups*.

**corn, waxy**  See *maize*.

**coronary thrombosis**  See *atherosclerosis*.

**corrinoids** (corrins)  Name given to chemical structure based on four pyrrole nuclei joined in a macro ring with three bridge carbon atoms and six conjugated double bonds. It is the basic structure of the cobalamins without the cobalt and side-chains. See *vitamin $B_{12}$*.

**cossettes**  Thin chips of sugar beet into which it is shredded for hot-water extraction of the sugar.

**cottonseed**  Of double use in the food field; the oil is valuable as a cooking oil, or for margarine when hardened, and the protein residue is a valuable animal feedingstuff.

**courgettes**  Italian marrows, Italian squash or zucchini (USA), a variety of gourd with small fruits. See *gourds*.

**Courlose**  Trade name (British Celanese Ltd) for sodium carboxymethylcellulose.

**cow manure factor**  Vitamin $B_{12}$.

**cozymase**  See *nicotinamide adenine dinucleotide*.

**C-peptide**  See *pro-insulin*.

**C3 plants**  Type of plants in which, during photosynthesis, the carbon dioxide is combined with ribulose diphosphate to produce two 3-carbon acids.

**C4 plants**  Type of plants in which, during photosynthesis, the carbon dioxide results in the formation, initially, of a 4-carbon compound, compared with 3-carbon compounds in C3-type plants. The procedure concentrates the carbon dioxide and the reaction is faster and more efficient than C3 photosynthesis.

**crabs**  Shellfish of the suborder Brachyura of the Order Decapoda and family, Lithodidae.

Large spider crab, *Maia squinado*, common on the south coast of England, 6 inches across, occasionally used as food.

Edible crab, *Cancer pagurus*, found in shallow water among rocks; can grow up to 12 lb weight.

Analysis of edible portion per 100 g: protein 20 g, fat 5 g carbohydrate 0, kcal 130 (0.55 MJ), Fe 1.3 mg, vitamin $B_1$ 0.1 mg, vitamin $B_2$ 0.15 mg, nicotinic acid 2.5 mg.

**cran**  Measure for herrings containing 37½ gallons or about 800 herrings.

**cranberry**  Fleshy, acid fruit of *Vaccinium oxycoccus* resembling cherry; commonly used for cranberry sauce.

Composition per 100 g: 3.5 g carbohydrate, 15 kcal (0.06 MJ), 1 mg iron, 12 mg vitamin C.

**crawfish**  See *lobster*.

**crayfish**  The English crayfish, *Astacus torrentium*, was almost entirely wiped out by disease in 1887, and crayfish for food are all imported, *Astacus fluviatilis*. See *lobster*.

**cream**  Fatty part of milk. In the United States usually designated light cream, with 20–25% fat, and heavy cream, with about 40% fat. In the UK cream contains not less than 18% fat; double cream or thick cream, 48%; clotted cream, not less than 48%; whipping cream, not less than 35%.

**cream, bitty**  Cream on the surface of milk appears as particles of fat released from fat globules when the membrane is broken down by lecithinase from *Bacillus cereus*, the spores of which have resisted destruction during pasteurisation.

**cream, clotted**  This usually has a higher fat content that double cream, which legally is 48% fat. Double cream is floated in a shallow layer on a layer of skim milk and scalded. The clotted cream at 63% fat is then skimmed off. This is Devonshire cream and contains 29.5% water, 4% protein, 2.8% lactose, 0.67% ash. Cornish cream is similar but is prepared by scalding the double cream alone, not floated on a layer of milk. See also *cream*.

**cream, Cornish**  See *cream, clotted*.

**cream, Devonshire**  See *cream, clotted*.

**creaming quality**  As applied to fats, is the ability to absorb air during mixing.

**cream line index**  The cream line or layer usually forms about 6% of the total depth of milk. The cream line index is the ratio between the percentage cream layer and the percentage fat in the milk. It is used as a test of the milk, and in ordinary bulk pasteurised milk is about 1.7.

**cream of tartar** Potassium hydrogen tartrate, used with sodium bicarbonate as baking powder because it acts more slowly than tartaric acid and gives a more prolonged evolution of carbon dioxide. This is tartrate baking powder; similarly, phosphate baking powder contains calcium acid phosphate or sodium hydrogen pyrophosphate.

Also used to 'invert' sugar in making boiled sweets, which see.

**cream, plastic** Term used for a cream containing as much fat as butter (80–83%) but as a dispersal of fat in water, whereas butter is water in fat. Prepared by intense centrifugal treatment of cream; crumbly, not greasy, in texture; used for preparation of cream cheese and whipped cream.

**cream, sleepy** Cream that will not churn to butter in the normal time.

**cream, synthetic** Name given to (a) emulsion of vegetable oil, milk or milk powder, egg yolk and sugar, and (b) emulsion of water with methyl cellulose, monoglycerides, and other synthetic materials.

**creatine** Methyl guanidine derivative of acetic acid. Essential part of the energy release system of muscle, as creatine phosphate, or phosphagen; possesses an energy-rich bond which is released when energy is required for muscular contraction.

The anhydride of creatine is creatinine, in which form it is found in urine. Meat extract contains a mixture of the two, derived from the creatine that was present in the fresh muscle. Creatine plus creatinine is used as an index of quality of commercial meat extract, and as a measure of extract present in manufactured products, such as soups.

**creatinine** Anhydride of creatine, which see.

**cress** *Lepidium sativum*. Seed leaves eaten raw with mustard leaves (mustard and cress: see *mustard*).

Winter or land cress, *Barbarea verna*, is a rarely grown salad plant.

**Creta Praeparata** Official British Pharmacopoeia name for prepared chalk, made by washing and drying naturally occurring calcium carbonate. The form in which calcium is added to flour (14 oz per 280 lb sack).

**cretinism** Underactivity of the thyroid gland (hypothyroidism) in children, resulting in poor growth and mental retardation. Hypothyroidism in adults is myxoedema. Can result from a dietary deficiency of iodine. See also *goitre*; *thyroid gland*.

**crispbreads** Name given to a flour and water wafer, originally Swedish and made from rye flour, but may be made from wheat flour. They have a much lower water content than bread and some brands are richer in protein because of added wheat gluten.

Although popularly believed to be an aid in slimming, they provide more energy than the same weight of ordinary bread, since they contain less water.

**cristal height**　A measure of leg length taken from the floor to the summit of the iliac crest. Cristal height as a proportion of total height increases with age in children, and a reduced rate of increase is an indication of undernourishment.

**croûtons**　Small diced or shaped pieces of bread fried in fat.

**crowdies**　See *milks, fermented*.

**crude fibre**　See *fibre, crude*.

**crude protein**　See *protein, crude*.

**crumb-softener**　See *polyoxyethylene*; *superglycerinated fats*.

**crumpets**　See *dough cakes*.

**crustacea**　Includes crabs, lobsters, prawns, scampi, shrimps.

**cryodesiccation**　Freeze-drying.

**cryogenic freezing**　Freezing with extremely cold freezants such as liquid nitrogen or solid carbon dioxide.

**Cryovac**　Trade name of thermoplastic resin wrapping film; can be heat-shrunk on to foods.

**cryptoxanthin**　Yellow colouring matter in certain vegetables such as yellow maize, and in the seeds of *Physalis*, the Chinese Lantern. A hydroxy derivative of carotene; converted into retinol in the body.

**crystallin**　Protein of the lens of the eye.

**CSM**　Corn–soya–milk; protein-rich baby food (20% protein) made in the USA from 68% precooked maize (corn), 25% defatted soya flour and 5% skim milk powder, with added vitamins $B_1$, $B_2$, $B_6$, $B_{12}$, nicotinic acid, pantothenic acid, folic acid, vitamins A, D and E, and calcium carbonate.

**CTC machine**　Two contrarotating toothed rollers that rotate at different speeds and provide a Crushing, Tearing and Curling action – used in breaking up leaves of tea to form small particles.

**Cubs**　Trade name (Nabisco Foods Ltd) for a breakfast cereal made from wheat.

**cucumber**　Fruit of *Cucumis sativus*, a member of the gourd family.

Analysis per 100 g: protein 0.6 g, fat 0.1 g, kcal 10 (40 kJ), Ca 7 mg, Fe 0.2 mg, vitamin $B_1$ 0.02 mg, vitamin $B_2$ 0.03 mg, nicotinic acid 0.1 mg, vitamin C 6 mg.

**cucurbits**　Term used for vegetables of the Cucurbitaceae; see *gourds*.

**cumin seed**　Dried fruit of *Cuminum cyminum* (parsley family); contains about 10% fixed oil and 2–4% essential oil, largely cuminal. Used in curry powder and for flavouring cordials.

**curaçao**  Liqueur made from the rind of Seville oranges and brandy or gin; 30% alcohol, 30% sugar.

**curds**  Clotted protein formed when fresh milk is treated with rennet; the fluid left is whey, which see.

**curd tension**  A measure of the toughness of the curd formed from milk by the digestive enzymes, and used as an index of the digestibility of the milk. The sample is coagulated with rennin and the force needed to pull a knife-blade through the curd is measured in grams under standardised conditions. Ideal score is zero, below 20 satisfactory; cow's milk 46; diluted with equal volume of water 20; reconstituted spray-dried milk 10; reconstituted roller-dried milk 5; evaporated milk 3; human milk 1.

**curing of meat**  Method of preservation by treating with salt and sodium nitrate (and nitrite), which serves to inhibit growth of pathogenic organisms while salt-tolerant bacteria develop. During the pickling process the nitrate is converted into nitrite, which combines with the muscle pigment, myoglobin, to form the red-coloured nitrosomyoglobin characteristic of pickled meat products.

**currants**  Fruit of *Ribes* species; white, red and black (see also *blackcurrants*).

Analysis per 100 g: Redcurrants: protein 1.1 g, carbohydrate 4.4 g, water 83 g, kcal 20 (85 kJ), Fe 1.2 mg, vitamin C 40 mg.

White currants: protein 1.3 g, carbohydrate 5.6 g, water 83%, kcal 25 (100 kJ), Fe 1 mg, vitamin C 40 mg.

**currants, dried**  Made by drying the small seedless black grape grown in and around Greece and in Australia; usually dried in bunches on the vine or after removal from the vine on supports.

Name derived from Raisins of Corauntz (Corinth).

For analysis, see *fruit, dried*. See also *muscatels*; *raisins*; *sultanas*.

**curry**  Mixture of several spices, including turmeric, coriander, cardamom, cinnamon, cumin, fenugreek, ginger, mustard, chilli, cloves and pepper. Reported to contain up to 75–100 mg iron per 100 g but a large part of this is due to contamination.

There is also a curry plant (*Murraya koenigii*) containing a number of alkaloids.

**custard**  May refer to custard powder, which see, or to egg custard. Egg custard is composed of milk and egg cooked together.

**custard apple**  One of a number of species of tropical American trees of the family Anonaceae. Sour sop, *Anona muricata*, white fibrous flesh, less sweet than the others, fruit may weigh up to 8 lb; sweet sop (*A. squamosa*) also known as 'true' custard apple, popular in West Indies; bullock's heart (*A. reticulata*), buff-coloured flesh.

Analysis per 100 g: 22 g carbohydrate, 1 g protein, 90 kcal (0.4 MJ), 0.5 mg Fe, 0.1 mg vitamin $B_1$, 0.08 mg vitamin $B_2$, 0.8 mg nicotinic acid, 30 mg vitamin C.

**custard powder**  Usually maize starch, coloured and flavoured.

**cyanocobalamin**  Vitamin $B_{12}$.

**cyanogen(et)ic glycosides**  Cyanhydrins combined via a glycosidic linkage with one or two sugars. Very widely distributed in plants; toxic through liberation of the cyanide.

**cycasin**  Methylazoxymethanol β-glucoside. Toxic substance in the Cycads.

**cyclamate**  See *cyclo-hexyl-sulphamate, sodium*

**cyclic AMP**  See *adenosine nucleotides*.

**cyclitols**  Cyclic sugars such as inositols, quercitols and tetritols.

**cyclo-hexyl-sulphamate, sodium**  A non-nutritive sweetener, 30 times as sweet as sugar, also used as the calcium salt; synthesised 1937.

Useful in low-calorie foods. Also called cyclamate and Sucaryl (trade name). Unlike saccharine, it is stable to heat.

**Cymogran**  Trade name (Allen & Hanbury's Ltd) for protein-rich food low in phenylalanine for feeding patients with phenylketonuria.

**cysteine**  A sulphur-containing non-essential amino acid – amino-thiol propionic acid. Cystine is formed when two molecules of cysteine are reduced and linked via the $-S-S-$ bond. Cysteine is used as a dough 'improver'.

**cystic fibrosis**  An inborn error of metabolism which causes a disturbance of the exocrine glands, with failure to secrete pancreatic enzymes, so that food is incompletely digested and absorbed. Treated by feeding predigested protein or adding dried pancreatin to the diet.

**cystine**  The double molecule of reduced cysteine, linked via the $-S-S$ bond; forms about 12% of hair protein, keratin.

**cytochromes**  Pigments present in every type of living cell (except the strictly anaerobic bacteria); act as an intermediate hydrogen acceptor in passing hydrogen along the chain from the substrate to oxygen, the ultimate hydrogen acceptor. When they accept the hydrogen, they change to the reduced form, and are re-oxidised by the enzyme cytochrome oxidase, which passes the hydrogen farther along the chain.

**cytochrome P450**  Part of the detoxication system of the body; at least four enzymes are involved – cytochromes P450 and $b_5$, together with their reductases. About ten forms of P450 occur in the liver and the system as a whole is referred to as mixed function oxidases; can deal with a variety of substrates, including drugs and food additives.

**cytokinins**   Substances that stimulate cell division – cytokinesis – and control development of plants; found in seed embryos, developing fruits and buds. They are derivatives of the purine base adenine.

**cytosine**   See *nucleic acids*; *pyrimidines*.


# D


*d-*   Obsolete prefix indicating dextrorotatory, now replaced by (+); see *optical activity*.

D-   A prefix to chemical names, especially sugars and amino acids, indicating their structure. When the first hydroxyl group of a sugar is on the same side as the alcohol group, it is the D-form, on opposite sides it is the L- form. Both L- and D- glucose exist.

In the case of amino acids L-alanine is related to the sugar L-glyceraldehyde and follows the same nomenclature. The other amino acids follow alanine. All the naturally occurring amino acids are L-; synthetic are DL-; few D- amino acids are found in nature.

Small capital L- and D- are not to be confused with *l*- and *d*-, which are the old terms for (+) and (−); see *optical activity*.

**D-araboascorbic acid**   See *ascorbic acid*.

**dadhi**   See *milks, fermented*.

**Daltose**   Trade name (Cow & Gate Ltd) of a carbohydrate preparation consisting of maltose, glucose and dextrin for infant feeding.

**damson**   Small dark-blue plum, *Prunus damascena*.

Analysis per 100 g: protein 0.5 g, water 70 g, carbohydrate 8.6 g, kcal 35 (150 kJ), Fe 0.4 mg, vitamin $B_1$ 0.1 mg, nicotinic acid 0.25 mg.

**dandelion greens**   The leaves of the weed, *Leontodon taraxacum*, used sometimes as a salad.

Analysis per 100 g: protein 2.4 g, fat 0.6 g, Ca 135 mg, Fe 2.8 mg, kcal 40 (0.17 MJ), carotene 3000 µg, vitamin $B_1$ 0.17 mg, vitamin $B_2$ 0.13 mg, nicotinic acid 0.7 mg, vitamin C 25 mg.

**dark adaptation**   The change that takes place in the retina of the eye to assist vision in dim light. In dark adaptation a pigment, visual purple or rhodopsin, is formed from retinal (vitamin A aldehyde) and a protein. This is bleached in bright light. When body stores of retinol are inadequate, poor dark adaptation – night blindness – results. This is the earliest indication of vitamin A deficiency.

**dasheen**   West Indian name for taro, which see.

**DATEM** Diacetyl tartaric esters of mono and diglycerides; emulsifiers used to strengthen bread doughs and delay staling of the bread.

**date-plum** See *persimmon*.

**date** Fruit of date palm, *Phoenix dactylifera*, known as far back as 3000 BC. Three types: 'soft' (about 80% of dry matter is invert sugars); 'semi-dry' (about 40% of dry matter is invert sugars and about 40% is sucrose); 'dry' (20–40% of dry matter is invert sugars, 40–60% sucrose).

General analysis per 100 g: 15 g water, 9 g dietary fibre, 2 g protein, 65 g sugars, 250 kcal (1 MJ), 1.5 mg iron, small amounts of most of the B vitamins.

**DBD process** See *dry-blanch-dry process*.

**DE** Dextrose equivalent value, which see.

**decimal reduction time (D value)** Duration of heat treatment required to reduce number of micro-organisms to one-tenth of initial value; temperature shown as subscript, e.g. $D_{121}$ – time at 121°C.

**defibrinated blood** See *blood, defibrinated*.

**degumming agents** Used in refining of fats to remove mucilaginous matter consisting of gum, resin, proteins and phosphatides. Include hydrochloric and phosphoric acids, and phosphates.

**dehydration** Scientific term for drying, but tends to be used for factory-dried materials as distinct from wind-dried.

**dehydroacetic acid** Also sodium salt (DHA-S). Active against moulds but not a permitted additive.

Chemically can be regarded as the condensation product of acetic and acetoacetic acids, or 3-acetyl-6-methyl-1-pyran-2,4 dione.

**dehydroascorbic acid** Oxidised form of vitamin C which can readily be reduced to the ordinary form, and is therefore biologically active.

**dehydrocanning** A process in which 50% of the water is removed from a food before canning. The advantages are that the texture is retained by the partial dehydration and there is a saving in bulk and weight.

**dehydrocholesterol** See *vitamin D*.

**dehydrofreezing** Process for preservation of fruits and vegetables by evaporation of one-half to two-thirds of the water before freezing. The texture and flavour are claimed to be superior to those resulting from either dehydration or freezing alone, and rehydration more rapid than with dehydrated products.

**dehydrogenases** Enzymes that carry out oxidations in the living cell by removing hydrogen from the substrate. They can only function by passing this hydrogen on to another substance, called the intermediate hydrogen acceptor. It is ultimately passed on to oxygen to form water.

There are specific dehydrogenases for each substrate – e.g. succinic dehydrogenase, lactic, malic, glucose, etc.

See also *intermediate hydrogen carrier*; *oxidases*.

**dehydrogenation** See *intermediate hydrogen carrier*; *oxidases*; *oxidation*.

**dehydroretinol** Formerly termed vitamin A$_2$.

**Delaney Amendment** Provision within the United States Federal Food, Drug and Cosmetic Act which states that no food additive shall be deemed to be safe after it is found to induce cancer when ingested by man or animals (at any dose level).

**Demerara sugar** See *sugar*.

**demersal fish** Those found living on or near the bottom of the sea, including cod, haddock, whiting and halibut, which contain little oil, 1–4%.

**denaturation** (1) A reversible change in proteins that precedes coagulation (which see); the solubility is reduced and free −SH groups appear. Denaturation can be effected by changes in pH, heat, ultraviolet irradiation and violent agitation.

There is no change in nutritive value, but pharmacological activity is often lost.

(2) When the term is applied to alcohol, it means the addition of denaturing agents, such as methyl violet and pyridine (as in methylated spirits) to render it unpleasant and so prevent its consumption.

**dendritic salt** A form of ordinary table salt, sodium chloride, with the crystals branched or star-like (dendritic) instead of the normal cubes. The advantages claimed are the lower bulk density, rapid solution, and unusual capacity for absorbing moisture before becoming wet.

**deodorisation** Generally applied to the removal of flavour (as in deodorised fish meal) but more specifically to the deodorisation of fats during refining. Superheated steam is bubbled through the hot oil under vacuum, when most of the flavoured substances are distilled off.

**depectinisation** Removal of pectins from fruit pulp to produce a clear thin juice instead of a viscous, cloudy liquid; achieved by the use of enzyme preparations.

**Derbyshire neck** See *goitre*; *iodine*.

**desferrioxamine** An iron-chelating agent used medicinally to reduce iron content of the body.

**desmosine** A complex cross-linked compound involving four lysyl residues formed, together with isodesmosine, in connective tissue.

**desoxyribonucleic acid** See *nucleic acids*.

**detoxication**   Destruction of a toxic compound, or, more usually, alteration of a chemical group to produce a non-toxic product.

In the body detoxication is effected by oxidation, reduction, hydrolysis; or by combination (conjugation) with glycine, glucuronic acid, glutamine, cysteine; or by methylation. For example, the toxic substance benzoic acid is excreted in the urine as a complex with glycine, namely hippuric acid.

**deuterium**   Or heavy hydrogen; isotope of hydrogen with atomic weight 2. The isotope of atomic weight 3 is tritium.

**devitalised gluten**   See *gluten*.

**dewberry**   A large variety of blackberry, but different in flavour.

**dewpoint**   Measure of moisture in air; the temperature at which the air becomes saturated when cooled (deposits dew).

**dexedrine**   See *anorectic drugs*.

**dextran**   A polysaccharide composed of linked fructose units; unwelcome in the sugar factory but valuable clinically for blood transfusion (plasma extender). Produced by the action of *Betacoccus arabinosus* on sugar.

**dextrin, limit**   See *limit dextrin*.

**dextrins**   Mixture of soluble compounds formed by partial breakdown of starch by heat, acid or enzymes (complete breakdown yields maltose). Formed when bread is toasted.

Nutritionally equivalent to starch; industrially used as adhesives in the sizing of paper and textiles, and as gums.

See also *amylases*.

**dextrorotatory**   See *optical activity*.

**dextrose**   Alternative name for glucose. Commercially the term 'glucose' is often used to mean corn syrup (a mixture of glucose, sugars and dextrins) and pure glucose is called dextrose.

**dextrose equivalent value**   Term used to indicate the degree of hydrolysis of starch into glucose syrup (which see). It is defined as the total reducing sugar content expressed as dextrose, calculated as a percentage of the dry solids content (i.e. the higher the DE the more sugar and the less dextrins are present).

Liquid glucoses are commercially available ranging from 2 DE to 65 DE. A complete acid hydrolysis converts all the starch into glucose but produces bitter degradation products.

Glucose syrups above 55 DE are termed 'high conversion' (of starch); 35–55, regular conversion. Below 20 the products of hydrolysis are maltins or maltodextrins.

**DFD meat**   Dark, firm, dry; condition of meat when pH remains high through lack of glycogen (which would form lactic acid); poses a microbiological hazard.

**DHA**   Docosohexaenoic acid – long chain marine fatty acid – 22 carbon atoms, 6 double bonds, omega-3 series.

**dhals**   Indian term for split peas of various kinds, e.g. pigeon pea

(*Cajanus indicus*), khesari (*Lathyrus sativus*), red dahl or Massur dahl is the lentil (*Lens esculenta*).

**dhool** Name given to leaves of tea up to the stage of drying.

**diabetes, alloxan** See *alloxan*.

**diabetes mellitus (sugar diabetes)** A metabolic disorder involving inability to metabolise glucose properly, so, if untreated, blood glucose levels rise after a meal to abnormal levels and some overflows into the urine.

Type I occurs in youth (juvenile diabetes) and is due to poor secretion of insulin so requires insulin injections. Type II generally arises in middle age and is non-insulin dependent (NIDD) and is due to resistance of the tissues to insulin. It can sometimes be treated by restricting the consumption of simple sugars or by the use of oral drugs which can stimulate insulin secretion and/or enhance the insulin sensitivity of the tissues (sulphonyl ureas and biguanides).

See also *insulin*; *sugar tolerance*.

**diabetes, renal** The appearance of glucose in the urine without undue elevation of the blood sugar. It is due to a reduction of the renal threshold which allows the blood glucose to be excreted. See also *phlorrhizin*.

**diabetes test** See *glucose tolerance*.

**di-acetate, sodium and calcium** Used to inhibit the growth of moulds in foods. Permitted in the USA but not the UK. Chemical formula $CH_3COONaCH_3COOH \cdot \frac{1}{2}H_2O$ (equimolecular compound of acetic acid and sodium acetate).

**diacetyl** $CH_3COCOCH_3$. The flavour-aroma agent in butter, formed during the ripening stage by the organism *Streptococcus lactis cremoris*. Added as a synthetic compound to margarine as 'butter flavour'.

**dialysis** Separation of small molecules from larger in solution by virtue of their different rates of diffusion through a membrane. Membranes are natural, such as pig bladder, or artificial, such as cellulose derivatives or collodion.

The solution is usually placed in a bag of the membrane and this immersed in water. The small molecules diffuse out into the water, leaving the larger molecules inside the bag. This is a frequent method of separating proteins from solutions of salts.

See *membranes, semi-permeable*.

**diaphorase** A flavoprotein enzyme in the cell respiratory system; its function is to accept hydrogen from NADPH.

**diastase** See *amylases*.

**diastatic activity** Of flour; a measure of its ability to produce maltose from its own starch under the influence of its own diastase. This sugar is needed for the growth of the yeast during fermentation. Measured as 'maltose figure'. See also *amylograph*.

**dicoumarin**  Toxic substance found in spoiled sweet clover; causes haemorrhage (haemorrhagic sweet clover disease) by interfering with the synthesis of prothrombin in the liver, i.e. has an anti-vitamin K action. Used clinically to prevent postoperative thrombosis.

**dietary fibre**  See *fibre, dietary*.

**dietetic foods**  Foods prepared to meet the particular nutritional needs of persons whose normal processes of assimilation or metabolism are modified, or for whom a particular effect is to be obtained by a controlled intake of foods or certain nutrients. They may be formulated for persons suffering from physiological disorders or for healthy people with additional needs.

**diethyl pyrocarbonate**  Pyrocarbonic acid diethyl (trade name Baycovin). Preservative for wines, soft drinks and fruit juices at a level of 50–300 ppm. Breaks down within a few days to ethanol and carbon dioxide; does not inhibit moulds.

**diet-induced thermogenesis**  See *specific dynamic action*.

**dietitian, dietician**  According to the US Department of Labour, Dictionary of Occupational Titles – one who applies the principles of nutrition to the feeding of individuals and groups; plans menus and special diets; supervises the preparation and serving of meals; instructs in the principles of nutrition as applied to the selection of foods. See also *nutritionist*.

**diets**  See under individual entries: *Hay diet*; *Karell diet*; *Kempner diet*; *ketogenic diet*; *Lenhartz diet*; *Meulingracht diet*; *Salisbury cure*; *salt-free diets*; *Sippy diet*.

**diets, therapeutic**  See *therapeutic diets*.

**differential cell count**  See *leucocytes*.

**digester**  Alternative name for autoclave or pressure cooker.

**digestibility**  The proportion of a foodstuff absorbed from the digestive tract into the bloodstream, normally 90–95%. It is measured as the difference between intake and faecal output, allowance being made for that part of the faeces which is not derived from undigested food residues (such as shed lining of the intestinal tract, bacteria, residues of digestive juices).

Digestibility measured in this way is referred to as 'true digestibility', as distinct from the approximate measure of 'apparent digestibility', which is simply the difference between intake and output.

**digestion**  The breakdown of a complex into its constituent parts. Most frequently refers to the digestion of food, which means the breakdown by the digestive enzymes of proteins to amino acids, starch to glucose, fats to glycerol and fatty acids – these simple breakdown products are then absorbed into the bloodstream.

Digestion is also applied to the acid hydrolysis of a protein; the Kjeldahl digestion is the complete breakdown of nitrogenous compound to ammonia by sulphuric acid.

See also *intestinal juice*; individual digestive enzymes.

**digestive juices** See *bile*; *gastric secretion*; *intestinal juice*; *pancreatic juice*.

**dihydrochalcones** See *neohesperidin dihydrochalcone*.

**Dijon mustard** French mustard, see *mustard*.

**dilatation of fats** When fats change from solids to liquid at the same temperature there is an increase in volume. Measurement of this increase, dilatometry, may be used to estimate the amount of solid fat present in a mixture at any given temperature. The precise measure is the difference between the volumes of solid and liquid fat measured in microlitres per 25 g of fat.

**dill** Dried ripe fruit of *Anethum graveolens* (Parsley family); leafy tops also used. Contains 15% fixed oil and 2–4% essential oil containing carvone, limonene and terpenes. Used in pickles and soups.

**diose** See *disaccharides*.

**dipeptide** See *peptides*.

**diphenyl** This, and orthophenylphenol (OPP), are used for treatment of fruit after harvesting to prevent mould growth. Permitted in citrus fruits, diphenyl up to 100 ppm, OPP up to 70 ppm. Apples, pears and pineapples may contain 10 ppm, peaches 20 ppm, and melons 125 ppm of OPP.

**diphosphopyridine nucleotide** See *nicotinamide adenine dinucleotide*.

**diphosphothiamin** See *cocarboxylase*.

**dipsa** Foods that cause thirst. Dipsetic – tending to produce thirst.

**dipsesis** Also dipsosis. Extreme thirst, craving for abnormal kinds of drinks. Dipsomania – imperative morbid craving for alcoholic drink.

**dipsogen** Thirst-provoking agent.

**direct extract** See *meat extract*.

**disaccharide intolerance** Impaired ability to digest maltose, sucrose or lactose, which may be inherited. Generalised lactose intolerance may be an adaptation to the absence of milk from the diet, and can be secondary to various inflammatory and degenerative diseases of the small intestine.

Treatment is by omitting the offending sugar from the diet.

**disaccharides** Sugars composed of two monosaccharide molecules combined, with the elimination of a molecule of water. For example, glucose, $C_6H_{12}O_6$, plus fructose, $C_6H_{12}O_6$, produces sucrose, $C_{12}H_{22}O_{11}$. Conversely, when a disaccharide is hydrolysed, either by acid or enzymically, a molecule of water is added and two monosaccharides result.

Also known as dioses or disaccharoses.

**disaccharose**   See *disaccharides*.

**disc mill**   One or more revolving circular plates between which substances, e.g. foodstuffs, are ground. The discs are separated by projecting teeth or pins, used to grind grain, fruit, sugar, chocolate, pastes, etc.

**distillers' solubles**   See *spent wash*.

**DIT**   Diet-induced thermogenesis. See *specific dynamic action*.

**diuresis**   Loss of water from the body as urine.

**diuretics**   Substances that increase the secretion of urine; include organic mercury compounds, xanthines (therefore also coffee and tea) and substances that alter the alkaline reserve of the blood, such as urea, potassium nitrate, potassium chloride.

**djenkolic acid**   A sulphur-containing amino acid found in the djenkol bean, *Pithecolobium lobatum* (grown in parts of Sumatra). Similar to cysteine in structure; it is metabolised but, being relatively insoluble, any djenkolic acid that escapes metabolism can crystallise in the kidney tubules and cause damage.

**DNA**   Desoxyribonucleic acid. See *nucleic acids*.

**dockage**   Name given to foreign material in wheat which can be readily removed by a simple cleaning procedure.

**docosanoids**   Long chain polyunsaturated (essential) fatty acids with 22 carbon atoms: docosapentaenoic (clupanodic – 5 double bonds) and docosahexaenoic (6 db) of the omega-3 series, and docosatetraenoic (adrenic–4 db) and docosapentaenoic (5 db) of the omega-6 series.

**dolomite**   Calcium magnesium carbonate.

**Do-Maker process**   For continuous breadmaking. Ingredients are automatically fed into continuous dough mixer, the yeast suspension being added in a very active state.

**dough cakes**   Term includes crumpets, muffins and pikelets, all made from flour, water and milk; batter is raised with yeast and baked on a hot plate. Crumpets have sodium bicarbonate added to the batter; muffins are thick and well aerated, less tough than crumpets; pikelets are made from crumpet batter that has been thinned down.

**Douglas bag**   Inflatable bag for collecting expired air. Energy usage can be determined from the oxygen and carbon dioxide analysis, i.e. by indirect calorimetry. See also *spirometer*.

**DPN**   See *nicotinamide adenine dinucleotide*.

**dragees**   Sugar confectionery made by applying multiple layers of coatings of coloured and flavoured sugary and chocolate mixtures to a confectionery centre. Silver dragees are coated with silver leaf.

**dripping**   Unbleached and untreated fat from the fatty tissues or bones of sheep or oxen.

**drupes**   Botanical name for fruit that is a single seed, surrounded by stony and fleshy pericarp, e.g. apricot, cherry, plum.

**dry-blanch-dry process**   A method of drying fruit so as to retain the bright colour and flavour; it is faster than drying in the sun and preserves flavour and colour better than hot air drying.

The material is dried to 50% water at about 82°C, blanched for a few minutes, then dried at 68°C over a period of 6–24h to 15–20% water content.

**dryers**   See *Birs dryer; fluid bed dryer; pneumatic dryers; roller dryer; rotary louvre dryer; spray dryer*.

**'dry frying'**   Frying without the use of fat by using an anti-sticking agent of silicone or a vegetable extract.

**dry ice**   Solid carbon dioxide; has a temperature of −79°C; used to refrigerate foodstuffs in transit, for carbonation of liquids, and for cold traps in the laboratory.

Sublimes from the solid stage to a gas without liquefying; latent heat at subliming temperature 246 BTU per pound; available refrigeration per pound nearly twice that of ice.

**drying, azeotropic**   See *azeotrope*.

**drying oil**   Highly unsaturated oil that absorbs oxygen and, when in thin films, polymerises to form a skin. Linseed and tung oil are examples of drying oils used in paints and in the manufacture of linoleum.

Nutritionally these oils are similar to edible fats, but when polymerised, are toxic.

See also *iodine value*.

**Du Bois formula**   See *surface area*.

**ductless glands**   See *hormones*.

**dulcin**   Synthetic material, paraphenetylurea (paraphenetolcarbamide), 250 times as sweet as sugar but not permitted in foods. Discovered 1883; also called sucrol and valzin.

**dulcite**   Dulcitol.

**dulcitol**   A six-carbon sugar-alcohol formed by reduction of galactose. Occurs in Madagascar manna (*Melampyrum nemorosum*), and also known as melampyrin, dulcite and galacticol.

**dulse**   Name given to two different edible seaweeds, *Rhodymenia palmata* and *Dilsea carnosa*; both purplish-brown; used in soups and jellies.

**dun**   In salted fish refers to the brown discoloration caused by mould growth.

***Dunaliella bardawil***   A red sea alga discovered in 1980 in Israel, extremely rich in (100 times more) beta-carotene than most other natural sources.

**dunst**   Very fine semolina (i.e. starch from the endosperm of the wheat grain) approaching the fineness of flour. Also called break middlings (not to be confused with middlings, which is the branny offal).

**duodenum**   First part of the small intestine, between the stomach and the jejunum. Pancreatic juice and bile are secreted into the intestine and the major part of digestion takes place there.

**durian**   Fruit of tree *Durio zibethinum* (Malaysia and Indonesia); each weighs 2–3 kg, soft, cream-coloured pulp (smell considered disgusting to the uninitiated). Analysis per 100 g edible part: 2.5 g protein, 1.5 g fat, 30 g carbohydrate, 125 kcal (500 kJ), 0.3 mg thiamin, 0.3 mg riboflavin, 1 mg niacin, 40 mg vitamin C.

**durum wheat**   A hard type of wheat of the species *Tricitum durum* (most bread wheats are *Tricitum vulgare*); largely used for the production of semolina intended for the preparation of macaroni.

**Dutching**   See *cocoa, Dutch*.

**Dutch oven**   Semicircular metal shield which may be placed close to an open fire; fitted with shelves on which food is roasted. It may also be clamped to the fire bars.

**D value**   See *decimal reduction time*.

**dynamic equilibrium**   Name given to the process in living organisms in which tissues are continually degraded to their constituents and resynthesised so that the structure remains constant. All protein structures in the body, for example, are in equilibrium with a 'metabolic pool' of amino acids.

**Dyox**   Trade name for chlorine dioxide used to treat flour. See *aging*.

**dyspepsia**   Any pain or discomfort associated with eating. Dyspepsia may be a symptom of gastritis, peptic ulcer, gall-bladder disease, etc., or, if there is no structural change in the intestinal tract, it is called 'functional dyspepsia'. Treatment includes a bland diet.

# E

**EAA index**   Essential amino acid index. See *protein quality*.

**earth nut**   Very small variety of truffle, *Conopodium denudatum*, also called pig nut and fairy potato. Also another name for peanut, which see.

**eau-de-vie de miel**   Or honey brandy, made by distilling mead (which, in turn, is made by fermenting honey).

**Eck fistula**   See *fistula*.

**ectomorph**   Description given to a tall, thin individual, possibly with underdeveloped muscles. See also *endomorph*; *mesomorph*.

**ecuelle**   Device for obtaining peel oil from citrus fruit. Consists of a shallow funnel lined with spikes on which the fruit is rolled by hand. As the oil glands are pierced, the oil and cell sap collect in the bottom of the funnel.

**eddo**   West Indian name for taro.

**edema**   See *oedema*.

**Edifas**   Trade name (Imperial Chemical Industries); Edifas A – methyl ethyl cellulose; Edifas B – sodium carboxymethylcellulose.

**Edosol**   Trade name (Trufood Ltd) for a low-sodium milk substitute.

Analysis per 100 g: protein 30.3%, fat 26.4%, carbohydrate 37.9%, Ca 846 mg, Fe 0.6 mg, sodium 43 mg (dried milk, sodium 400 mg), kcal 510 (2.1 MJ).

**EDTA**   See *ethylenediamine tetraacetic acid*.

**eel**   Long thin fish, *Anguilla anguilla,* inhabits rivers but breeds in the sea. Eaten cooked, smoked and jellied. Analysis per 100 g edible part: 17 g protein, 12 g fat, 180 kcal (700 kJ), 100 mg calcium, 1 mg iron, 800 μg retinol, 0.2 mg riboflavin, 3 mg niacin.

Conger eel, *Conger myriaster*.

**EFA**   Essential fatty acids, which see.

**egg**   Hens' eggs are graded according to quality and size (European Economic Community).

Quality: A – fresh; A extra – packed less than 7 days ago; B – less fresh than A, preserved or refrigerated; C – fit for food manufacture only.

Sizes: Grade 1, 70 g and over, then grades 2 to 6 at 5 g intervals, with grade 7 under 45 g.

Analysis whole egg per 100 g: 12 g protein, 11 g fat, 150 kcal (0.60 MJ), 50 mg Ca, 2 mg Fe, 150 μg retinol, 0.1 mg vitamin $B_1$, 0.5 mg vitamin $B_2$, 0.1 mg nicotinic acid, 2 μg vitamin D, 1.6 mg vitamin E.

Yolk per 100 g: 16 g protein, 31 g fat, 340 kcal (1.4 MJ), 130 mg Ca, 6 mg Fe, 400 μg retinol, 0.3 mg vitamin $B_1$, 0.5 mg vitamin $B_2$, 0.02 mg nicotinic acid, 5 μg vitamin D, 5 mg vitamin E.

White per 100 g: 9 g protein, trace fat, 36 kcal (0.15 MJ), 5 mg Ca, trace Fe, 0.4 mg vitamin $B_2$, 0.1 mg nicotinic acid.

Useful in food preparation to thicken sauces and custards, as an emulsifier, to hold air in meringues and sponges, and as a binder in croquettes.

**egg albumen**   See *egg-white*.

**egg, dehydrated**   Analysis per 100 g: 43 g protein, 43 g fat, 500 kcal (2 MJ), 190 mg Ca, 8 mg Fe, 500 μg retinol, 0.35 mg vitamin $B_1$, 1.2 mg vitamin $B_2$, 0.2 mg nicotinic acid, 6 μg vitamin D, 6 mg vitamin E.

**egg plant**   See *aubergine*.

**egg proteins**   What is generally referred to as egg protein is a mixture of individual proteins, including ovalbumin, ovomucin, ovoglobulin, conalbumin and vitellin. Egg-white contains 10.9% protein, mostly ovalbumin; yolk contains 16% protein, mainly two phosphoproteins – vitellin and vitellenin.

**egg substitute** Name formerly used for golden raising powder. See *baking powder*.

**egg-white** 87.8% water, 10.8% protein, 0.6% ash. Composed of outer layer of thin white, layer of thick white, richer in ovomucin, and inner layer of thin white surrounding the yolk. Eggs vary in ratio of thick to thin white, depending on the individual hen. Higher percentage of thick white desirable for frying and poaching (helps the egg to coagulate into small firm mass instead of spreading); thin white produces larger volume of froth when beaten than does thick.

Proteins are ovomucin, ovalbumin, ovomucoid, ovoglobulin and conalbumin.

**egg-white injury** See *biotin*.

**EH** Equilibrium humidity, which see.

**eicosanoids** Derivatives of eicosenoic acids – polyunsaturated fatty acids with 20 carbon atoms, i.e. eicosatetraenoic (4 double bonds) and pentaenoic (5) of the omega-3 series and dihomo-γ-linolenic (3) and arachidonic (4) of the omega-6 series.

Eicosanoids include prostaglandins, prostacyclins, thromb-exanes, leukotrienes (involved in wound healing, inflammation, allergy, blood platelet aggregation, etc.).

**eicosenoic acids** Derived from C20 polyunsaturated fatty acids.

**einkorn** A type of wheat, the wild form of which, *Triticum boeoticum*, was probably one of the ancestors of all cultivated wheats. Still grown in some parts of S. Europe and Middle East, usually for animal feed.

The name einkorn, 'one seed', derives from the single seed found in each spikelet.

**eiweiss milch** See *protein milk*.

**elastin** Insoluble protein uniting muscle fibres in meat, not changed on heating; the cause of tough meat. See also *albuminoids*; *connective tissue*.

**electronic heating** See *high-frequency heating*.

**electrophoresis** The movement of electrically charged particles under the influence of a current. The electric charge on proteins is sufficient to make them migrate at a rate depending on the protein itself, and electrophoresis on paper, gels, etc., is a convenient analytical tool for separating proteins.

**electropure process** Method of pasteurising milk by passing a low-frequency, alternating current.

**elemental diets** Same as formula diet, which see.

**elements, minor** See *trace elements*.

**ELISA** Enzyme-linked immunosorbent assay; enzyme assay using antibodies or antigens conjugated with an easily assayed enzyme; combines specificity of antibodies with sensitivity of spectrophotometer.

**elute** To wash off or remove. Rather specifically applied to the removal of adsorbed chemicals from the substance that has adsorbed them, as in chromatography.

**elvers** Young of European eel, about 5 cm in length.

**Embden groats** See *groats*.

**Embden–Meyerhof–Parnas scheme** Name for the first series of steps in the breakdown of glucose in the tissues, as far as pyruvic acid, i.e. the glycolytic part as distinct from the subsequent oxidation. See *glucose metabolism*.

**emblic** Berry of the S.E. Asian malacca tree, *Emblica officinalis*; similar in appearance to the gooseberry. Also known as Indian gooseberry. Rich source of vitamin C – 600 mg per 100 g.

**emmer** A type of wheat known to be used more than 8000 years ago; tetraploid (4 sets of 7 chromosomes). Wild emmer is *Triticum dicoccoides* and true emmer is *T. dicoccum*. Nowadays usually grown for animal feed.

**Emprote** Trade name (Eustace Miles Foods Co., Bucks.) for a dried milk and cereal preparation consumed as a beverage. 33% protein.

**emulsifying agents** Fatty substances that are soluble in fat and water (lipophilic and hydrophilic) and enable water-fat emulsions to be formed. These include substances such as gums, egg yolks, albumin, casein, soaps, agar, lecithin, glycerol monostearate, alginates, Irish moss, that aid the uniform dispersion of oil in water, i.e. form emulsions like margarine, ice-cream, salad cream, etc. Stabilisers (which see) maintain these emulsions in a stable form. Also used in baking to aid to smooth incorporation of fat into the dough and to keep the crumb soft.

**emulsifying salts** Sodium citrate, sodium phosphates and sodium tartrate, used in the manufacture of milk powder, evaporated milk, sterilised cream and processed cheese.

**emulsin** Mixture of glycosidase enzymes in bitter almond which decompose the glucoside amygdalin to benzaldehyde, glucose and hydrocyanic acid.

**emulsion** An intimate mixture of two immiscible liquids, one being dispersed in the other in the form of fine droplets. For example, oil and water. They will stay mixed only as long as they are stirred together unless an emulsifying agent (which see) is added to stabilise the emulsion.

**emulsoids**  See *colloids, lyophilic*.

**endergonic**  Used of reactions (in living tissues) that require a supply of energy, such as the synthesis of complex molecules.

**endive**  A species of chicory, *Cichorium endivia*; the curly leaves are eaten as a salad – blanched to debitter. Called chicory in the USA.

Analysis per 100 g: water 94 g, protein 1.8 g, carotene 2000 μg, vitamin C 12 mg.

**endocrines**  See *hormones*.

**endomorph**  In relation to body build, means short and stocky. See *ectomorph*; *mesomorph*.

**endomysium**  See *muscle*.

**endopeptidases**  Enzymes that split peptide bonds inside the protein molecule; i.e., according to the older nomenclature, they are proteinases, such as pepsin, trypsin and chymotrypsin.

**endosperm**  The inner and greater part of cereal grains. In wheat comprises about 83% of the grain, mainly starch, and is the source of semolina (which see).

Contains only about 10% of the thiamin, 35% of the riboflavin, 40% of the nicotinic acid, 50% of the pyridoxine and pantothenic acid of the whole grain.

**endotoxins**  Toxins produced by bacteria as integral part of the cell, so cannot be separated; unlike exotoxins, they do not usually stimulate antitoxin formation but the antibodies produced act directly on the bacteria; they are relatively stable to heat.

**enema**  See *nutrient enemata*.

**Energen rolls**  Trade name (Energen Foods Co. Ltd) for a light bread roll of wheat flour plus added wheat gluten.

Analysis per 100 g: protein 44 g, fat 4.1 g, carbohydrate 45.7 g, Ca 47 mg, Fe 4 mg, kcal 390 (1.63 MJ).

**energy**  Defined as the ability to do work. Exists in several forms, such as chemical energy in fuels and food; kinetic, potential, light and heat energy. Measured in joules; since various forms of energy are interconvertible, often measured as heat in calories or British thermal units.

Total chemical energy in a food, as released in the bomb calorimeter, is gross energy. After allowance is made for the losses in the faeces the remainder is digestible energy. After allowance is made for loss in the urine (e.g. urea from dietary proteins) the remainder is metabolisable energy. Finally, after allowing for the loss by specific dynamic action, the remainder is net energy.

Available energy in foods is calculated by use of the following factors: protein 17 kJ/g, fat 37 kJ/g, carbohydrate (calculated as monosaccharide) 16 kJ/g, alcohol 29 kJ/g.

Energy expenditure of average adult man: basal 1700 kcal (7.1 MJ) per day; light work, total 2300 kcal (9.7 MJ); medium work 3000 kcal (12.6 MJ); heavy work 3500 kcal (14.7 MJ).

See also *Atwater factors*; *phosphate bond, energy-rich*; *Rubner factors*.

**energy conversion factors** The amount of energy available in foodstuffs. When this was expressed in calories, the factors were slightly different, depending upon whether allowances were made for absorption (see *Atwater factors*; *Rubner factors*). With the change to the joule it was recognised that conversion factors for calculating the metabolisable energies of foods are relatively inaccurate, and until better values become available the following are used; protein 17 kJ/g, fat 37 kJ/g, carbohydrate (as monosaccharide) 16 kJ/g, ethyl alcohol 29 kJ/g, sugar alcohols 10 kJ/g, organic acids 13 kJ/g.

**energy-rich phosphate** See *phosphate bond, energy-rich*.

**enfleurage** Method of extracting essential oils from blossoms, by placing them on glass trays covered with purified lard or other fat, which eventually becomes saturated with the oil.

**ennoblement** See *enrichment*.

**enocianina** Desugared grape extract used to colour fruit flavours. Prepared by acid extraction of skins of red grapes; bluish when neutralised, turns red on acidifying.

**enolase** Enzyme that catalyses the conversion of 2-phosphoglyceric acid to phospho-enol-pyruvic acid, with the formation of an energy-rich phosphate bond. Important in the breakdown of glucose.

**en papillote** French method of cooking in closed container, parchment paper case. See also *sous-vide*.

**enrichment** Term applied to addition of nutrients to foods. Although often used interchangeably, the term fortification is used of legally imposed additions, and enrichment means the addition of nutrients beyond the levels originally present. See also *nutrification*; *restoration*.

**ensete** See *banana, false*.

**enteral nutrition** Tube feeding with liquid diet into stomach or intestinal tract.

**enterogastrone** Hormone found in the small intestine which inhibits both motor and secretory activity of the stomach. Its secretion is stimulated by fat; hence, fat in the diet inhibits gastric activity.

**enterokinase** An ingredient of the intestinal juice which activates the trypsinogen and chymotrypsinogen of the pancreatic juice to form trypsin and chymotrypsin, the active enzymes.

**entoleter**   Machine used to disinfest cereals and other foods. The material is fed to the centre of a high-speed rotating disc carrying studs so that it is thrown against the studs and the impact kills any insects and destroys their eggs.

**enzyme**   Catalyst produced by living cells. Composed of protein and destroyed by heat and protein coagulation; responsible for most of reactions carried out in living tissues.

Some are composed of two parts: the apoenzyme, the protein which is inactive alone; and its prosthetic group, a small non-protein molecule normally derived from a vitamin. This differs from a coenzyme, which readily dissociates from the enzyme protein (e.g. pyridoxal phosphate, biotin, thiamin pyrophosphate), while a prosthetic group is covalently bound (e.g. flavin mononucleotide and flavin adenine dinucleotide).

**enzyme activation tests**   Used for the diagnosis of malnutrition for vitamins ($B_1$, $B_2$ and $B_6$) which function as coenzymes (prosthetic groups).

The enzymes that can be so used exist *in vivo* as a mixture of the (inactive) apoenzyme and the (active) holoenzyme. When body reserves of the vitamin are low, the coenzyme is present in inadequate amounts. Testing the system before and after adding extra vitamin to the reaction mixture (activation) indicates whether the original levels were abnormally low. In adequately nourished subjects there can be up to 20% activation after adding the vitamin; greater stimulation is indicative of malnutrition.

Tests can be carried out on red blood cells for thiamin (transketolase), riboflavin (glutathione reductase) and vitamin $B_6$ (aspartate or alanine aminotransferase).

**enzyme activators**   A number of small molecules can increase the activity of enzymes – these may be substrates, precursors or coenzymes such as adenine nucleotides and nicotinamide nucleotides or mineral salts, especially Ca, Mg, Cu, Mo, Zn, etc.

**enzyme, allosteric**   An enzyme consisting of multiple protein subunits can show allosteric kinetics – a change in the affinity for its substrate, and, hence, in the activity observed, as a result of changes in configuration in response to the binding of either substrates or other small molecules collectively known as allosteric effectors (they may be either activators or inhibitors).

**enzyme induction**   Synthesis of new enzyme protein in response to some stimulus such as a hormone or a substrate (e.g. drug or food additive).

**enzyme inhibition**   Many compounds can inhibit enzymes. Reversible inhibition is common with a number of physiological compounds, including products of the reaction or pathway, and coenzymes such as adenine and nicotinamide nucleotides. Inhibition by non-physiological compounds (drugs, food additives, etc.) may be reversible or irreversible; reversible inhibition may be competitive with respect to substrate, non-competitive or uncompetitive.

**enzyme repression**  Reduction in synthesis of enzyme protein in response to some stimulus such as a hormone or the presence of large amounts of the end-product of a pathway.

**EPA**  Eicosapentaenoic acid – long chain marine fatty acid – 20 carbon atoms, 5 double bonds, omega-3 series.

**epicarp**  See *flavedo*.

**epinephrine**  See *adrenaline*.

**epoxy-**  Prefix denoting an oxygen atom attached to two different atoms in a molecule.

**Epsom salts**  Magnesium sulphate; acts as a purgative because the osmotic pressure of the solution causes it to retain water in the intestine and so increase the bulk of the faeces.

**Equal**  Trade name (USA) for aspartame.

**equilibrium humidity**  The relative humidity of the atmosphere with which the substance under consideration is in equilibrium.

**equilibrium, nitrogen**  See *nitrogen balance*.

**erepsin**  Name given to a mixture of enzymes contained in the intestinal juice, including aminopeptidases and dipeptidases.

**ergocalciferol**  See *vitamin D*.

**ergosterol**  Sterol isolated from yeast; when treated with ultraviolet light, is converted to vitamin $D_2$ (ergocalciferol). This is the method of manufacture of the vitamin.

**ergot**  Fungus that grows on grasses and cereal grains; the ergot of medical importance is *Claviceps purpurea* that grows on rye. The consumption of infected rye is harmful, causing the disease known as St Anthony's Fire, and can be fatal.

The active principles in ergot are alkaloids, ergotinine, ergotoxine, ergotamine, ergometrine, etc. Hydrolysis of all of these produces lysergic acid, which is therefore believed to be the active component. Its effect is to increase tone and contraction of smooth muscle, particularly of the pregnant uterus. For this reason ergot is used in obstetrics, but pure ergonovine maleate and ergotonine tartrate are preferable.

**ergothioneine**  Betaine of thiolhistidine; occurs in red blood cells, liver and kidney, and is constituent of ergot.

**ergotism**  Poisoning due to a mould infection of rye (see *ergot*). Occurs from time to time among peoples eating rye bread. Last outbreak in the UK was 1925 in Manchester, when there were 200 cases. Symptoms appear when as little as 1% of ergotised rye is included in the flour.

**eriodictin**  See *vitamin P*.

**erucic acid**  *Cis*-13-docosenoic acid (22-carbon monounsaturated fatty acid) found in *Brassica napus* (rape seed) and *B. junca* and *B. nigra* (mustard seed). Can constitute 30–50% of the oil in some varieties. Causes fatty infiltration of heart muscle in experimental animals among other changes, and the amount of hardened rape seed oil used in margarines is consequently limited (EEC suggested maximum is 5%; Sweden 2%). See *rape*.

**erythorbic acid**  D-isomer of ascorbic acid with only slight anti-scorbutic activity; also called D-araboascorbic acid. Slight biological effect – may be only by protecting the vitamin C – but it is as powerful an antioxidant as vitamin C and used in foods for that purpose.

**erythroamylose**  Old name for amylopectin.

**erythrocytes**  Red blood cells. See *blood, red cells*.

**erythropoiesis**  Development of the red blood cells; takes place in the bone marrow.

**erythrosine BS**  Red colour permitted in foods in most countries. Disodium or potassium salt of 2,4,5,7-tetraiodofluorescein. (In the USA called Red No. 3.)
 Used in preserved cherries, sausage and meat and fish pastes; unstable to light and heat.

**erythrotin**  Obsolete name for vitamin $B_{12}$.

**escalopes**  Thin pieces of meat or fish.

**esculin**  See *aesculin*.

**essential amino acid index**  See *protein quality*.

**essential amino acid pattern, provisional**  The quantities of the essential amino acids considered desirable in the diet.

**essential amino acids**  See *amino acid*.

**essential fatty acids**  Name originally given to a group of three fatty acids, linoleic (18:2 ω6), γ-linolenic (18:3 ω6) and arachidonic (20:4 ω6) – originally called vitamin F. See *linoleic acid* for nomenclature. Arachidonic can be synthesised in the body from linoleic so is not strictly an essential fatty acid (EFA)
 Several other fatty acids have some EFA activity in that they cure some but not all of the symptoms of EFA deficiency in experimental animals.
 Deficiency does not occur in human beings except babies in abnormal circumstances; signs of deficiency – eczema, scaly skin with oozing into body folds, changes in hair texture. Minimum requirement thought to be about 1% of total energy intake, equivalent to 260 mg per MJ.

**essential oils**  Volatile, odorous oils found in plants. They bear no relation to the edible oils, since they are not glycerol esters.

They are inflammable, soluble in alcohol and ether but not water; used for flavouring foods. Examples are oil of spearmint, oil of bitter almonds, oil of citronella, spirits of turpentine. See also *terpenes*.

**ester**  Chemical name of compound of acid and alcohol, e.g. ethyl alcohol and acetic acid yield ethyl acetate – an ester.

Fats are esters of the trihydric alcohol glycerol, and long-chain acids such as stearic or oleic.

See also *flavours, synthetic*; *waxes*.

**esterases**  Name given to a group of enzymes that attack simple esters rather than fats; may be of low specificity as esterase itself, which attacks all simple esters, or of more specific nature, such as cholinesterase.

**ester value**  Same as saponification value.

**ethanolamine**  2-aminoethanol; $HOCH_2CH_2NH_2$. Widely distributed in plant and animal tissues as component of phospholipids; intermediate in catecholamine and phospholipid metabolism. Used as softening agent for hides, as dispersing agent for agricultural chemicals and as paring (peeling) agent for fruits and vegetables.

**ethanol**  Systematic chemical name for ethyl alcohol; see under *alcohol*.

**ethyl alcohol**  See under *alcohol*.

**ethyl carbamate**  See *urethane*.

**ethylene**  A gas of the formula $CH_2CH_2$, of interest in its use to assist the ripening of fruits: e.g. 0.4% accelerates the ripening of pears; 0.05% will convert green lemons to yellow in one week at 30–40°C.

**ethylene diaminetetra-acetic acid**  Also called versene and sequestrol; forms a stable complex with metal ions and so removes them from activity. See *chelating agents*.

**ethyl formate**  $HCOOC_2H_5$.

Fumigant – used against raisin moth, dried fruit beetle, fig moth, etc.

Flavour – ingredient of lemon and strawberry flavour and artificial rum and arrack.

Chemical intermediate – in synthesis of vitamin $B_1$, sulphadiazine, etc.

**euglobulin**  The name given to that fraction of serum globulin which is precipitated by dialysis of blood serum against distilled water. The name implies that this fraction is a typical globulin by reason of its insolubilty in water.

**eukeratins**  See *keratin*.

**Euler's yeast coenzyme**  Nicotinamide adenine dinucleotide.

**eutectic ice**  The solid formed when a mixture of 76.7% water and

23.3% salt (by weight) is frozen. It melts at $-21\,°C$; 3 lb eutectic ice has the refrigeration effect equivalent to 1 lb solid carbon dioxide; particularly useful in icing fish on board trawlers.

**eutrophia**   Normal nutrition.

**evaporation, flash**   A short, rapid application of heat so that a small volume (about 1%) is quickly distilled off carrying with it the greater part of the volatiles. The flash distillate is collected separately from the later distillate and added back to the concentrate to restore the flavour; applied to products such as fruit juices.

**evening primrose**   *Oenothera biennis*, source of α-linolenic acid, 8% of total fatty acids.

**Evian water**   Non-gaseous, slightly mineralised; diuretic.

**exergonic**   Energy-supplying reactions, such as oxidation of foodstuffs.

**exopeptidases**   Enzymes that split peptide bonds near the terminal units, i.e. at the ends of the protein chain. According to the older nomenclature, they were peptidases, such as aminopeptidase, carboxypeptidase and dipeptidases of the digestive juices.

**exotoxins**   Toxic substances produced by bacteria which diffuse out of the cells; stimulate antibodies which specifically neutralise them; generally heat-labile and inactivated in 1 hour at $60\,°C$. Exotoxins include those produced by botulism, tetanus and diphtheria organisms.

**expansion ring**   In relation to cans, refers to the concentric rings stamped into the ends of the can to allow bulging during heat processing without straining the seams unduly.

**expeller cake**   Oilseed after removal of most of the oil by pressing: a valuable source of protein. (Cotton, coconut, groundnut, sunflower, sesame, etc.)

**extensograph**   Instrument for measuring the stretching quality of a dough as an index of its baking quality; the dough is stretched in cylindrical form.

**extensometer**   Instrument used to measure the stretching strength of a dough as an index of its baking quality. A ball of fermenting dough is fixed on two pins which are moved apart to stretch the dough. See also *alveograph*.

**extraction rate**   Refers to the yield of flour obtained from wheat in the milling process. 100% extraction (or straight-run flour) is wholemeal flour containing all of the grain; lower extraction rates are the whiter flours from which more of the bran and the germ are excluded, down to a figure of 72% extraction, which is the normal white flour of commerce.

'Patent' flours are of lower extraction rate, 30–50%, and so comprise mostly the endosperm of the grain.

Analysis per 100 g, 72% extraction, fortified; protein 11.5 g, fat 1.4 g, carbohydrate 75 g, 340 kcal–1.5 MJ, fibre 4 g, Fe 2 mg, Ca 140 mg, vitamin $B_1$ 0.3 mg, vitamin $B_2$ 0.03 mg, niacin 2 mg.

80% extraction (fortified); protein 12.5 g, fat 1.8 g, carbohydrate 70 g, 320 kcal–1.4 MJ, fibre 7 g, Fe 3.2 mg, Ca 130 mg, vitamin $B_1$ 0.4 mg, vitamin $B_2$ 0.07 mg, niacin 4 mg.

100% extraction, protein 13 g, fat 2 g, carbohydrate 64 g, 310 kcal–1.3 MJ, fibre 8.5 g, Fe 4 mg, Ca 40 mg, vitamin $B_1$ 0.5 mg, vitamin $B_2$ 0.1 mg, niacin 6 mg.

**extract of malt** See *malt*.

**extract of meat** See *meat extract*.

**extract of yeast** See *yeast extract*.

**extremophiles** Name given to micro-organisms that can grow under extreme conditions of heat or cold, acid or alkali, high concentrations of salt or under high pressure.

**extrinsic factor** Vitamin $B_{12}$; see under *pernicious anaemia*.

# F

**factor 3** See *selenium*.

**factor I** Obsolete name for vitamin $B_6$.

**factor U** Cabagin, anti-ulcer factor reported in cabbage leaves, believed to be methyl sulphonium salt of methionine. See also *folic acid*.

**factor W** Obsolete name for biotin.

**factor X** Obsolete name for vitamin $B_{12}$.

**factor Y** Obsolete name for vitamin $B_6$.

**FAD** See *flavine adenine dinucleotide*.

**faeces** Composed of undigested food residues, remains of digestive secretions not reabsorbed, bacteria from the intestinal tract, cells and mucus from the intestinal lining, substances excreted into the intestinal tract. Average 100 g per day. Principal pigment, stercobilin.

**faggot** (1) Small bundle of parsley, thyme, marjoram and bay leaf tied together with cotton and added to the dish being cooked. Also known as bouquet garni.

(2) Dish of liver, chopped, seasoned and baked.

**fair maids** Cornish name for pilchards (thought to be corruption of Spanish fumade = smoked).

**FAO** Food and Agriculture Organisation of the United Nations.

**Farex** Trade name (Glaxo Laboratories) of an infant cereal food.

Analysis per 100 g: protein 12.9 g, fat 2.3 g, carbohydrate 73 g, Ca 900 mg, Fe 24 mg, kcal 350 (1.4 MJ), vitamin $B_1$ 1.4 mg, vitamin $B_2$ 1.6 mg.

**farfals** See *alimentary pastes*.

**farina**  General term for starch. More specifically in the UK refers to potato starch; in the USA is defined as the starch obtained from wheat other than durum wheat; starch from the latter is semolina.

**farina dolce**  Italian flour made from dried chestnuts.

**farinograph**  An instrument for measuring the physical properties of a dough. It measures the time taken for the dough to attain standard consistency in a high-speed mixer, the time it can maintain this consistency and the extent to which the dough falls on further mixing.

**Farlene**  Trade name (Farley's Infant Food, Plymouth) for a high-protein baby food in the form of a dried powder. Composed of wheat flour, high-protein wheat flour, soya, peas, milk, wheat gluten and egg, fortified with vitamins and minerals.

Analysis per 100 g: protein 25 g, fat 5.5 g, carbohydrate 61.5 g, kcal 390 (1.6 MJ), Ca 0.8 g, Fe 12 mg, vitamin A 840 µg, vitamin $B_1$ 0.8 mg, vitamin $B_2$ 0.6 mg, nicotinic acid 15 mg, vitamin C 70 mg, vitamin D 18 µg.

**fast foods**  General term used for a limited menu of foods that lend themselves to production line techniques; suppliers tend to specialise in products such as hamburgers, pizzas, chicken or sandwiches.

**fat, blood**  About 590 mg per 100 ml plasma; 150 mg neutral fat, 160 mg cholesterol, 200 mg phospholipid.

**fat-extenders**  Substances that permit a reduction of fat content without altering the texture; used in baked products, e.g. glyceryl monostearate.

**fat, neutral**  The triglyceride fats; used in distinction from other lipids, as, for example, in blood, where the subdivision is neutral fat, cholesterol and phospholipid.

**fats**  (1) Chemically fats are substances which are insoluble in water but soluble in organic solvents such as ether, chloroform and benzene, and are actual or potential esters of fatty acids. The term includes triglycerides, phospholipids, waxes and sterols; also termed lipids.

(2) In the more general use the term 'fats' refers to the neutral fats which are mixtures of esters of fatty acids with glycerol, i.e. triglycerides.

**fats, high-ratio**  Shortenings with a greater proportion of mono- and diglycerides, i.e. superglycerinated (see also *superglycinerated fats*). These shortenings disperse more readily into doughs, and allow the use of a higher ratio of sugar to flour than with ordinary shortening. See also *flour, high-ratio*.

**fats, hydrogenated**  See *hydrogenated oils*.

**fat-soluble vitamins**  Vitamins A, D, E and K; occur in food in solution in the fats. Are stored in the body to a greater extent than the water-soluble.

The distinction into fat-soluble and water-soluble is of historical interest and is convenient for chapter headings in textbooks, but otherwise has no significance.

**fat spread, low**   Not more than 40% fat (compared with standard 80%).

**fat spread, reduced**   Not more than 60% fat (compared with standard 80%).

**fats, yellow**   Term applied to butter, margarine and similar fat-containing breadspreads.

**fatty acids**   Organic acids consisting of carbon chains with a carboxyl group at the end. Simplest is formic acid, HCOOH, then acetic acid, $CH_3COOH$, propionic, butyric, etc.

Longer-chain fatty acids include those found in soap, such as stearic, palmitic and oleic.

They may be saturated fatty acids, in which every carbon atom carries its full quota of hydrogen atoms, or unsaturated, in which there is a shortage of hydrogen atoms compensated for by a double instead of a single bond linking two adjacent carbon atoms. Such double bonds are susceptible to the addition of oxygen and, hence, unsaturated fatty acids (and unsaturated fats made from them) are less stable than fully saturated ones. Fats with a large number of double bonds, i.e. highly unsaturated, readily oxidise to resin-like consistency and are the so-called 'drying oils' such as linseed and tung oil, used in paints.

**fatty acids, essential**   See *essential fatty acids*.

**fatty acids, free**   (1) Liberated from triglycerides when subjected to hydrolytic rancidity; therefore determination of FFA is an index of quality of fats.

(2) See also *non-esterified fatty acids*.

**favism**   Acute haemolytic anaemia induced in genetically sensitive people by eating broad beans, *Vicia faba*. The genetic disease is a deficiency of the enzyme glucose-6-phosphate dehydrogenase in the red blood cells, which are often vulnerable to the toxins, vicine and convicine, in the beans. The deficiency is said to affect some 100 million people of all races, especially in Mediterranean and Middle Eastern countries, and is rare or virtually absent in N. European nations.

**fecula**   Name given to foods which are almost solely starch; prepared from roots and stems by grating, e.g. tapioca, sago and arrowroot. See under separate entries.

**Fehling's solution**   See *Fehling's test*.

**Fehling's test**   For reducing substances, mostly used to distinguish reducing from non-reducing sugars. Depends upon the reduction of blue cupric hydroxide to yellow cuprous oxide on heating the alkaline solution.

Fehling's solution A is copper sulphate, and solution B is alkaline tartrate; mixed immediately before use to prevent deterioration. See also *Benedict's test*.

**fennel** *Foeniculum vulgare* (parsley family): seeds contain 10% fixed oil and 6% essential oil, containing anethole, fenchone and terpenes. Leaves used in fish dishes and sauces.

**fenugreek** *Trigonella feonumgraecum*. Leguminous plant eaten as vegetable, seeds used for flavouring. Consumed by women in Orient to help gain weight.

Analysis of seeds per 100 g: 29 g protein, 5 g fat, 50 g carbohydrate, 355 kcal (1.46 MJ), 180 mg Ca, 22 mg Fe, 0.4 mg vitamin $B_1$, 0.3 mg vitamin $B_2$, 1.5 mg nicotinic acid.

**Ferguzade** Trade name (Ferguzade Ltd) for a glucose beverage.

**ferment** As a noun, the old name for enzyme. As a verb, to carry out the process of fermentation.

**fermentation** Anaerobic metabolism. Used generally of alcohol fermentation of sugars, also production of lactic acid, citric acid, etc., by micro-organisms.

**fermented milks** See *milks, fermented*.

**fermentograph** Instrument for measuring the gas-producing power of a dough. The fermenting dough is contained in a balloon immersed in water and as gas is produced the balloon expands and rises in the water, the rise being measured continuously.

**ferric ammonium citrate** Form in which iron is sometimes added to foods. Occurs as brown-red scales (16.5–18.5% iron) and as green scales (14.5–16% iron).

**ferritin** A ferric hydroxide–phosphate–protein complex (containing 23% iron) present in the cells of the intestinal mucosa, liver, spleen and bone marrow, as a storage form of iron. See also *haemosiderin*.

**ferrum redactum** See *iron, reduced*.

**FFA** Free fatty acids. See *fatty acids, free*.

**fibre, crude** Term given to indigestible part of foods, defined in the UK Fertiliser and Feedingstuffs Act of 1932 as the residue left after successive extractions with petroleum ether, 1.25% sulphuric acid and 1.25% sodium hydroxide minus ash, carried out under closely specified conditions. Dietary fibre (see *fibre, dietary*) bears no real relation to crude fibre and its estimation involves a series of specified separation procedures.

**fibre, dietary** Term applied to structural parts of plant tissues which are not digested by human digestive enzymes although partly metabolised by bacteria in the intestine to form short chain fatty acids which do provide a source of energy – includes cellulose, hemicellulose, lignin, pectins and gums; previously termed roughage or bulk.

The amount of dietary fibre in a food depends on the method of analysis (e.g. Southgate or Englyst method which can include enzyme-resistant starch (see *starch, enzyme-resistant*). The fibre fractions of different foods vary considerably in composition and in their physiological effects.

**fibrin**   (1) See *fibrinogen*.

(2) Discarded name for one of the muscle proteins, once called 'albumin' and 'fibrin'.

**fibrinogen**   One of the proteins of the blood plasma which is responsible for the clotting of blood. Under the influence of thrombin it is converted to fibrin, which is deposited as strands that trap the red cells and form the clot. See also *blood, defibrinated*; *coagulation, blood*.

**fibronectin**   A protein (alpha$_2$-glycoprotein) found in plasma; has a very short half-life and serves as an index of undernutrition.

**fibrous proteins**   See *albuminoids*.

**ficin**   Proteolytic enzyme from the fig.

**fig**   *Ficus carica*; eaten fresh, dried (when they contain 50% sugars) and preserved; have mild laxative properties, e.g. syrup of figs is a medicinal preparation.

Analysis per 100 g: 1.3 g protein, 11 g carbohydrate, 50 kcal (0.2 MJ), 1 mg Fe, 25 µg vitamin A, 0.05 mg vitamin B$_1$, 0.05 mg vitamin B$_2$, 0.4 mg nicotinic acid, 2 mg vitamin C.

Dried figs: 4 g protein, 63 g carbohydrate, 270 kcal (1.1 MJ), 200 mg Ca, 4 mg Fe, 30 µg vitamin A, 0.1 mg vitamin B$_1$, 0.08 mg vitamin B$_2$, 1.7 mg nicotinic acid, zero vitamin C.

**FIGLU test**   See *formiminoglutamic acid test*.

*Filix mas*   Male fern; contains organic acids, including filicic acid, which have a selective action on, and therefore used in treatment for, tapeworm.

**filled milk**   See *milk, filled*.

**film yeasts**   See *yeasts*.

**filth test**   Name given to a test originated in the USA for determining the contamination of a food with rodent hairs and insect fragments as an index of the hygienic handling of the food.

**filtrate factor**   See *pantothenic acid*.

**fines herbes**   A mixture of chopped parsley, chervil, chives and tarragon.

**fining agents**   Substances used to clarify liquids by precipitating and carrying down suspended matter, e.g. egg albumin, casein, bentonite, isinglass, gelatin, etc.

**Finnan haddock**   Smoke-cured haddock. (Findon in Scotland.)

**fireless cooker**   See *haybox cooking*.

**fire point**   Term used with reference to frying oils; the temperature at which the fat will sustain combustion. It ranges between
340 and 360°C for different fats. See also *flash point*; *smoke
point*.

**firkin**   A quarter of a barrel of beer, i.e. 9 imperial gallons; also
56 lb of butter.

**firming agents**   Fresh fruits contain insoluble pectins as a firm gel
around the fibrous tissues and keep the fruit firm. Breakdown of
cell structure allows conversion of pectin to pectic acid, with loss
of firmness. Addition of calcium salts (chloride or carbonate)
forms calcium pectate gel which protects the fruit against
softening; these are known as firming agents.

Alum is sometimes used to firm pickles.

See also *pectin*.

**fish**   The composition of all non-fatty fish, such as cod, hake,
haddock, flatfish, is similar. See *codfish*; see also *fish, fatty*.

**fish, fatty**   Anchovies, herring, mackerel, salmon, sardines –
containing about 15% fat (varying from 5 to 20% throughout
the year) and containing 10–40 μg vitamin D per 100 g, as
distinct from white fish, which contain 1–2% fat and only a trace
of vitamin D.

**fish fingers**   (fish sticks USA). Shaped fish fillets covered with
breadcrumbs; approximately 50% fish. Analysis per 100 g when
fried: 14 g protein, 13 g fat, 17 g carbohydrate, 180 kcal (750 kJ).

**fish ham**   Japanese product made from a red fish such as tuna or
marlin, pickled with salt and nitrite, mixed with whale meat and
pork fat and stuffed into a large sausage-type casing.

**fish meal**   Surplus fish, waste from filleting (fish-house waste) and
fish unfit for human consumption are dried in vacuum, by
steam, or hot air, and powdered.

The resultant fish meal is a valuable source of protein as
animal feedingstuff, or, after deodorisation, as human food,
since it contains about 70% protein of biological value up to 0.75.

That made from white fish is termed white fish meal, as
distinct from the oily type. The latter is sometimes of very poor
quality and is then used as fertiliser.

**fish paste**   A spread made from ground fish and cereal. In the UK
legally contains not less than 70% fish.

**fish protein concentrate**   Deodorised, decolorised, defatted fish
meal also known as fish flour. Cheap source of protein for
enrichment of foods.

Approximately 75% protein; biological value 0.75.

**fish sausage**  Japanese product made from chopped fish fillet, spiced, flavoured, plus fat and starch, and the whole packed into sausage casing.

**fistula**  A short-circuiting connection. For example, an Eck fistula is a surgical joining of the portal vein to the inferior vena cava, so that the liver is short-circuited. Used as an experimental technique for examining the function of the liver.

**flambé**  To light spirit poured over a dish, e.g. brandy on the Christmas pudding.

**flash evaporation**  See *evaporation, flash*.

**flash-pasteurisation**  Process in which the material is held at a higher temperature than in normal pasteurisation, but for a shorter period. There is less development of the cooked flavour in the shorter period.

For milk, ordinary pasteurisation involves heating to 60°C for 30 seconds; in the flash process 74°C for only a few seconds.

See also *pasteurisation*.

**flash point**  With reference to frying oils, the temperature at which the decomposition products can be ignited, but will not support combustion. When they will support combustion, this is the fire point. Cottonseed oil: smoke point 232°C, flash point 330°C, fire point 363°C. These points are lowered by the presence of free fatty acids.

Flash point varies with different fats, and ranges between 290 and 330°C.

**flash 18**  A method of canning foods (Swift & Co., USA) under pressure 18 pounds per square inch above atmospheric pressure. The food is sterilised at 121°C and then canned at that temperature, not requiring further heat.

The advantages claimed are improved taste and texture compared with conventional canning, and the possibility of using large containers without overheating the food.

**flatogens**  Substances that cause gas production, flatulence, in the intestine. Those identified include raffinose, stachyose and verbascose in a variety of beans.

**flat sours**  Bacteria that render canned food sour, without gas production, i.e. the ends of the can are not swelled out but remain flat. They are thermophilic, facultative anaerobes, which attack carbohydrates with the production of acids, lactic, formic, acetic, but without gas formation.

Economically they are the most important of the thermophilic spoilage agents; some species can grow slowly at 25°C and thus spoil products after long storage periods. Type species is *Bacillus stearothermophilus*.

**flatulence**  Production of gas in the intestine – hydrogen, carbon

110

dioxide and methane. Possibly caused by a variety of foods, including beans, Brussels sprouts, cabbage, cauliflower, onions, radishes, melon, avocado, which contain indigestible carbohydrates which are fermented by the bacteria in the intestine.

**flatus** Gas production in the intestinal tract, arising either from the stomach (released by mouth) or the colon (released rectally). Undigested sugars (stachyose, raffinose and verbascose) serve as substrate for intestinal bacteria, with the production of methane, carbon dioxide and hydrogen.

**flavanols** See *flavonoids*.

**flavanones** See *flavonoids*.

**flavedo** The coloured outer peel layer of citrus fruits, also called the epicarp or zest. It contains the oil sacs and numerous yellow plastids (green in the unripe fruit, containing chlorophyll; yellow in the ripe fruit, containing carotene and xanthophyll).

**flavin** Also called quercitron. Colour obtained from the quercitron bark (species of oak, *Quercus tinctoria*); legally permitted in food in most countries. Insoluble in water but soluble in alkalies to give yellow colour, changed to brown in air.

**flavin adenine dinucleotide** (FAD) Coenzyme in cellular oxidation consisting of the vitamin riboflavin, attached to two phosphate molecules, and ribose and adenine. See *flavoproteins*.

**flavins** Derivatives of iso-alloxazine, as in riboflavin (the 6,7 dimethyl derivative).

**flavone** See *flavonoids*.

**flavonoids** Compounds widely distributed in nature as pigments in flowers, fruit, vegetables and tree barks.

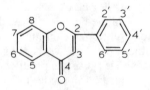

Structurally the flavone nucleus consists of a benzenoid ring fused to gamma-pyrone carrying a second benzenoid ring and bearing a number of hydroxyl groups. Flavonoids are flavone glycosides with rhamnose or rhamnoglucose attached at position 3 or 7.

Flavonoids divided into flavonols – hydroxyl group replaces H in flavone nucleus; flavonones – one double bond reduced in the 2=3 position; flavanals – hydroxyl group in place of the O and reduction of double bond at 4 and reduction of 2=3 double bond; isoflavones – benzenoid ring attached to C3 instead of C2.

**flavonols**  See *flavonoids*.

**flavoproteins**  A group of oxidising enzymes composed of conjugated proteins containing riboflavin (vitamin $B_2$) as the prosthetic group. There are two classes, those containing flavin mononucleotide, and those containing adenineflavin dinucleotide. The protein itself differs in each specific enzyme.

Examples: amino acid oxidase (which oxidises amino acids to ketonic acids), cytochrome reductase (part of the oxidation chain in the cell), diaphorase and Warburg's yellow enzyme (also part of the oxidation chain).

**flavour**  See *organoleptic*.

**flavour potentiator**  Substance that enhances the flavours of other substances without itself imparting any characteristic flavour of its own, e.g. monosodium glutamate, ribotide, as well as small quantities of sugar, salt and vinegar.

**flavour profile**  Method of judging flavour of foods by examination of a list of the separate factors into which the flavour can be analysed – the so-called character notes.

**flavours, synthetic**  Mostly mixtures of esters, e.g. banana oil – ethyl butyrate and amyl acetate; apple oil – ethyl butyrate, ethyl valerianate, ethyl salicylate, amyl butyrate, glycerol, chloroform and alcohol; pineapple oil – ethyl and amyl butyrates, acetaldehyde, chloroform, glycerol, alcohol.

**flipper**  See *swells*.

**Florence oil**  Name given to high grade of olive oil.

**Florentine**  (1) Thin biscuits with nuts and dried fruit coated with chocolate. (2) Garnished with spinach.

**floridean starch**  A glucosan resembling glycogen, obtained from red algae (*Florideae*).

**flour**  Generally refers to the ground wheat berry, although also used for other cereals and applied to powdered dried materials such as fish flour (deodorised dried fish), potato flour, etc.

The ground wheat berry yields wholemeal flour (100% extraction); whiter flours are obtained by separation of the bran and the germ from the starchy endosperm (see *extraction rate*).

The white flour as used in the ordinary white loaf is 70–72% extraction fortified to contain not less than 0.24 mg vitamin $B_1$, 1.6 mg nicotinic acid, and 1.65 mg iron per 100 g plus 14 oz of Creta Praeparata (chalk) per 280 lb sack of flour.

See also *aging*; *extraction rate*; *wheatmeal, national*.

**flour, agglomerated**  A dispersible form, easily wetted, produced by agglomerating the fine particles in steam; particles are greater than 100 μm diameter so the flour is dust-free.

**flour, aging**  See *aging*.

**flour, bleaching**  See *aging*.

**flour enrichment**  The addition of certain vitamins and minerals to flour.

UK, mg per 100g: vitamin $B_1$ 0.24, vitamin $B_2$ not added, nicotinic acid 1.6, Fe 1.65, Ca 14oz per 280lb sack as Creta.

USA, mg per 100g: vitamin $B_1$ 0.44–0.56, vitamin $B_2$ 0.26–0.33, nicotinic acid 3.6–4.4, Fe 2.9–3.7, calcium not specified.

**flour, enzyme inactivated**  Flour in which enzymes, specifically alpha-amylase, have been inactivated by heat to prevent degradation when the flour is used as a thickening agent in gravies, soups, etc.

**flour, extraction rate**  See *extraction rate*.

**flour, high-ratio**  Flour of very fine and more uniform particle size, treated with chlorine to reduce the gluten strength. Used for making cakes, since it is possible to add up to 140 parts of sugar to 100 parts of this flour, whereas only half this quantity of sugar can be incorporated into cakes with ordinary flour. See *flour strength*.

**flour improvers**  See *aging*.

**flour, national**  See *wheatmeal, national*.

**flour, patent**  See *extraction rate*.

**flour, self-raising**  Flour to which have been added chemicals that produce carbon dioxide in the presence of water and heat; the dough is thus aerated without prolonged fermentation. Usually 'weaker' flours are used. See *flour strength*.

Chemical agents used: sodium carbonate (3lb 4oz per 280lb sack); calcium acid phosphate or sodium pyrophosphate (4⅓ lb); or a mixture of these two. Legally, self-raising flour must contain not less than 0.4% available carbon dioxide.

See *baking powder*.

**flour strength**  A property of the flour proteins enabling the dough to retain gas during fermentation to give a 'bold' loaf. 'strong' flour is higher in protein content, has greater elasticity and resistance to extension, and greater ability to absorb water. A 'weak' flour gives a loaf that lacks volume. See also *extensometer*; *farinograph*.

**flour, whole meal**  See *flour*.

**fluid balance**  See *water balance*.

**fluid bed dryer**  A bed of solid particles is supported on a cushion of hot air jets (fluidised) and the material may be conveyed in this way, while being dried. The method achieves intimate mixing without mechanical damage: it is applicable to particles of a size sufficiently small to become impervious when packed closely and sufficiently large to float on an air cushion (as distinct from fine powders), e.g. cereals, tabletting granules, salt, coffee and dried vegetables.

**flummery**   Old English pudding made by boiling down the water from soaked oatmeal until it becomes thick and gelatinous. Similar to frumenty (which see).

**fluorescence**   The ability to absorb light at one wavelength and radiate part of it at another wavelength. Is used analytically for quantitative measurement by fluorimetry, the intensity of fluorescence being proportional to the amount of material present. For example, vitamin $B_2$ and thiochrome, prepared from vitamin $B_1$, fluoresce.

**fluoridation**   See *fluorine*.

**fluorimetry**   See *fluorescence*.

**fluorine**   An element of the same family as chlorine, bromine and iodine (the halogens). Although it ordinarily occurs in small amounts in plants and animals, it is not thought to be essential to either and no deficiency symptoms have ever been produced.

   Drinking water ranges in fluoride content between 0.05 and 14 parts per million, and water containing concentrations around 1 ppm helps to protect teeth from decay, although the mechanism of this effect is unknown. Quantities of this order are added to drinking water in enlightened areas to confer this protection. In larger amounts it causes chalky white patches to appear on the surface of the teeth, known as mottled enamel. Excessive doses are toxic and give rise to fluorosis.

**FMN**   Flavine mononucleotide.

**foam-mat drying**   A method of drying food. The liquid concentrate is whipped to a foam with the aid of a foaming agent, spread on a tray and dried in a stream of warm air. It reconstitutes very rapidly with water because of the fine structure of the foam. It has the further advantage that the foam-dried materials hold less water at a given relative humidity than do spray-dried foods and are less liable to cake.

**folacin**   See *folic acid*.

**folic acid**   Or folacin. A vitamin: generic descriptor for a group of substances essential for the synthesis of purines and pyrimidines and so for nucleic acid synthesis, and all processes of cell division. Functions by serving as a carrier of one-carbon units; deficiency signs include megaloblastic anaemia.

   The active principle is tetrahydrofolic acid or folinic acid (tetrahydropteroyl glutamic acid). The numerous chemical derivatives gave rise to various names over the years of their elucidation – citrovorum factor (CF) and leucovorin (5-formyl tetrahydroglutamic acid), rhizopterin, SLR (*Streptococcus lactis* R) factor, Wills factor, vitamin M, vitamin Bc, factors U, R and S – all of which consist of pteroyl glutamic acid with up to six additional glutamyl residues.

   Occurs in liver, kidneys, green leafy vegetables and yeast.

**folinic acid**   See *folic acid*.

**fondant**   Minute sugar crystals in a saturated sugar syrup; used as the creamy filling in chocolates and biscuits and for decorating cakes. Prepared by boiling sugar solution with addition of confectioners' glucose or an inverting agent and cooling rapidly while stirring.

**food**   Generally substances usable by the body to supply energy, build and replace tissue or participate in such reactions. Defined by FAO/WHO Codex Alimentarius Commission as any substance, whether processed, semi-processed or raw, which is intended for human consumption and includes drink, chewing gum and any substance that has been used in the manufacture, preparation or treatment of food but does not include cosmetics, tobacco or substances used only as drugs.

**food phosphate factor**   Term applied to the resistance of bacteria to thermal destruction; defined as the ratio between the resistance to heat when present in a food and the resistance when in phosphate buffer (at pH 6.98). The protective action of the ingredients of food renders the bacteria more resistant than in buffer.

**food poisoning**   May be due to (1) contamination with harmful bacteria; (2) toxic chemicals; (3) allergic reaction to certain proteins; (4) chemical contamination.

  The commonest bacterial contamination is due to salmonellae, staphylococci and *Clostridium welchii*. Staphylococcal poisoning causes rapid symptoms within 2–4 hours of abdominal cramp, nausea, vomiting and diarrhoea; recovery is rapid.

  Salmonellae produce an endotoxin which is not destroyed by cooking and causes acute gastroenteritis after 12–24 hours. It is not often fatal but nausea, vomiting and diarrhoea may persist several weeks.

  Very rarely food poisoning is due to *Clostridium botulinum*, i.e. botulism, which see.

**food scientist**   One who studies the basic chemical and physical, biochemical and biophysical properties of foods and their constituents.

**Food Standards Committee**   Advisory body to Ministry of Agriculture, Fisheries and Food in UK.

**food technologist**   One who applies food science to the preservation, processing and preparation of foods, and to their packaging, storage and transportation.

**food yeast**   See *yeasts*.

**foots**   See *soapstock*.

**forbidden fruit**   Grapefruit, *Citrus paradisi*.

**Force** Trade name (Fincken and Co. Ltd) for a breakfast cereal made from wheat flakes. Not fortified with added vitamins; natural content 0.07 mg vitamin $B_1$ and 0.07 mg vitamin $B_2$ per 100 g.

**forcemeat** A highly seasoned stuffing made from chopped or minced veal or pork or sausage meat mixed with onion and a range of herbs (from French, *farce*, stuffing).

**formiminoglutamic acid test** (FIGLU) Test for vitamin $B_{12}$ deficiency based on the enhanced excretion of formiminoglutamic acid in the urine following a test dose of histidine.

**Formula 21** 'Slimming' preparation (Greenwood Laboratories Ltd) composed of methyl cellulose and glucose, with flavour and colour, plus vitamin $B_1$ 1.1 mg, vitamin $B_2$ 2.7 mg, nicotinic acid 10.9 mg, reduced iron 10.9 mg, Ca 675 mg per oz.

**formula diet** Composed of purified substances that are readily absorbed and leave a minimum residue in the intestine (glucose, amino acids or peptides, mono and diglycerides).

**Fortifex** Protein-rich baby food (30% protein) developed in Brazil; made from maize, defatted soya flour with added vitamins A, $B_1$, $B_2$, calcium carbonate and methionine.

**fortification** See *enrichment*.

**four ale** Originally sold at fourpence per quart. Four ale bar is the public bar.

**fovantini** See *alimentary pastes*.

**FPC** Fish protein concentrate.

**fractional test meal** Method of examining secretion of gastric juices of patients. The stomach contents are sampled at intervals via a stomach tube after a test meal of gruel. It is usual to test for total and free acidity, and in addition peptic activity may be measured.

**frail** Rush basket for raisins, figs, etc.; also quantity of raisins, usually about 75 lb (34 kg).

**frangipane (or i)** Originally a jasmine perfume, which gave its name to an almond cream flavoured with the perfume. The term is used for cake-filling made from eggs, milk and flour with flavouring, and also for the pastry filled with an almond-flavoured mixture.

**frankfurters** See *sausage*.

**frappé** Egg-white and sugar syrup whipped until so aerated that the density reaches 5 lb per gallon.

**Frederickson's classification** System of classifying hyperlipid-aemias according to types of plasma lipoproteins which are elevated.

**freeze concentration** Concentration of a liquid by freezing out pure ice, leaving a more concentrated solution; of interest in the concentration of fruit juices, vinegar and beer.

**freeze drying**   A method of drying in which the material is frozen and subjected to high vacuum. The ice sublimes off as water vapour without melting. Materials dried in this way are damaged little, if at all. Also termed lyophilisation.

Freeze-dried food is very porous, since it occupies the same volume as the original and so rehydrates rapidly. There is less loss of flavour and texture than with most other methods of drying. Controlled heat may be applied to the process without melting the frozen material – this is accelerated freeze drying.

**freezerburn**   A change in the texture of frozen meat, fish and poultry during storage due to sublimation of the ice.

**French dressing**   Temporary emulsion of oil and acid, in distinction to mayonnaise, which is a stable emulsion. Heavy French dressing is a similar product stabilised with pectin or vegetable gum.

**frenching**   Breaking up the fibres of meat by cutting, usually diagonally or in a criss-cross pattern.

**French mustard**   See *mustard*.

**freons**   See *refrigerants*.

**fricassée**   See *cooking*.

**frigi-canning**   A process of preserving food by controlled heating, sufficient to destroy the vegetative form of micro-organisms (and possibly to damage spores sufficiently to prevent germination) followed by sealing aseptically and storing at a low temperature but not at freezing point.

**fromage frais**   Low fat, acid-ripened, soft cheese, 0–8% fat, 20% solids; French, similar to the German quarg.

**Froment**   Trade name (John H. Heron Ltd) for a wheat germ preparation.

Analysis per 100 g: protein 28.5 g, fat 7.7 g, carbohydrate 44.4 g, kcal 360 (1.5 MJ), vitamin $B_1$ 0.45 mg, vitamin $B_2$ 0.2 mg, vitamin E 8 mg, Fe 2.7 mg.

**fructofuranose**   Fructose formulated as the five-membered furan ring.

**fructopyranose**   Fructose formulated as the six-membered pyranose ring.

**fructosan**   A complex built up of units of fructose, e.g. inulin.

**fructose**   A six-carbon sugar – $C_6H_{12}O_6$ – differing from glucose in containing a ketonic group (on C2) instead of an aldehyde group (which glucose has on C1).

Found as the free sugar in some fruits and in honey and combined with glucose as sucrose. Prepared by the hydrolysis of inulin from the Jerusalem artichoke. Alternative names fruit sugar and laevulose; 173% as sweet as sucrose.

Fructose rotates polarised light to the left (hence the name laevulose), in distinction from glucose, which rotates polarised light to the right.

See also *invert sugar.*

**fructose syrups** (high-fructose glucose syrups)  Glucose syrups containing more than 10% fructose produced by enzymatic or alkali conversion; can be 35% glucose, 45% fructose and 5–10% maltose, and then they are as sweet as sucrose, with viscosity similar to that of 67% sucrose solution; used in soft drinks, canned fruits, jams and preserves and bakery products. Also termed isosyrups.

**fruit**  Fleshy seed-bearing part of plants (including tomato, usually called a vegetable). Contain negligible protein and fat; carbohydrate varies from 3% in melon to 25% in banana. Carbohydrate occurs as glucose, fructose, sucrose, starch, pectin and cellulose. Cellulose adds bulk to the diet; pectin gives jellying power to fruit.

During ripening of fruit starch changes to sugars. Fruits are a good source of potassium and vitamin C, and some are a useful source of carotene and iron.

**fruit, canned**  The fruit is usually canned in a sugar solution (see *syrup*) and, hence, the energy content is greater than that of the fresh fruit.

Analysis per 100 g of, for example, fresh peaches (without stones): 9 g carbohydrate, 37 kcal (0.15 MJ); canned, 17.2 g carbohydrate, 66 kcal (0.27 MJ).

Vitamin loss is about 50%, e.g. peaches lose half of the carotene, vitamins $B_1$ and $B_2$, nicotinic acid and vitamin C in canning.

**fruit cordials**  See *soft drinks.*

**fruit, dried**  Dried figs, dates, prunes and raisins, all have similar analyses.

Protein 2.5 g, fat 0.6 g, 250 kcal (1 MJ), Ca 70 mg, Fe 2.7 mg, vitamin A 20 μg, vitamin $B_1$ 0.1 mg, vitamin $B_2$ 0.1 mg, nicotinic acid 1.5 mg, vitamin C nil – per 100 g.

**fruit drinks**  See *soft drinks.*

**fruit squash**  See *soft drinks.*

**frumenty**  Whole wheat stewed in water for 24 hours until the grains have burst and set in a thick jelly, then boiled with milk.

**frying**  Involves rapid evaporation of water. In the case of meat nearly all the extractives are left in the meat and the losses are smaller than in roasting. (See also *connective tissue.*) About 10–20% loss of vitamin $B_1$, 10–15% loss of vitamin $B_2$ and nicotinic acid.

Fish loses 20% vitamin $B_1$.

**fudge**  Caramel in which crystallisation of the sugar (graining) is deliberately induced by the addition of fondant (saturated syrup containing sugar crystals).

**fuga**  Japanese puffer fish, *Fuga* species. See *tetraodontin poisoning*.

**Fuller's earth**  An adsorbent clay, calcium montmorillonite, or bentonite; adsorbs both by physical means and by ion extraction. Used to bleach oils, clarify liquids and absorb grease. Named after Reverend Thomas Fuller.

**fumeol**  Refined smoke with the bitter principles removed; used for preparing 'liquid' smokes for dipping foods such as fish to give them a smoked flavour. See also *smoking*.

**fungal protein**  Mould mycelium; see *moulds*.

**fungi**  Sub-division of Thallophyta, plants without differentiation into root, stem and leaf; cannot photosynthesise, all are parasites or saprophytes. Varieties of *Penicillium, Aspergillus*, etc., are the cause of deterioration in foods in the presence of oxygen and relative humidity of at least 70%. On the other hand, varieties of *Penicillium* such as *P. cambertii* and *P. rocquefortii* are desirable in certain cheeses.

Among the edible fungi are mushrooms, *Agaricus campestris*.

Experimentally, varieties such as *Graphium, Fusarium* and *Rhizopus* are grown on waste carbohydrates as a potential food; their fibrillar structure offers textural advantages in foods manufactured from them.

**furcellaran**  Danish agar. An anionic, sulphated polysaccharide extracted from the red alga, *Furcellaria fastigiata*, structurally similar to carrageenan; used as a gelling agent.

**fusel oil**  Alcoholic fermentation produces about 95% alcohol and 5% fusel oil – a mixture of organic acids, higher alcohols (propyl, butyl and amyl), aldehydes and esters.

Present in low concentration in wines and beer, and higher concentration in pot-still spirit. On maturation of the liquor the fusel oil changes and imparts the special flavour to the spirit.

**fussol**  Monofluoroacetamide – a systemic insecticide for treating fruit.

**fustic**  Colouring matter obtained from the tree *Chlorophora tinctoria* or *Maclura tinctoria*. Two colour agents present, morin, sparingly soluble in water but soluble in alcohol, and maclurin, more soluble. Both are yellow but altered by alkali and metals.

**F value**  Unit of measurement used to compare relative sterilising effects of different procedures; equal to 1 minute at 121.1 °C.

# G

**gaffelbitar** 'Semi-preserved' herring product in which microbial growth is checked by the addition of salt at a concentration of 10–12%, and sometimes by the addition of benzoic acid as preservative.

Anchovy is a similar product.

**galacticol** Dulcitol, which see.

**Galactomin** Trade name (Trufood Ltd) for preparation free from lactose and galactose used for patients suffering from lactose intolerance.

**galactosaemia** Inherited inability to metabolise the sugar galactose beyond the formation of its phosphate. Unless galactose is excluded from the diet, the subject suffers mental retardation, growth failure, vomiting and jaundice. Special baby foods are therefore prepared entirely free from lactose.

**galactose** A six-carbon sugar differing from glucose only in the position of the hydroxyl group on C4.

It occurs mainly linked with glucose to form lactose (milk sugar), and is also present in the galactolipids of nerve tissue. Has 32% of the sweetness of sucrose.

See also *cerebrosides*.

**galantine** A dish of white meat or poultry, boned, rolled, cooked with herbs, glazed with aspic jelly and served cold.

**galenicals** Crude drugs, infusions, decoctions and tinctures prepared from medicinal plants.

**gallates** Salts and esters of gallic acid, found in many plants. Used in making dyes and inks, and medicinally as an astringent.

Propyl, octyl and dodecyl gallates are legally permitted antioxidants; 100ppm permitted in fats and vitamin oils, 80ppm in butter-fat for manufacturing, 1000ppm in essential oils for flavouring.

**gall-bladder** Organ situated in the liver which stores the bile manufactured by the liver.

**gallimaufry** Medieval chicken stew with bacon, mustard and wine.

**gallon** Imperial gallon is 4.546 litres (=10lb of water at 17°C). US gallon is 3.7853 litres; Imperial gallon = 1.2 US gallons.

**gall-stones** (cholelithiasis) Concretions composed of cholesterol, bile pigments and calcium salts, formed in the gall-bladder or bile duct when the bile becomes supersaturated.

**game** Non-domesticated (i.e. wild) animals and birds.

**game chips** Thin slices of fried potato chips – crisps in England, chips in USA.

**gammon** Hind legs of bacon pig, cured while still part of carcass.

Ham is the same part of the pig but cured after removal from the carcass.

**garbanzo**   Chickpea (*Cicer arietinum*).

**garlic**   Bulb of *Allium sativum* (lily family) with pungent odour when crushed. This is due to diallyl thiosulphinate, ammonia and pyruvic acid liberated from an odourless precursor, alliin (allyl-cysteine sulphoxide) by the enzyme alliinase. Diallyl disulphide derived from diallyl thiosulphinate is responsible for the characteristic odour of garlic.

**garum**   See *liquamen*.

**gas storage, controlled (modified)**   Storage of fruits and vegetables and pre-packed red meat in a controlled atmosphere in which a proportion of the oxygen is replaced by carbon dioxide, sometimes with the addition of other gases. In modified atmosphere storage (MA) the control is less precise.

**gastrin**   Polypeptide hormones (I and II) secreted in stomach which stimulate secretion of gastric HCl and pancreatic enzyme output.

**gastric secretion**   Gastric juice consists of the enzymes pepsin, rennin and lipase, together with mucin and hydrochloric acid. The acid is secreted by the parietal cells at a strength of $0.16\text{N} = 0.5-0.6\%$ acid.

The pepsin is secreted by the chief cells, and the mucin by the mucous cells. Pepsin requires an acid medium to function and breaks down proteins to proteoses.

The sole function of rennin is to coagulate milk. The small amount of lipase present splits only a very small proportion of the fat. See also *fractional test meal*.

**gastrin**   Hormone secreted by the pyloric antrum of the stomach under the influence of certain foods (especially meat) and by distension of the stomach. The gastrin enters the blood stream and stimulates the secretion of gastric juice.

**gastro-intestinal tract**   Term covering the whole of the digestive tract, from the mouth to the anus. Average length 4.5 metres (15 feet).

**gavage**   Process of feeding liquids by stomach tube. Also feeding excessive amount (hyperalimentation).

**gean**   Scottish name for fruit of *Prunus avium avium*; also wild cherry, sweet cherry and mazzard.

**gefilte fish**   Also spelled 'gefilte' and 'gefültte'. Literally, German for stuffed fish. The dish is of Russian or Polish origin, where it is commonly referred to as Jewish fish. The whole fish is served and the filleted portion chopped and stuffed back between the skin and the backbone. More frequently today, the fish is simply chopped into a pulp and made into balls.

In the UK has been legally referred to as 'fish cutlets in fish sauce' instead of a fish cake.

**gel** A sol or colloidal suspension that has set to a jelly.

**gelatin** Water-soluble protein prepared from collagen by boiling with water, or from bones (see *ossein*). There are several grades used for different purposes, e.g. 40 mesh for confectionery; crumble gelatin for meat canning; sheet gelatin for table jellies; 10 mesh for pharmaceutical capsules.

As a protein it is of poor nutritive value, since it lacks tryptophan.

**gelatin, Chinese** Agar.

**gelatin sugar** Glycine.

**gelometer** See *Bloom gelometer*.

**generic descriptor** See *vitamin*.

**genetic disease** In connection with food, the inherited inability to metabolise certain dietary factors, often with harmful results. See *alcaptonuria*; *galactosaemia*; *phenylketonuria*; *tyrosinosis*.

**gentiobiose** Two molecules of glucose joined 1,6-β.

**Gentleman's relish** Paste for anchovies, butter, cereal, salt and spices developed UK nineteenth century; also called patum peperium.

**Gerber test** Test for fat in milk. When sulphuric acid and milk are mixed, heat develops, the organic matter dissolves, but not the fat. This separates, aided by the addition of amyl alcohol. The reaction is carried out in a Gerber bottle with a thin, graduated neck, in which the fat collects, and is measured. Used for routine analyses of milk.

**germ, wheat** The embryo or sprouting portion of the wheat berry, comprising about 2.5% of the seed. Contains 64% of the thiamin, 26% of the riboflavin, 21% of the pyridoxine and most of the fat of the wheat grain, and is discarded when the grain is milled to white flour.

**ghee** Clarified butter fat made by heating and separating the water; made from milk of cow, buffalo, goat or sheep.

Widely used in India; does not go rancid as quickly as butter; Egyptian equivalent is samna.

**gherkin** *Cucumis anguira*. Young green cucumber of small variety, used for pickling.

**gibberellic acid** Originally found in the fungus *Gibberella fujikuroi* growing on rice. About 30 gibberellins are known; they are plant growth hormones which cause stem extension and allow mutant dwarf forms of plants to revert to normal size, induce flower formation, break bud dormancy; used to accelerate germination of barley for brewing purposes; affect the synthesis of DNA.

**gin**  Spirit containing 31% alcohol flavoured with juniper berries and other flavours; 220 kcal (0.9 MJ) per 100 ml. Name derived from French *genièvre*, meaning juniper; originally known as Geneva, Schiedam and Hollands, since it is Dutch in origin.

**ginger**  Rhizome of *Zingiber officinale*; used as a flavouring; pungency due to non-volatile compounds, including gingerol, zingerone and shogool. Preserved ginger made from young fleshy rhizomes boiled with sugar and packed in syrup.

Analysis per 100 g: 2.5 g protein, 0.8 g fat, 11 g carbohydrate, 2.1 g fibre, 63 kcal (0.26 MJ), 2.5 mg Fe, 0.8 mg nicotinic acid, 4 mg vitamin C.

**ginger paralysis**  See *Jamaica ginger paralysis*.

**GIP**  Gastric inhibitory peptide (glucose-dependent insulino-tropic polypeptide); hormone produced from mucosa of duodenum and jejunum in response to absorbed fat and carbohydrate that stimulates the pancreas to secrete insulin.

**gipping (of fish)**  Partial evisceration to remove intestines but not pyloric caeca which contains enzymes responsible for the characteristic flavour of herring when it is subsequently salted.

**Glamorgan sausage**  A dish based on Caerphilly cheese, bread crumbs and egg, fried in sausage shape (traditional Welsh dish).

**Glasgow magistrate**  Term for red herrings, which see.

**gliadin**  One of the proteins of wheat; gliadin and glutenin compose what is generally called gluten, the protein mixture which is the basis of dough formation. Gliadin is the protein responsible for coeliac disease.

**globins**  Basic proteins that differ from histones, since they are rich in histidine, deficient in isoleucine and contain average amounts of arginine and tryptophan.

Globins are simple proteins themselves (i.e. free from non-protein substances) but are often found as the protein portion of conjugated proteins, e.g. globin from haemoglobin.

**globulins**  Class of proteins that are heat-coagulated and soluble in dilute solutions of salts; they differ from albumins in being insoluble in water. They occur in blood, i.e. serum globulins, in milk, i.e. lactoglobulins; and edestin from hemp seed and amandin from almond are also globulins.

**glossitis**  See *ariboflavinosis*.

**glucagon**  Hormone secreted by the pancreas which causes an increase in blood sugar probably by increasing the breakdown of liver glycogen.

**glucaric acid**  Alternative name for saccharic acid, the dicarboxylic acid derived from glucose.

**glucide**  Name occasionally used for saccharin.

**glucitol** (glycitol)  Obsolete for sorbitol. See *glycitols*.

**glucoascorbic acid**  Homologue of ascorbic acid containing an extra CHOH group. Acts as an antagonist to the vitamin; its administration can cause scurvy in animals that do not normally require the vitamin in the diet.

**glucocorticoid**  Obsolescent term for the steroid hormones of the adrenal cortex which affect carbohydrate metabolism. See *adrenal glands*.

**glucofuranose**  Glucose formulated as the five-membered furan ring.

**glucomannan**  A polysaccharide consisting of repeating units of β-1,4-linked glucose and mannose; found in the konjac root.

**gluconeogenesis**  Formation of glucose and glycogen from non-carbohydrate sources via glucose.

**gluconic acid**  Also termed dextronic acid, maltonic acid and glycogenic acid. Formed by oxidation of the hydroxyl group on the first carbon of glucose.

**glucono-delta-lactone**  Lactone of gluconic acid; slowly liberates acid at a controlled rate; used in chemically leavened bread, i.e. to liberate carbon dioxide from bicarbonate instead of using yeast (see *bread, aerated*). Also used in bland-flavoured sherbets and to reduce fat-absorption in products such as doughnuts.

**glucopyranose**  Glucose formulated as the six-membered pyran ring.

**glucosaccharic acid**  Alternative name for saccharic acid.

**glucosamine**  Amino derivative of glucose. Constituent of many complex polysaccharides.

**glucosan**  A complex of glucose molecules, e.g. starch, cellulose and glycogen. Inulin is a complex of fructose molecules and is a fructosan. The general name for the polysaccharide complexes made up from simple hexose units is hexosans.

**glucose**  Also known as dextrose, grape sugar and blood sugar.

A simple six-carbon sugar (hexose) $C_6H_{12}O_6$, occurring naturally in plant tissues and formed by the hydrolysis of starch. It is the major product of the digestion of carbohydrates in the intestine and is the form in which the carbohydrate is absorbed into the bloodstream. During digestion sucrose is hydrolysed to glucose and fructose, lactose to glucose and galactose, and starches and maltose to glucose.

Normal levels in blood lie between 4.5 and 5.5 mmol/l (80–100 mg per 100 ml), any surplus being converted to glycogen and stored as such in the liver and muscles. Glycogen is broken down to glucose when required for energy.

Energy is liberated by the oxidation of glucose to carbon dioxide and water at the rate of 3.9 kcal per g or 686 kcal per gram-mol.

Used in the manufacture of confectionery, since its mixture with fructose prevents sucrose from crystallising (see *boiled sweets*) and it is 74% as sweet as sucrose.

See also *glucose metabolism*; *glucose syrups*.

**glucose, liquid**   See *glucose syrups*.

**glucose metabolism**   Process through which glucose is broken down in living tissues to provide energy. The overall reaction follows the equation:

$$C_6H_{12}O_6 + 6O_2 = 6CO_2 + 6H_2O + 3.9 \, kcal \text{ per gram of glucose}$$

but in detail the process involves about 20 stages.

The first series of stages does not require oxygen and is referred to as glycolysis or glucose fermentation. The glucose is converted through a number of sugar phosphates to three-carbon sugars (trioses) and then to pyruvic acid.

The latter is oxidised in a series of reactions known as the Krebs or tricarboxylic acid cycle ultimately to carbon dioxide and water. The energy is liberated from the glucose at certain of these stages.

Surplus blood glucose is stored in the muscles as glycogen, and when energy is required, the latter is first converted to glucose and then follows the metabolic pathway outlined above.

**glucose oxidase**   Enzyme that specifically oxidises glucose to gluconic acid, with the formation of hydrogen peroxide. Used for quantitative determination of glucose, including urinary glucose excreted in diabetes, and to remove traces of glucose from foodstuffs (e.g. to remove glucose from egg and so prevent Maillard reaction during storage).

Originally isolated from the mould *Penicillium notatum* and called notatin.

**glucose syrups**   Purified, concentrated, aqueous solutions of nutritive saccharides from starch (Codex definition). Prepared by hydrolysis of maize starch (or potato starch) by enzymes, acid or a combination of the two. Usually 70% w/w total solids – glucose, maltose and oligomers of glucose of three, four or more units.

Used as a sweetening agent in sugar confectionery; also termed corn syrup, corn starch hydrolysate, starch syrup, confectioners' glucose and uncrystallisable syrup.

See also *dextrose equivalent value*.

**glucose tolerance**   The ability of the body to deal with a large dose of glucose; used as a test for diabetes mellitus.

The fasting subject ingests 50 g or 75 g of glucose and the blood sugar is measured at intervals. In the normal individual the fasting sugar level is approximately 5 mmol/l (80–100 mg per

100 ml), rises to about 7.5 mmol, and returns to the starting level within 1–1½ hours. In diabetics the sugar rises to higher levels and takes longer to return. The plotted results form a glucose-tolerance curve.

**glucose tolerance factor**   See *chromium*.

**glucose-$T_m$**   Term used in measuring the efficiency of the kidneys; it is the maximum rate of reabsorption of glucose by the kidney tubules.

**glucosides**   Complexes of substances with glucose. General name for such complexes with other sugars is glycosides.

**glucosinolates**   Thioesters including in the molecule thiocyanates, isothiocyanates, nitriles, oxazolidine-2-thione occurring widely in plants of the family Crucifera, genus *Brassica* (e.g. Brussel sprouts, cabbage, watercress, radishes). Broken down by the enzyme myrosinase in the same plant to yield, among other products, mustard oils which are responsible for the pungent flavour (especially in mustard and horseradish). One of these, progoitrin, is goitrogenic.

**glucostatic mechanism**   Theory that appetite depends on the difference between arterial and venous levels of glucose; when the difference falls to 8 mg per 100 ml, the hypothalamus is stimulated and hunger results.

**glucuronic acid**   The acid derived from glucose by the oxidation of the group on C6. Many toxic substances are excreted from the body combined with glucuronic acid as glucuronides. It is also present in various complex polysaccharides.

**glutamic acid**   A dicarboxylic non-essential amino acid; amino-glutaric acid. Involved in transamination reactions; its amide is glutamine.

The sodium salt, monosodium glutamate, MSG, originally called Aginomoto, is used to enhance flavour of savoury dishes and is often added to canned meats and soups.

**glutamine**   Amide of the amino acid glutamic acid; formed by the addition of ammonia to glutamic acid.

Occurs in plants, where it appears to function as a storage depot for ammonia, and as part of the urea cycle in animals.

**glutathione**   A tripeptide of glycine, glutamic acid and cysteine; occurs in animal tissues and believed to function as an oxi-dation–reduction system.

**glutathione peroxidase**   Selenium-containing enzyme that pro-tects tissue from oxidative damage and prevents accumulation of free radicals.

**glutathione reductase**   Enzyme is red blood cells which has riboflavin (flavine adenine dinucleotide) as co-factor; reactiva-tion of this enzyme with added riboflavin serves as measure of riboflavin nutritional status.

**glutelins**   Proteins insoluble in water and neutral salt solutions but soluble in dilute acids and alkalies, e.g. wheat glutenin.

**gluten**   The protein complex in wheat, and to a lesser extent rye, which gives dough the viscid property that holds gas when it rises. None in oats, barley, maize. It is a mixture of gliadin and glutelin.

In the undamaged state with extensible properties it is termed vital gluten; when overheated, these properties are lost and the product is termed devitalised gluten.

**gluten-free foods**   Formulated without any wheat or rye protein (although the starch may be used) for subjects suffering from coeliac disease, which see.

**glutose**   A hexose sugar carrying a keto group on C3; not metabolised and non-fermentable.

**glycaemic index**   Rate of rise in blood sugar level (area under curve for 2 hours following ingestion of 50 g of available carbohydrate) relative to glucose taken as 100.

**glycaemic index (of a food)**   Degree to which the food increases blood glucose in proportion to glucose itself.

**glycamines**   Derivatives of sugar alcohols in which the $CH_2OH$ group is replaced by $CH_2NH_2$, e.g. ethanolamine and ribamine (part of vitamin $B_2$).

**glycation**   Linking of reducing sugar with receptive amino acid (as in Maillard reaction); accumulates in long living proteins (such as crystallins, elastin, myelin) causing functional changes. See *haemoglobin, glycated*.

**glycerides**   Esters of glycerol with fatty acids. As glycerol possesses three hydroxyl groups, it can combine with three molecules of fatty acid to form a triglyceride or simple fat.

If all three molecules of fatty acid are the same, a simple triglyceride is formed, e.g. tristearin, triolein; mixed glycerides may be formed such as distearo-olein and stearo-oleo-palmitin.

See also *fats*; *glycerol*; *superglycerinated fats*.

**glycerides, partial**   See *acetoglycerides*; *superglycerinated fats*.

**glycerine**   See *glycerol*.

**glycerol**   A trihydric alcohol, chemically 1,2,3-propane triol, $CH_2OHCHOHCH_2OH$, popularly called glycerine.

Simple or neutral fats are esters of glycerol with three molecules of fatty acid, i.e. triglycerides.

Glycerol is a clear, colourless, odourless, viscous liquid, sweet to taste; it is made from fats by alkaline hydrolysis (saponification). Used as a solvent for flavours, as a humectant to keep foods moist, and in cake batters to improve texture and slow down staling.

See also *glycerides*; *superglycerinated fats*.

**glycerose**  Simple, three-carbon sugar, derived from the corresponding alcohol, glycerol. Formula $CHOCHOHCH_2OH$.

**glyceryl lactostearate**  Also known as lactostearin. Formed by glycerolysis of hydrogenated soya bean oil followed by esterification with lactic acid, which results in a mixture of mono- and diglycerides and their lactic mono esters. Used as an emulsifier in shortenings.

**glyceryl monostearate**  See *superglycerinated fats*.

**glycine**  A non-essential amino acid, chemically amino acetic acid, $CH_2NH_2COOH$. Clinically used as a buffer for gastric acidity.

Has 70% of the sweetness of sucrose and is sometimes used mixed with saccharine as a sweetening agent.

**glycinin**  Globulin protein in soya bean.

**glycitols**  Compounds with the general formula $CH_2OH(CHOH)_nCH_2OH$; sugar alcohols, including sorbitol, xylitol, mannitol; also used previously as an alternative name for sorbitol itself.

**glycocholic acid**  See *bile*.

**glycocoll**  Obsolete name for the amino acid glycine.

**glycogen**  Storage form of carbohydrate in the animal body, in the liver and muscles. Composed of glucose units; is synthesised from the blood sugar and broken down to blood sugar as required. Sometimes referred to as animal starch.

In an adult the glycogen stored in the muscles is about 250 g and in the liver about 100 g.

Since glycogen is rapidly broken down to glucose immediately an animal is killed, meat and animal liver do not contain glycogen; the only dietary sources are oysters, cockles, mussels, scallops, clams, whelks and winkles that are eaten virtually alive and contain about 5% glycogen.

**glycogenesis**  Synthesis of glycogen from glucose, as, for example, occurs in the muscle where glucose is stored as glycogen; facilitated by insulin.

**glycogenolysis**  Breakdown of glycogen to glucose when this is required for the production of energy.

**glycoleucine**  Obsolete name for norleucine.

**glycolysis**  There are two parts to the total breakdown of glucose. The first is anaerobic and called glucose fermentation or glycolysis. This ends at the formation of pyruvic acid. The second part is an oxidation and the series of reactions is the Krebs tricarboxylic acid cycle, or the citric acid cycle. This completes the breakdown to carbon dioxide and water. See also *glucose metabolism*.

**glycoproteins**  Group of proteins conjugated with carbohydrates such as uronic acids, polymerised glucosamine-mannose, etc., including mucins and mucoids; found in the vitreous humour of the eye, cornea, cartilage, gastric mucosa. See also *mucoproteins*.

**glycosides** Compounds consisting of a sugar attached to another molecule. When glucose is the sugar, they are called glucosides. A wide variety occur in plants and some are useful medicinally, such as digitalis and rutin.

**glycosuria** Appearance of glucose in the urine, as in diabetes and after the administration of drugs that lower the renal threshold. See also *phlorrhizin*.

**glycyrrhiza** Liquorice, *Glycyrrhiza glabra*. Extract of root long used to flavour medicines because of sweet taste due to calcium and potassium salts of glycyrrhizic acid.

**glycyrrhizin** Triterpenoid glycoside extracted from liquorice root; 50–100 times as sweet as sucrose but with liquorice flavour. Used to flavour tobacco and pharmaceutical substances, and as foaming agent in some non-alcoholic beverages.

**GMS** Abbreviation for glyceryl monostearate. See *superglycerinated fats*.

**goitre** Enlargement of the thyroid gland, seen as a swelling in the neck, due to deficiency of iodine in the diet and to the presence of 'goitrogens' in certain foods such as Brassicas and peanuts.

Supplementation with an iodide often prevents the condition; hence the use of iodised salt.

See also *cretinism*; *thyroid gland*.

**goitrogens** Substances found in foods (especially of the *Brassica* species but including also groundnuts, cassava and soya bean) which interfere with normal functioning of the thyroid gland and can cause goitre in animals. They include glucosinolates (progoitrin), which prevent the synthesis of thyroxine in the thyroid gland, and thiocyanates, which interfere with the uptake of iodine. Progoitrin is converted into active goitrin – 5-vinyloxazolidine-2-thione. It is not clear that these substances are a cause of goitre in human beings.

**golden berry** See *gooseberry, Cape*.

**gold thioglucose** Chemical used to cause obesity in experimental animals by stimulation of the appetite through damage to the hypothalamus.

**Good Manufacturing Practice (GMP)** Part of food and drink control operation aimed at ensuring that products are consistently manufactured to a quality appropriate to their intended use (detailed in *Good Manufacturing Practice – A Guide to its Responsible Management*, Institute of Food Science and Technology, 1987).

**gooseberry**   Berry of shrub, *Ribes grossularia*.

   Analysis per 100 g: protein 1 g, fat 0.4 g, kcal 42 (0.18 MJ), Ca 22 mg, Fe 0.5 mg, carotene 90 µg, vitamin $B_1$ 0.04 mg, vitamin $B_2$ 0.02 mg, nicotinic acid 1 mg, vitamin C 33 mg.

**gooseberry, Cape**   Edible fruit of *Physalis peruviana*, also called golden berry.

   Analysis per 100 g: carbohydrate 9 g, protein 2 g, 48 kcal (200 kJ), 600 µg carotene, approximately 30 mg vitamin C.

**gooseberry, Indian**   See *emblic*.

**gossypol**   Yellow toxic pigment found up to 2–4% dry weight in some varieties of cottonseed (hexahydroxy di-isopropyl dimethyl (binaphthalene) dicarboxyaldehyde). When included in chicken feed, it causes discoloration of the yolk, but has not been found to be toxic to man.

**gourds**   Vegetables of the family Cucurbitaceae, including cucumber, marrow, pumpkin, squash, gourd and melon.

   Calabash or bottle gourd (*Lagenaria vulgaris*), ash gourd (*Benincasa hispida*), snake gourd (*Trichosanthes anguina*), cucumber (*Cucumis sativus*), vegetable marrow (*Cucurbita pepo*), pumpkin (*Cucurbita moschata*), squash (*Cucurbita maxima*), coocha or chayote (*Sechium edule*), cantaloupe melon (*Cucumis melo*), water melon (*Citrullus vulgaris*).

   All contain more than 90% water and about 1% protein and have little food value apart from vitamin C at 10 mg per 100 g. In addition, yellow pumpkin contains 900 µg carotene per 100 g. Melons are sometimes grown for their seeds, which contain 20–40% oil and 20% protein.

**Graham bread**   Whole-wheat bread in which the bran is very finely ground. Graham cakes are made from wholemeal flour and milk. The name is that of a miller of wholemeal flour who advocated its use in the USA (Treatise on Bread and Bread Making, 1837).

**Gram-negative, Gram-positive**   Bacteria fall into two groups, depending on whether or not they retain crystal-violet dye after staining and decolorising with alcohol. Named after Danish botanist Gram.

**grams, Indian**   Name given to small dried peas, e.g. green gram (*Phaseolus aureus*), black gram (*Phaseolus mungo*), red gram (*Cajanus indicus*). See *legumes, food*.

**granadilla**   See *passion fruit*.

**granita**   See *sherbet*.

**grape**   Fresh fruit of a large number of varieties of *Vitis vinifera*. One of the oldest cultivated plants (ancient Egypt 4000 BC).

   Can be grouped as dessert grapes, wine grapes and varieties

that are used for drying to produce raisins, currants and sultanas. Contain only 3–4 mg vitamin C per 100 g.

See also *Phylloxera*.

**grapefruit** Fruit of *Citrus paradisi*; thought to have arisen as a sport of pomelo or shaddock (*Citrus grandis*), a coarser citrus fruit, or as a hybrid between pomelo and sweet orange. 35–45 mg vitamin C per 100 g.

The pith contains naringin, which is very bitter (see separate entry). Name said to have arisen because the fruit is borne on the tree in clusters (like grapes!).

**Grapenuts** Trade name (Alfred Bird and Sons Ltd) for a breakfast cereal made from wheat.

Analysis per 100 g: protein 11.7 g, fat 3.0 g, carbohydrate 75 g, Ca 50 mg, Fe 5 mg, kcal 360 (1.5 MJ).

**grape sugar** Alternative name for glucose.

**GRAS** 'Generally regarded as safe.' Designation given to food additives when further evidence is required before the substance can be classified more precisely (US usage).

**grass tetany** Magnesium deficiency in cattle. See *magnesium*.

**gratin** Gratin is French term for the thin brown crust formed on top of foods that have been covered with butter, breadcrumbs or cheese and heated under the grill or in the oven.

Au gratin is the term used when cheese is used.

Gratin is also the name given to a fireproof dish, and the verb is gratiner.

**gray (Gy)** The SI unit for ionising radiation instead of the rad – the gray is equivalent to 1 J/kg (=100 rad).

**green butter** See *vegetable butters*.

**green S** Food colour also known as Wool green S and Brilliant acid green BS; sodium salt of di-(*p*-dimethyl-aminophenyl)-2-hydroxy-3,6-disulphonaphthyl-methanol anhydride.

**grill** To cook by radiant heat; some of the fat is lost. Barbecues cook by grilling.

**grissini** Italian 'finger rolls' or stick bread 6–18 inches long.

**grist** Cereal for grinding.

**grits, corn** See *hominy*.

**groats** Oats from which the husk has been entirely removed; when crushed, Embden groats result.

**groundnut** See *peanut*.

**GTF** Glucose tolerance factor. See *chromium*.

**guacamole** Mexican dish or sauce based on very ripe avocado; used as hors d'oeuvre or a 'dip'.

**guanine** See *nucleic acids*; *purines*.

**guarana** Dried paste prepared from the seeds of the climbing shrub *Paullinia cupana* (South America); rich in caffeine; used in South America as a beverage similar to cocoa.

**guar gum** Cyamopsis gum; from the cluster bean, *Cyamopsis tetragonoloba*. Member of Leguminosae, used in India as livestock feed. The gum is a water-soluble, galactomannan; used in 'slimming' preparations, since it is not digested by digestive enzymes, and in experimental treatment of diabetes, since it delays gastric emptying and prevents a rapid rise in blood sugar.

**guava** Fruit of *Psidium guajava*, tropical shrub (Central and South America), eaten raw or preserved as guava jelly.

Analysis per 100 g: water 80 g, protein 1 g, fat 0.4 g, carbohydrate 13 g, kcal 60 (0.25 MJ), Fe 1 mg, carotene 60 µg, vitamin $B_1$ 0.05 mg, vitamin $B_2$ 0.04 mg, nicotinic acid 1.0 mg, vitamin C 200 mg.

**gum acacia** See *gum arabic*.

**gum arabic** Exudate from the stems of several species of acacia, also known as gum acacia (best product comes from *Acacia senegal*). Used as thickening agent, as stabiliser often in combination with other gums, in gum drops and soft jelly gums and to prevent crystallisation in sugar confectionery.

**gumbo** Okra, which see.

**gum, British** Dextrin – partly hydrolysed starch.

**gum, chewing** Based on chicle, the partially evaporated milky juice of latex of the Sapodilla tree, plus sugar, balsam of Tolu and flavour.

**gums** Substances that can disperse in water to form a viscous, mucilaginous mass. Used in food processing to stabilise emulsions (such as salad dressings, processed cheese), as a thickener and in sugar confectionery.

Extracted from seeds (guar gum, locust, quince, psyllium), sap or exudates (gum arabic, karaya (or sterculia), tragacanth, ghatti, bassora or hog gum, shiraz, mesquite, anguo) and seaweeds (agar, kelp, alginate, Irish moss) or they may be made from starch or cellulose (dextrins and methyl-, carboxymethyl-, etc. cellulose) or they may be synthetic, such as vinyl polymers.

Most of these (apart from dextrins) are not digested and have no food value.

**gum tragacanth** Obtained from the trees of *Astralagus* species; used as stabiliser.

**gur** Mixture of sugar crystals and syrup, brown, toffee-like, made by evaporation of juice of sugar cane; also called jaggery.

**gut sweetbread** See *pancreas*.

**GYE** Guiness Yeast Extract; see *yeast extract*.

**gyle** Alcohol solution formed in the first stage of vinegar production, 6–9% alcohol. Subsequent fermentation with *Acetobacter* converts the alcohol to acetic acid.

**gynaminic acid** See *sialic acid*.

**gynolactose** See *allolactose*.

**haem** The iron-containing pigment which, in combination with protein, forms the haemoglobin of the red blood cell. (The iron is in the ferrous state.)

**haemagglutinins** (hemagglutinins) See *lectins*.

**haematin** Formed by the oxidation of haem, the non-protein part of haemoglobin; the iron is oxidised from the ferrous to the ferric state.

**haemin** The hydrochloride of haematin, derived from haemoglobin. The crystals are readily recognisable under the microscope and used as a test for blood.

**haemoglobin** Red colouring matter of the red blood cell – 94% protein (globin) and 6% iron-containing pigment, haem. Combines reversibly with oxygen for transport to the tissues and carbon dioxide for transport away from tissues.

In iron-deficiency anaemia there is a deficiency of haemoglobin and impaired oxygenation.

**haemoglobin, glycated (glycosylated)** Haemoglobin linked via its lysine to glucose; used to indicate abnormally high blood sugar levels in control of diabetes over the preceding 2–3 months. Normally 3–6% of haemoglobin is glycated, can be 20% in uncontrolled diabetes.

**haemoglobinometer** Instrument to measure the amount of haemoglobin in blood by direct colorimetry or after conversion to another coloured compound.

**haemopoietic factor** See *intrinsic factor*.

**haemosiderin** Long-term reserve (storage form) of iron – colloidal iron hydroxide combined with protein and phosphate; probably formed by agglomeration of ferritin, the short-term storage form. See also *siderosis*.

**Haff disease** Acute paroxysmal myoglobinuria suffered by fishermen around the Koenigsberg Haff in Eastern Germany; attributed either to a toxin in the seawater which entered the fish, or to thiaminase in raw or incompletely cooked fish.

**Hagberg test** Measure of alpha-amylase activity of flour derived from the change in viscosity of flour paste.

**haggis** Traditional Scottish dish. Made from liver, heart and lungs of sheep, cooked with suet, oatmeal and seasoning, then filled into a bag made from sheep's stomach and boiled for several hours.

Said to have been originated by the Romans when campaigning in Scotland; when breaking camp in an emergency, the food was wrapped in the sheep stomach.

Analysis per 100 g: 11 g protein, 22 g fat, 19 g carbohydrate, 2.5 g fibre, 325 kcal (1300 kJ).

**hake** See *codfish*.

**half-life** In the field of radioactive isotopes this term means the period of time in which half of the original material has decomposed.

In biochemistry it refers to the time taken for half of the body tissue in question to be replaced. The tissues are continuously being degraded and rebuilt even in the mature adult, and the half-life is used as a quantitative measure of this 'dynamic equilibrium'. The half-life of human liver and serum proteins is 10 days, and of the total body protein 80 days.

**halibut liver oil** One of the richest natural sources of vitamins A and D; contains 5 g vitamin A and 8 mg vitamin D per 100 g.

**halophilic bacteria** Able to grow in high concentrations of salt (25%). Colon group of bacteria are inhibited at 8–9% salt, *Clostridia* at 7–10%, food poisoning staphylococci at 15–20%, *Penicillium* 20%; film-forming yeasts can grow in 24% brine.

**Halphen test** Test for the presence of cottonseed oil in other oils and fats.

**halva** Also spelled halwa, halawa and chalva. A sweetmeat composed of an aerated mixture of glucose, sugar and crushed sesame seeds; because of the seeds, the sweet contains 25% fat.

**halverine** Name sometimes given to low-fat spreads with less than the statutory amount of fat in a margarine.

**ham** The whole hind leg of the pig removed from the carcase and cured individually; sometimes the process is secret.

Hams cured or smoked in different ways have different flavours – York, Bradenham, Suffolk and Westphalian hams.

Analysis per 100 g after cooking: protein 16 g, fat 40 g, carbohydrate nil, kcal 435 (1.8 MJ), Fe 2.5 mg, vitamin $B_1$ 0.5 mg, vitamin $B_2$ 0.2 mg, nicotinic acid 3.5 mg.

**Hammarsten's casein** Casein prepared by the method of Hammarsten. Fat-free milk diluted with water and precipitated with acetic acid. Washed three times with water by decantation; dissolved in ammonium hydroxide and reprecipitated, this repeated twice. The final precipitate washed with alcohol and ether and finally extracted with ether in a Soxhlet.

**hammer mill** Mill in which material is powdered by impact from a set of hammers; a continuous process.

**Hansa can** An all-aluminium can (developed in Germany) with easily opened ends.

**hardening of oils** See *hydrogenated oils*.

**hardness of water** See *water hardness*.

**hashish** See *Indian hemp*.

**haslet** (harslet) Old English country dish made from pig's offal (heart, liver, lungs and sweetbread) cooked in small pieces with seasoning and flour. (Named from old French from Latin *hasta* (spear), implying that it was cooked over a spit.)

**hasty pudding** Made from flour, milk, butter and spices, which, since they were usually readily available, could be quickly made into the pudding for unexpected visitors. Made in the USA with maize (corn) flour instead of wheat flour.

**Hausa groundnut** *Kerstingiella geocarpa*; member of legume family grown in West Africa; 20% protein, 60% fat.

**haybox cooking** The food is cooked for only a short time, then placed in a well-lagged container, the haybox, where it remains hot for many hours and so cooking continues without further use of fuel. Also known as the fireless cooker.

**Hay diet** A system of eating based on the fallacy that carbo-hydrates and proteins should not be eaten at the same meal. Since protein, in the absence of adequate carbohydrate, is oxidised to provide energy and therefore not available for tissue building, this diet is not only faddish but foolish.

**haze** Term in general use in brewing to indicate cloudiness of the beer. Chill haze appears at 0°C and disappears at 20°C; permanent haze remains at 20°C but there is no fundamental difference. Due to gums derived from the barley, leucoantho-cyanins from the malt and hops, and glucose, pentoses and amino acids.

**HDL** High-density lipoproteins. See *lipids, plasma*.

**headcheese** Chopped, cooked edible parts of meat or meat products, also known as mock brawn.

**health foods** Substances whose consumption is advocated by various reform movements, including vegetable foods, whole grain cereals, food processed without chemical additives, foods grown on organic compost, 'magic' foods (honey, molasses, yogurt, etc.) and pills and potions.

**heart sugar** Inositol.

**heat exchanger** Equipment for heating or cooling liquids rapidly by providing a large surface area and turbulence for the rapid and efficient transfer of heat. Used for continuous pasteurisa-tion and also for the subsequent cooling.

**heat of combustion** Energy released by complete combustion, as, for example, in the bomb calorimeter. Values can be used to predict energy available physiologically only if an allowance is made for material not oxidised in the body. For example, the end products of protein oxidation in the body are carbon dioxide, water and urea; the latter contains non-available energy.

**hedonic scale** Term used in tasting panels where the judge indicates the extent of his like or dislike for the food.

**heifer** Young cow that has never had a calf.

**hemataminic acid** See *sialic acid*.

**hematin** See *haematin*.

**heme** See *haem*.

**hemicelluloses** Complex carbohydrates composed of polyuronic acids combined with xylose, glucose, mannose and arabinose. Found together with cellulose and lignin in plant cell walls; most gums and mucilages belong to this group of compounds.

**hemoglobin** See *haemoglobin*.

**hemosiderin** See *haemosiderin*.

**heparin** Substance isolated from liver, lung, muscle, heart and blood which prevents blood coagulation by acting as an anti-prothrombin and an antithrombin. *In vivo* disappears rapidly from the blood stream, but *in vitro* 10 mg prevents the coagulation of 100 ml of blood.

**hepatoflavin** Name given to substance isolated from liver, shown later to be riboflavin.

**herbs** Not clearly distinguished from spices, except that they usually refer to the whole of the soft-stemmed aromatic plant, while spices are only part of the plant.

**Hermesetas** Trade name (Crookes-Anestan Ltd) for saccharin tablets.

**herring family** Herring is *Clupea harengus*; young herrings are sild. Sprat is *Clupea sprattus*; young are brislings. Pilchard is *Clupea pilchardus*; young are sardines. Kippers, bloaters and red herrings are salted and smoked herrings; bucklings are hot-smoked herrings. Gaffelbitar are preserved herring.

For analysis, see *fish, fatty*.

**hesperidin** At one time called vitamin P, since it affects the fragility of the capillary walls. Found in the pith of the unripe orange and other citrus fruits; chemically a complex of glucose and rhamnose with the flavonone hesperin.

**Hess test** A test for capillary fragility in scurvy. A slight pressure is applied to the arm for 5 minutes and a shower of petechiae appear on the skin below the area of application.

**heterosides** See *holosides*.

**heterotrophes** See *autotrophes*.

**Hexamic acid** A synthetic sweetening agent; trade name (Abbott Laboratories) for cyclohexyl sulphamic acid (the free acid of cyclamate); 27 times as sweet as sugar. Used in effervescent drinks.

**hexamine** Hexamethylene tetramine or methenamine used in conjunction with benzoic acid and benzoates to preserve marinated or semi-preserved fish products where pH is above 4.5.

**hexoestrol** Synthetic oestrogenic hormone; does not occur naturally. See *oestrogens*.

**hexosans** The general name for complex polysaccharides built up from simple units of hexose sugars. See *fructosan*; *glucosan*.

**hexose** A six-carbon sugar such as glucose and fructose.

**hexose monophosphate shunt** An alternative pathway in the metabolism of glucose to the Embden–Meyerhof–Parnas pathway.

The glucose-6-phosphate formed in the main route can be converted to phosphogluconic acid, then to pentose phosphate and to sedoheptulose-7-phosphate. The latter then joins the main pathway.

Since pentoses are formed, it is also referred to as the pentose cycle and the direct oxidative pathway.

**hexuronic acid** The acid derived from a hexose sugar by the oxidation of the group on C6. The hexuronic acid derived from glucose is glucuronic acid.

**HFCS** High-fructose corn syrup. See *fructose syrups*.

**HF heating** High-frequency heating.

**high-frequency heating** See *irradiation*.

**high-ratio fats** See *fats, high-ratio*.

**high-ratio flour** See *flour, high-ratio*.

**high-ratio shortenings** See *fats, high-ratio*.

**hindle wakes chicken** Very old English method of cooking chicken, corruption of hen de la wake (feast), fourteenth century, Flemish introduction; stuffed with fruit and spices, including prunes.

**hiochic acid** Growth factor isolated 1956 in Japanese rice wine (saké) and later shown to be identical with mevalonic acid, which see.

**H ion** See *pH*.

**hirudin** Blood anticoagulant found in the buccal glands of the leech. Functions by interfering with thrombin.

**Hi-soy** Trade name (British Arkady) for full-fat soya flour.

**histamine** Compound formed from decarboxylation of the amino acid histidine, and also found in beer, chocolate, sauerkraut, and wines in small amounts.

Has effect of constricting smooth muscle of the bronchioles such as occurs in asthma (hence the use of antihistamines in its treatment); lowers blood pressure by dilating the blood vessels; stimulates secretion of gastric acid; and used as test for achlorhydria.

**histidine** An amino acid essential to the growing rat but not to adult man. It is assumed that it is essential to the growing child. Chemically, amino iminazole propionic acid.

Decarboxylation produces histamine.

**histohaematin**  Or myohaematin, earlier name for cytochrome, which see.

**histones**  Proteins soluble in water but insoluble in dilute ammonia; yield precipitates with solutions of other proteins; on hydrolysis yield large quantities of arginine and lysine. For example, scombrone from mackerel sperm, thymus histone.

**HMS**  See *hexose monophosphate shunt*.

**HMT**  Hexamethylene tetramine. Preservative permitted in some countries.

**hogget**  One-year-old sheep.

**hogshead**  For beer or cider contains 54 gallons; for wine contains 52½ gallons.

**holocellulose**  Mixture of cellulose and hemicellulose in wood, the fibrous residue that remains after the extractives, the lignin, and the ash-forming elements, have been removed.

**holoenzyme**  An enzyme protein together with its coenzyme or prosthetic group.

**holosides**  Name given to complexes of sugars (or osides) that yield only sugars on hydrolysis. As distinct from heterosides, which yield other substances as well as sugars on hydrolysis, e.g. tannins, anthocyanins, nucleosides.

**hominy**  Prepared maize kernels. Lye hominy – pericarp and germ removed by soaking in caustic soda. Pearled hominy – degermed hulled maize.

Corn grits are ground hominy.

**homocysteine**  The demethylated form of the amino acid methionine, $SHCH_2CH_2CHNH_2COOH$. Does not occur in foods and is not of nutritional importance, but of great biochemical interest as an intermediate in cell reactions. The non-essential amino acid cystine is made from the essential methionine via homocysteine.

**homogenisation**  Emulsions usually consist of a suspension of globules of varying size. Homogenisation reduces these globules to a smaller and approximately equal size.

In homogenised milk the smaller globules adsorb more of the milk protein, which is a stabiliser, and the cream does not rise to the top.

**homogeniser, ultrasonic**  See *ultrasonic homogeniser*.

**homoiotherms**  Animals that maintain constant body temperature irrespective of the surrounding temperature; also known as warm-blooded animals.

**honey**  Syrupy liquid manufactured by bees from the nectar of flowers (essentially sucrose). The flavour and colour depend on the flowers from which the nectar was obtained and the composition also varies with the source.

Average composition: water 18% (12–26%), invert sugars, i.e. glucose and fructose, 74% (69–75%), sucrose 1.9% (0–4%), ash 0.18% (0.1–0.8%), organic acid 0.1–0.4%.

If the ratio between fructose and glucose is high, there is a tendency for the honey to crystallise.

**honeydew honey** During periods of prolonged drought bees may supplement their nectar supplies with honeydew, the sweet fluid excreted on leaves by leaf-sucking insects. The resultant honey is dark with an unpleasant taste.

**hop** A perennial climbing plant, *Humulus lupulus*. The female flowers contain bitter resins and essential oils used in brewing beer. See *humulone*.

**Horchata de chufa** Aqueous extract of tiger nut used as a drink (Spain); see *tiger nut*.

**hordein** A protein in barley; one of the prolamines.

**hordenin** Alkaloid found in germinated barley, sorghum and millet which can cause hypertension and respiratory inhibition.

**Horlick's** Trade name (Horlick's Ltd) for a preparation of malted milk, for consumption as a beverage when added to milk.

Analysis per 100 g: protein 14.4 g, fat 8.0 g, carbohydrate 70.8 g, Ca 272 mg, Fe 1 mg, kcal 400 (1.7 MJ).

**hormones** Chemical agents produced in the body, also known as endocrines. Thyroxine and tri-iodothyronine from the thyroid, adrenaline from the adrenals, insulin from the pancreas and a variety of hormones from the pituitary gland. They are secreted directly into the blood stream from these ductless glands and act as chemical messengers which stimulate other tissues. See also *hormones, sex*; *oestrogens*.

**hormones, sex** Male hormones, or androgens, include testosterone and androsterone; female hormones, or oestrogens, include oestradiol, oestrone and progesterone. Chemically, all are steroid in structure.

The synthetic female hormones stilboestrol and hexoestrol are similar in biological activity but quite different chemically. Apart from clinical use the oestrogens have been widely used in chemical caponisation of cockerels and to enhance the growth rate of cattle.

See also *oestrogens*.

**horsemeat** Analysis per 100 g: protein 15 g, fat 3 g, kcal 94 (0.4 MJ), Ca 8 mg, Fe 1.8 mg, vitamin A nil, vitamin $B_1$ 0.05 mg, vitamin $B_2$ 0.08 mg, nicotinic acid 3.2 mg, vitamin C nil.

**horse radish** Root of *Armoracia lapathifolia*. Pungency due to volatile oil (including allyl isothiocyanate and butyl sulphocyanide) liberated by the enzyme myrosinase from the glucoside sinigrin. Used as a condiment.

**Hortvet freezing test**   Test for the adulteration of milk with water by measuring the depression of freezing point; normal range −0.53 to −0.55 °C.

**hot breads**   Americanese for waffles and pancakes.

**hot sauce**   A tomato sauce with hot flavour due to cayenne.

**Hot Springs Conference**   International Conference held in 1943 at which the Food and Agriculture Organization of the United Nations originated.

**Hovis**   Trade name (Rank-Hovis-McDougall Ltd) of a wheat germ-enriched loaf.

Analysis per 100 g: protein 9 g, fat 2.3 g, carbohydrate 47.6 g, Ca 107 mg, Fe 2.7 mg, kcal 237 (1 MJ), vitamin $B_1$ 0.29 mg, nicotinic acid 2.0 mg.

Phytic acid phosphorus 38% of total P (which is 200 mg per 100 g of the bread), compared with white bread, in which phytic acid P is 15% of total P (which is 80 mg per 100 g bread).

**Howard mould count**   Standardised microscopical technique for measuring mould contamination.

**HPLC**   High-performance liquid chromatography. See *chromatography*.

**HTST**   High-temperature–short time treatment; defined as sterilisation by heat from times ranging from a few seconds to 6 minutes; usually applied to flow sterilisation, in which the process time is less than about 1 minute.

**huckleberry**   Wild N. American berry, *Gaylussacia baccata* and other species (named after the French chemist Gay-Lussac). Similar to blueberry but larger seeds; used in tarts, pies and preserves.

**humble pie**   See *umbles*.

**humectant**   Substance that absorbs moisture and used to maintain the water content of materials like tobacco, glue, inks, baked products, soaps, textiles. For example, glucose syrup, invert sugar, honey, dried whey, glycerol, sorbitol. They allow the addition of sugar without adding more water and so prevent the growth of moulds.

**humidity**   Moistness of air. Weight of water per unit weight of air is absolute or specific humidity.

Saturation humidity is the absolute humidity of air which is saturated with water vapour at a given temperature.

Relative humidity is the degree of saturation; ratio of water vapour pressure in the atmosphere to water vapour pressure that would be exerted by pure water at the same temperature.

**humulone**   One of the two resins found in hops, the other being lupulone. Humulone is a mixture of humulone, cohumulone and adhumulone. The resins are responsible for the bitter flavour of the hops used in brewing.

**Hursting mill** Horizontal stone grinders once used for grain milling.

**husk, or hull** In reference to cereal grain, this is the outer woody cellulose covering. In wheat it is loosely attached and removed during threshing; in rice it is firmly attached.

High in fibre content and of limited use as animal feed.

**hyaluronic acid** See also *hyaluronidase*. The mucopolysaccharide which, in animal tissues, binds water in the interstitial spaces, and holds the cells together and acts as a shock-absorber in the joints; also present in the vitreous humour of the eye.

Its viscosity is reduced by the enzyme hyaluronidase, by which it is depolymerised.

**hyaluronidase** Group of carbohydrase enzymes that depolymerise mucopolysaccharides such as hyaluronic acid. Found in bee-sting, bacteria, testes, leeches.

Also known as spreading factor, because the enzyme breaks down the hyaluronic acid under the skin and permits the spread of substances there. For this reason it is used clinically to aid the absorption of drugs administered subcutaneously or intramuscularly, and to permit the subcutaneous injections of relatively large volumes of solution as, for example, in glucose feeding by this route.

**hydrocooling** Vegetables are washed in cold water, then, while still wet, subjected to vacuum. The evaporation of the water chills the vegetables for transport. The term is also applied to vegetables washed in ice water without the vacuum treatment.

**hydrogen acceptor** See *intermediate hydrogen carrier*.

**hydrogenated oils** Liquid oils can be hardened by hydrogenation. Treatment with hydrogen in the presence of a nickel catalyst causes 'saturation' of the double bonds of the fatty acid chain and a rise in melting point. Cottonseed, maize, sunflower and whale oils are commonly hardened and used in margarine and cooking fats.

**hydrogen carrier** See *intermediate hydrogen carrier*.

**hydrogen, heavy** Or deuterium; the isotope of hydrogen with atomic weight 2 instead of 1. Tritium has atomic weight 3.

**hydrogen-ion concentration** Measure of the acidity or alkalinity of a solution by the concentration of hydrogen ions present. See *pH*.

**hydrogen peroxide** Anti-microbial agent; can be used at 0.1% to preserve milk (Buddeised milk), but destroys vitamin C, methionine and tryptophan. Not permitted in the UK.

Formula $H_2O_2$, readily loses active oxygen, the effective sterilising agent, and so forms water.

**hydrogen swells** See *swells*.

**hydrolyse** To split a substance and add the OH and the H of the water to the two halves. For example, cane sugar, $C_{12}H_{22}O_{11}$, is hydrolysed to glucose, $C_6H_{12}O_6$, and fructose, $C_6H_{12}O_6$: proteins are hydrolysed to amino acids. Acid or alkali is usually needed as catalyst.

**hydrostatic steriliser** Continuous steriliser in which the process is carried out under sufficient depth of water to maintain the required pressure. Used for continuous sterilisation of canned foods on a large scale.

**hydroxybenzoic acid esters** Methyl, ethyl, propyl and butyl esters of hydroxybenzoic acid and their sodium salts; used as antifungal agents and preservatives. Also called paraben esters.

**hydroxycholecalciferol** See *vitamin D*.

**hydroxylysine** Amino acid found only in connective tissue proteins of animals; incorporated into the protein as lysine and then hydroxylated in the delta position.

**hydroxyproline** Amino acid found only in connective tissue proteins of animals; incorporated into the protein as proline and then hydroxylated. Peptides of hydroxyproline are excreted in the urine and the output is increased when collagen turnover is high, as in rapid growth or resorption of tissue.

**hydroxyproline index** Urinary hydroxyproline excretion is reduced in children suffering protein-energy malnutrition. The index is the ratio between hydroxyproline and creatinine per kg body weight and is low in malnourished children.

**5-hydroxytryptamine** Or serotonin; 3-(2-aminoethyl)-5-indolol. Formed from the amino acid tryptophan; found in blood, and in higher concentrations in the plantain; causes vasoconstriction and is a neurotransmitter.

**hygroscopic** Readily absorbing water, as when table salt becomes damp. Materials such as calcium chloride and silica gel absorb water so readily that they are used as drying agents.

**hyperalimentation**, (intravenous) Provision of unusually large amount of energy (usually intravenously).

**hypercalcaemia, idiopathic** Elevated levels of blood calcium believed to be due to hypersensitivity of some children to vitamin D. There is excessive absorption of calcium, with loss of appetite, vomiting, constipation, flabby muscles and deposition of calcium in the soft tissues and kidneys. It can be fatal in infants.

**hyperchlorhydria** Excess of hydrochloric acid in the stomach, due, not to higher concentration in the gastric juice, but to a greater volume of secretion.

**hyperglycaemia** Elevated blood glucose levels.

**hyperlipidaemias** (hyperlipoproteinaemias)  Common disorder of affluent communities, in which there is an increased level of the plasma lipids – phospholipids, triglycerides, free and esterified cholesterol and unesterified fatty acids. See *lipids, plasma*.

**hyperthyroidism**  Overactivity of the thyroid gland causing increased basal metabolic rate.

**hypertonic**  A solution more concentrated than isotonic, which see.

**hypervitaminosis**  Overdosage with vitamins. In most cases there is no ill-effect, but hypervitaminosis A and also D have ill-effects; overdosage with nicotinic acid causes flushing of the face and neck.

**hypoglycaemia**  Depressed levels of blood glucose.

**hypokalaemia**  A fall in the level of blood potassium. (Latin name *kalium*.)

**hypophysectomy**  Surgical removal of the pituitary gland (the hypophysis).

**hypoproteinaemia**  Total plasma protein level less than 5.5 g per 100 ml (normally 6.7–7.7).

**hyposite**  Little used word, from Greek, for low-energy food.

**hypothermia**  Low body temperature. Occurs among elderly far more easily than in younger adults, often with fatal results. Also used in connection with reduction of body temperature down to 28°C to permit surgery of heart and brain.

**hypothyroidism**  Underactivity of the thyroid gland. See *cretinism*; *thyroid gland*.

**hypotonic**  A solution more dilute than isotonic, which see.

**hypoxanthine**  See *nucleic acids*; *purines*.

# I

**ice cream**  A frozen confection made from fat, milk solids and sugar. Some European countries permit the use of non-milk fats and term the product ice cream; while if milk fat is used, it is termed dairy ice cream.

According to UK regulations, contains not less than 5% fat and 7% other milk solids; according to US regulations, 10% milk fat and 20% other milk solids. Stabilisers such as carboxymethylcellulose, gums and alginates are included, and emulsifiers such as polysorbate and monoglycerides. Mono- and diglycerides bind the looser globules of water and are added in 'non-drip' ice cream.

**ichthyosarcotoxins**  Toxins in fish.

**idli**  A mixture of cooked rice and black gram fermented with the aid of mould; eaten in the Far East.

**IEP**  Iso-electric point.

**IHD**  Ischaemic heart disease, which see.

**ileum**  Last portion of the small intestine, after the jejunum and before the small intestine joins the large intestine or colon.

**illipé butter**  See *vegetable butters*.

**immune system**  Series of defence mechanisms of the body. There are two major parts, humoral, mediated through antibodies (immunoglobulins), and cell-mediated, phagocytic cells (B and T type lymphocytes).

**immunoglobulins**  Specific antibodies produced in the blood in response to foreign proteins. Five classes, IgA, IgE, IgG, IgM and IgI; present in circulating blood as a result of previous stimulation and also present in breast milk to confer some immunity on the baby.

**IMP**  Integrating motor pneumotachograph. Apparatus for measuring energy expenditure indirectly from oxygen consumption. It meters the expired air and removes a proportion for analysis.

**improvers, flour**  See *aging*.

**inanition**  Exhaustion and wasting due to complete lack of or non-assimilation of food; a state of starvation.

**inborn errors of metabolism**  See *genetic disease*.

**Incaparina**  A protein-rich dietary supplement developed by the Institute of Nutrition of Central America and Panama (INCAP). One version consists of 38% cottonseed flour, 29% ground corn, 39% sorghum, 3% Torula yeast, 1% calcium carbonate and 1350μg vitamin A per 100g. Incaparina 9A includes 58% maize and 38% cottonseed flour; in formula 14 the cottonseed is replaced by soya. All versions contain 27.5% protein.

**index of nutritional quality**  (INQ)  An attempt to provide an overall figure for the nutrient content of a food or a diet. It is the ratio between the percentage of the recommended daily amount of each nutrient and the percentage of the RDA (which see) for energy.

**Indian corn**  Maize, which see.

**Indian hemp**  Or hashish, *Cannabis indica*; active principle unknown, stimulates and deranges the mental processes.

**Indian rice grass**  Perennial, growing wild in the USA, *Oryzopsis hymenoides*; tolerant to drought.

Seeds resemble millet, small, round, dark in colour, covered with white hairs. Used by North American Indians for flour; now used almost exclusively for forage.

**indican**  (1) Metabolic indican is 3-indoxylsulphuric acid excreted in urine of mammals and found in blood plasma; derived from tryptophan.

(2) Plant indican is 3-beta-glucosido-indole (indoxyl-glucoside) found in plants of *Indigofera* and some other species.

**indigo carmine**   Blue food colour, disodium salt of indigotin-5,5'-disulphonic acid. Indigotin is the colouring principle of natural indigo obtained from the indigo fern. Permitted food colour in most countries but its use is limited by its low stability and solubility.

**indoxyl**   See *indican*.

**induction period**   Frequently used in connection with fats. It is the lag period during which the fat shows stability to oxidation because of its content of antioxidants, natural or added, which are preferentially oxidised. After this induction period there is a sudden and large consumption of oxygen and the fat becomes rancid. See *antioxidants*.

**infra-red spectroscopy**   Spectroscopic method of measuring water, fat and protein in food or feed by scanning wavelengths 1200–2500 nm – region of electromagnetic spectrum where chemical bonding, CH (lipids), OH (water) and NH (proteins) vibrate strongly.

**inhibition, competitive**   With reference to enzymes, means inhibition by a substance chemically similar to the substrate, which competes with the true substrate for the active surface of the enzyme. Thus, malonic acid competitively inhibits succinic dehydrogenase, of which the true substrate is the chemically similar succinic acid.

The inhibition is reversed with a sufficiently high concentration of the true substrate.

Sulphanilamides act as bacteriostats, because they compete for a vitamin essential to the bacteria – namely para-amino benzoic acid.

**inorganic**   Denoting of mineral as distinct from animal and vegetable origin. Appart from carbonates and cyanides, inorganic chemicals are those that contain no carbon.

**inosite**   Obsolete name for inositol.

**inositol**   Essential nutrient for micro-organisms and many animals and so classed as a vitamin, although there is no evidence of its essentiality for man. Deficiency causes alopecia in mice and 'spectacle eye' (denudation around the eye) in rats.

Chemically hexahydrocyclohexane $(CHOH)_6$; there are nine stereoisomers of this compound but only one, meso- or myo-inositol, is of major interest. It occurs widely in plant and animal tissues as an essential part of the structure and in combination in phosphatides. Its hexaphosphoric acid ester is phytic acid, which see.

Obsolete names inosite and meat sugar. The insecticide

gammexane is hexachlorocyclohexane, and appears to function by competing with inositol.

**instant foods**  Dried foods that reconstitute rapidly when water is added, e.g. tea, coffee, milk, soups, precooked cereal products, potatoes, etc. Products may be agglomerated after drying to control particle size and improve solubility.

'Instant puddings' are formulated with pregelatinised starch and disperse rapidly in cold milk.

(Instant coffee was first prepared in 1906 by an Englishman, G. Washington, living in Guatemala, and marketed in 1909.)

**insulin**  Hormone that controls carbohydrate metabolism; secreted by the pancreas gland. Diabetes mellitus (which see) is due to underproduction or overdestruction of insulin. The hormone is a protein and is digested if given by mouth, so must be administered by injection.

Cannot be synthesised and is prepared from animal pancreas. There are four types used clinically: standard (quick-acting), protamin–zinc–insulin (12–24 hours), globin insulin (8–10 hours), and modified protamin insulin (28–30 hours).

See also *glucose tolerance*.

**interesterification**  Fats are mixtures of triglycerides with various fatty acids esterified to the glycerol. By dry heat at 45–95°C there is an exchange of the fatty acids between the glycerol molecules – interesterification – with a consequent change in physical properties of the fat. For example, lard is not a good creaming fat until it has been so treated.

**intermediate hydrogen carrier**  The oxidation of many substances in the living cell involves their loss of hydrogen. The hydrogen is passed on to an intermediate hydrogen acceptor, under the influence of an enzyme, and thence along a chain of acceptors to the ultimate hydrogen acceptor, which is oxygen (thus forming water).

For example, lactic acid is dehydrogenated (oxidised) to pyruvic acid, under the influence of a specific enzyme, and the hydrogen is passed on to coenzyme I (an intermediate hydrogen carrier), thence to cytochrome (another intermediate hydrogen carrier) and finally to oxygen.

**intermediate moisture foods**  Semi-moist, around 25% moisture (15–50%) with water activity reduced to less than 0.86 by the addition of substances such as glycerol, sorbitol, salt, certain organic acids so preventing the growth of micro-organisms.

**international units**  Used as a measure of the comparative potency of natural substances, such as vitamins, before they are obtained in sufficiently pure form to measure by weight.

An international unit (i.u.) is arbitrarily defined in terms of a reproducible standard, e.g. 1 i.u. of vitamin A was originally 1 μg of the purest then known preparation of carotene, later 0.6 μg of beta-carotene.

**intestinal juice** Also called succus entericus. Digestive juice produced by the intestinal glands lining the small intestine. Contains the enzymes 'erepsin' (aminopeptidase and dipeptidase), amylase, maltase, lactase, sucrase, lipase, esterase, nucleases, nucleotidase, and the activator enterokinase (activates trypsinogen and chymotrypsinogen of the pancreatic juice to trypsin and chymotrypsin).

**intestine** Loosely used to describe the whole of the gastrointestinal tract; more specifically that part after the stomach – comprising small intestine (duodenum, jejunum and ileum) and large intestine.

**intestine, small** That part lying between the stomach and the large intestine, comprising duodenum, jejunum and ileum. The site of the greater part of digestion of food and absorption of the products. Only water is absorbed in the large intestine.

**intolerance** (to foods) See *adverse reactions (to food)*.

**intravenous hyperalimentation** Supply of energy, either intravenously or by stomach tube, in amounts greater than normal requirements.

**intravenous nutrition** Slow infusion of solution of nutrients into veins by catheter.

**intrinsic factor** See *pernicious anaemia*.

**inulin** A polysaccharide composed of fructose units; produced in the dahlia tuber and Jerusalem artichoke as a storage carbohydrate. It is used as a test of renal function. See *kidney clearance test*. Also called dahlin and alant starch.

**inversion** Applied to sucrose, means its hydrolysis to glucose and fructose. See *optical activity*.

**invertase** Enzyme that splits sucrose into the invert sugars, glucose and fructose. Also known as sucrase or saccharase.

  Saccharases are widely distributed in plant tissues and the digestive juice of animals, and are of two types, glucosaccharases (in animals and the mould *Aspergillus*) and fructosaccharases (in yeast). They, respectively, attack the glucose and the fructose end of complex sugars. As sucrose is glucosefructoside, it is attacked by any of the saccharases.

**invert sugar** Mixture of glucose and fructose produced by hydrolysis of sucrose. (See *optical activity*.) 130% sweetness of sucrose. Important in the manufacture of sugar confectionery (see *boiled sweets*), since the presence of 10–15% of invert sugar prevents the crystallisation of cane sugar.

**in vitro**  Literally 'in glass'; used to indicate an observation made experimentally in the test-tube, as distinct from the natural living conditions, *in vivo*.

**in vivo**  In the living state, as distinct from *in vitro* – in the test-tube.

**iodine**  A trace element required at the level of 150 μg per day. It is part of the hormone thyroxine produced by the thyroid gland, and a prolonged shortage of iodide in the diet leads to goitre.

It is plentifully supplied by sea foods and by vegetables grown in soil containing iodide. In certain areas where the soil water is deficient in iodide, goitre occurs in defined geographical regions. For example, in England it occurred in Derbyshire, where it was known as Derbyshire neck, and in Oxfordshire; there are goitrous areas in most countries, e.g. Switzerland, USA, New Zealand.

Iodine is not essential to plant growth but is present in plants in amounts varying with the level in the soil.

See also *goitre*; *iodised salt*; *thyroid gland*.

**iodine number**  See *iodine value*.

**iodine, protein-bound**  See *thyroglobulin*.

**iodine solution, Hübl's**  Solution of iodine and mercuric chloride used to determine the iodine number of unsaturated compounds.

**iodine value**  Or iodine number; measure of the degree of unsaturation of a fat by the extent of the uptake of iodine (grams iodine per 100 g of fat) by the unsaturated double bonds in the fatty acid chain.

Examples of iodine values: butter 22–38, lard 54–70, coconut oil 8–10, cottonseed 104–114, linseed 170–202. Drying oils (which see) are highly unsaturated and have high iodine numbers, as linseed oil.

**iodised salt**  Usually 1 part of iodide in 25 000–50 000 parts of salt.

**iodophors**  Acidic solutions of iodine complexed with a non-ionic surface-active agent which release iodine when diluted with water and are effective antibacterial agents at relatively low temperatures.

**ion-exchange resins**  Various resins, such as Permutit, Zeocarb, Amberlite, Dowex, will adsorb ions under one set of conditions and release them under other conditions. The best-known example is in water-softening, where the calcium ions are removed from the hard water by the resin, and liberated from the resin by the addition of salt (regeneration).

The ion-exchange resins are used for purification of chemicals, metal recovery and analysis.

See also *Amberlite*.

**ionisation**   When a salt such as sodium chloride is put into solution, the NaCl splits into positively charged Na ions (cations) and negatively charged Cl ions (anions). Salts ionise readily; many organic compounds do not ionise. The degree of ionisation of an acid determines its strength (see *pH*).

Ionising radiation is that which ionises the air or water through which it passes, e.g. X-rays and gamma-rays.

**ionising radiation**   See *irradiation*.

**IQB**   Individual quick blanch. A method of blanching food by subjecting each particle to steam for a relatively short time and then accumulating the food in a deep bed until equilibration of temperature takes place.

**Irish moss**   Red seaweed, *Chrondrus crispus*; source of the polysaccharide carrageenan, which see.

**iron**   A mineral essential to the body; the average adult has 4–5 g of iron, of which 60–70% is present as haem in the circulating haemoglobin, and the remainder present in various enzymes (e.g. catalase, cytochrome oxidase), in muscle myoglobin or stored. About 15% of the iron is stored in the liver as ferritin, in other tissues as haemosiderin, and as the blood transport complex called transferrin (average blood level 50–180 μg of iron per 100 ml plasma.)

Iron balance: losses in faeces 0.3–0.5 mg per day, in sweat as skin cells 0.5 mg, traces in hair and urine, total loss 0.5–1.5 mg per day; diet contains 10–15 mg, of which 0.5–1.5 mg is absorbed.

Recommended intake 12 mg for adults, 15 mg during pregnancy and lactation and for adolescents, 7.5–10.5 mg for children, rising to 13.5 mg in 11–14-year-old group. Absorption aided by vitamin C and reduced by phosphate and phytic acid.

Content of foods: liver 6–14 mg per 100 g, cereal up to 9 mg, nuts 1–5 mg, eggs 2–3 mg, meat 2–4 mg. Added to flour so that it contains not less than 1.65 mg per 100 g. Fortified cereals provide 35% of the iron of British diets.

Prolonged deficiency gives rise to nutritional anaemia.

**iron ammonium citrate**   See *ferric ammonium citrate*.

**iron caseinate**   Preparation of iron and casein; also known as iron nucleo-albuminate.

**iron chink**   Machine used to behead and eviscerate salmon before canning (in the early days the work was done by Chinese labour).

**iron, reduced**   Metallic iron in finely divided form produced by reduction of iron oxide. The form in which iron is sometimes added to foods, such as bread. Latin name *ferrum redactum*.

**iron, storage**   See *ferritin*; *haemosiderin*.

**iron, transport**   See *siderophilin*.

**iron vitellinate**   Preparation of egg yolk and iron.

**irradiation**   With reference to foods, three main types of irradiation are used: ultraviolet, ionising and high-frequency (or microwave).

Ultraviolet irradiation (2100–2900 nm) is of interest, since it is used to sterilise the surface of foods, and convert ergosterol and 7-dehydrocholesterol to ergocalciferol (vitamin $D_2$) and cholecalciferol (vitamin $D_3$), respectively.

Ionising irradiation from radioactive isotopes or the linear accelerator destroys micro-organisms and insects, and also inhibits sprouting of potatoes. It is used at various levels of treatment.

(1) Radurisation refers to low doses adequate to reduce the numbers of spoilage organisms.

(2) Radicidation refers to doses sufficient to reduce the number of specified viable non-sporing pathogens below detectable levels.

(3) Radappertisation is treatment with doses sufficiently great to reduce the numbers of organisms below detectable levels (so-called commercial sterility) (see also *appertisation*).

(4) Radiopasteurisation is sufficient to destroy most pathogens (see *pasteurisation*).

Microwave heating employs high-energy electromagnetic radiation (commonly 2350 MHz, wavelength 12 cm) which generates heat throughout the food. It is used for domestic cooking, to reheat food in catering and to 'finish drying' some commercially manufactured foods.

**ischaemic heart disease**   Or coronary heart disease. Group of syndromes arising from failure of coronary arteries to supply sufficient blood to heart muscles; associated with atherosclerosis of coronary arteries.

**isinglass**   Protein membrane from the swim bladder of certain species of sturgeon; practically pure collagen. When specially prepared, is used to clarify beer as it slowly precipitates and carries with it any suspended particles.

**islets of Langerhans**   Areas of the pancreas from which the insulin is secreted.

**isoascorbic acid**   Erythorbic acid, which see.

**isodesmosine**   A complex cross-linked compound involving four lysyl residues formed, together with desmosine, in connective tissue.

**isoelectric point**   Proteins and amino acids carry both negative and positive charges on the molecule, and are therefore called

150

amphoteric. At a certain degree of acidity, depending on the particular protein or amino acid, the substance becomes electrically neutral, i.e. the isoelectric point.

Proteins are usually least soluble and therefore precipitated from solution at the IEP.

**isoenzymes** Name given to enzymes with the same catalytic function but different structures and therefore different properties, e.g. tissue lactic dehydrogenase contains at least five isoenzymes.

**isoflavones** See *flavonoids*.

**isoleucine** An essential amino acid, rarely limiting in foods. Chemically, aminomethyl valeric acid.

**isomalt** An approximately equimolar mixture of 6-*O*-alpha-D-glucopyranosyl-D-sorbitol and 1-*O*-alpha-glucopyranosyl-D-mannitol. Bulk sweetener, half the sweetness of sucrose. Only partly metabolised to produce approx. 2 kcal/g.

**isomaltose** Also termed brachyose. Differs from maltose in that the two glucose units are linked 1,6 instead of 1,4. Unlike maltose, isomaltose is not fermented by yeasts; it is a reducing sugar.

**isomaltulose** 6-*O*-glucosyl fructose (palatinose).

**isomerase** Name given to the enzyme used to convert glucose into fructose, although its primary specificity is conversion of D-xylose to D-xylulose.

**Isomerose** Trade name of high-fructose corn syrup (see *fructose syrups*): 70–72% solids, 42% fructose, 55% glucose, 3% polysaccharides.

**isomers** Molecules containing the same atoms but differently arranged. They can be quite different compounds or closely related, as citric and isocitric acids, leucine and isoleucine. See also *cis-trans isomerism*.

**iso-osmotic** See *isotonic*.

**isoprene** The unit that forms part of the structure of the terpenes and the carotenoids,

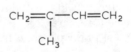

**isoriboflavin** An analogue of riboflavin containing the two methyl groups in the 5,6 instead of the 6,7 position. It competes with the vitamin and so inhibits growth.

**isosyrups** See *fructose syrups*.

**isotonic** Two solutions are iso-osmotic (isosmotic) when they have the same total osmotic pressure. They are isotonic, relative to a particular semi-permeable membrane, when their effective osmotic pressures are the same, i.e. the osmotic pressure of their non-permeating ions.

If two isotonic solutions are separated by a semi-permeable membrane, there is no net movement of water across the membrane. For example, human blood plasma is isosmotic with 0.945% sodium chloride, and isotonic with 0.935% sodium chloride, since part of the osmotic pressure of the blood is due to its proteins, which are non-permeating.

**isotopes** Elements with the same chemical properties, differing only in their atomic weights. Thus, carbon can exist as four isotopes, carbons 11, 12, 13 and 14. C12 and C13 are stable isotopes and detected by the mass spectrometer; C11 and C14 are radioactive, i.e. they continually break down with the emission of radioactive particles or radiation. These isotopes are detected through the radiation emitted.

Isotopes incorporated into physiological substances, such as amino acids, enable those substances to be traced in their reactions in the body.

See *labelled substances*; *irradiation*.

**isozymes** Isoenzymes.

**i.u.** International unit, which see.

# J

**JACNE** Joint Advisory Committee on Nutrition Education. (A UK working party that puts nutritional guidelines into popular language.)

**jaffarine** Name given to cross between grapefruit and tangerine, mandarin and orange and tangerine.

**jaggery** Coarse dark sugar made from the sap of the coconut palm; or raw sugar cane juice, used in India as sweetening agent – also known as gur.

Used also to prevent oxidative rancidity of fats, since it contains a natural antioxidant.

**jake paralysis** See *Jamaica ginger paralysis*.

**jak fruit** Tropical fruit that grows from the trunk and large boughs of *Artocarpus integrifolia, A. heterophyllus* and *A. integra*. Both pulp and seeds are eaten.

Analysis per 100 g, pulp: carbohydrate 10 g, protein 2.5 g, carotene 130 µg, vitamin $B_1$ 0.1 mg, nicotinic acid 0.4 mg.

Seeds: carbohydrate 30 g, protein 3.5 g.

**jam** Fruit preserve set to a gel by reaction between acid, pectin and added sugar. The solution of pectin in the fruit is caused to conglomerate by the sugar and forms a network of fibres enclosing liquid, i.e. a jelly. This only occurs under acid conditions, pH 2.5–3.5, optimum sugar concentration 67.5%. Normally 0.5–1% pectin used in jam manufacture.

Legally jam must contain not less than 68% soluble solids (or 65% if hermetically sealed). Minimum fruit content: blackberry, strawberry and greengage 38%; blackcurrant 25%; damson, redcurrant, strawberry-and-gooseberry 35%; gooseberry, raspberry, loganberry 30%; marmalade 20%. (UK regulations.)

See also *pectin*.

**Jamaica ginger paralysis** Polyneuritis caused by poisoning from an illicit extract of Jamaica ginger ('jake') affecting thousands of people in the USA in 1930. Due to triorthocresyl phosphate.

**Jamaica pepper** See *allspice*.

**jam, extra** Standard jam, with certain exceptions, contains a minimum of 35 g of fruit per 100 g; extra jam, with certain exceptions, contains 45 g.

**jejunum** Second portion of the small intestine, between the duodenum and the ileum.

**jelly** A colloidal suspension that has set; may be made from gelatin, pectin, agar, usually flavoured with fruit juice or synthetic flavour.

**jerked beef** Dried meat of South America, similar to biltong. See also *charqui*.

**jerky** Jerked (dried) meat.

**Jesuit's bark** Cinchona bark, source of quinine.

**Job's tears** Adlay, which see.

**jodbasedow** See *thyrotoxicosis*.

**jojoba oil** Liquid wax of long chain fatty acids (eicosenoic and docosenoic (erucic) acids) esterfied with eicosanol and docosanol alcohols from seeds of shrub *Simmondsia chinensis*. Of interest in cosmetics as replacement for sperm whale oil but also has food applications, e.g. coating agent for dried fruits.

**jonathan** Calcined, ground oat chaff used as adulterant for maize and other cereals (mid-nineteenth century).

**joule** Unit of energy; used to express energy content of foods and energy expenditure of man and animals. Gradually adopted as replacement for the calorie from about 1970, in accordance with International System of Units.

4.184 J = 1 calorie; 1000 J = 1 kJ = 0.239 kcal; 1000 kJ = 1 MJ.

**jowar** Indian name for sorghum (*Sorghum vulgare*) (great millet, kaffir corn, guinea corn). See under *sorghum*.

**Judas goat** Sheep cannot readily be driven to slaughter but will follow a goat. A Judas goat is used to lead the sheep to the killing pens.

**julienne**   Vegetables cut into thin, match-like strips. Also a clear, vegetable soup.

**junket**   Precipitated protein of milk (casein only) carrying the fat with it and leaving behind the clear whey. The precipitation is carried out with the enzyme rennin.

# K

$K_i$ **(enzyme)**   The $K_i$ of an enzyme inhibitor is an index of the potency of a given compound as an inhibitor of that enzyme; in practical terms it is the concentration of inhibitor which leads to 50% inhibition of the enzyme.

$K_m$ **(enzyme)**   The $K_m$ of an enzyme (Michaelis constant) is an index of its affinity for the substrate; in practical terms it is the substrate concentration that results in half maximum velocity of reaction.

**kaffir beer**   A beer brewed from kaffir corn grain (sorghum), kaffircorn malt, and various maize products.

**kaffir corn**   Variety of millet, which see.

**kamaboko**   Japanese fish paste made from surimi, sometimes with added starch.

**kaoliang**   Sorghum, Chinese sorghum, *Sorgum nervosum*; also name of drink made from.

**Karaya gum**   Obtained from East Indian trees of the genus *Sterculia*. Used as stabiliser, e.g. in frozen water ices; also used in combination with other stabilisers; sometimes used as a laxative.

Also called sterculia gum.

**Karell diet**   For patients with severe cardiac failure. It is a low-calorie fluid diet consisting of 800 ml milk given in four feeds; it provides 550 kcal (2.3 MJ), 28 g protein and 0.45 g (20 mEq.) of sodium and is given for only two or three days.

**Karl Fischer method**   Titrimetric method of determining small amounts of water, 0.5–1%, in fats or fatty foods.

**Karo Syrup**   Trade name (Corn Products Refining Co., USA) for a dextromaltose preparation made from maize starch, used as a carbohydrate modifier in milk preparations for infant feeding. Consists of a mixture of dextrin, maltose, glucose and sucrose.

**kasha**   See *buckwheat*.

**katadyn process**   See *oligodynamic*.

**katemfe**   *Thaumatococcus daniellii*. Intensely sweet African fruit, called katemfe in Sierra Leone and miraculous fruit of the Sudan (not the same as Miracle Berry). Active principle, protein named thaumatin; 1600 times as sweet as sucrose on weight basis; 100 000 times as sweet on molar basis.

**kathepsins**   See *cathepsins*.

**kcal**   Kilocalorie; see also *calorie*.

**kebab**   General name (Oriental) for meat, usually two or three kinds, grilled on charcoal; the pieces of meat are interspersed with vegetables.

**kebobs**   Indian dish; slices of mutton or fowl dipped in eggs and cooked on skewer.

**kedgeree**   Indian dish of rice, split pulse, onions, eggs, etc.; European dish of fish, rice, eggs, etc. (Hindustani, *khichri*).

**kefir**   See *milks, fermented*.

**Kellogg's Special K**   Trade name for an enriched breakfast cereal.
Analysis per 100 g: 19 g protein, 1 g fat, 73 g available carbohydrate, 360 kcal (1.5 MJ), 3.4 g dietary fibre, 1 g sodium, 13 mg iron, 1.2 mg thiamin, 1.7 mg riboflavin, 18 g niacin, 2.2 mg vitamin $B_6$, 2.8 µg vitamin D.

**kelp**   Any of several species of genus *Laminaria* – large brown seaweeds. Occasionally used as food or food ingredient but mostly the ash is used as a source of alkali and iodine. Sometimes claimed as a 'health' food with unspecified properties.

**Kempner diet**   Or rice diet. A diet low in salt, comprising rice, fruit, fruit juices, sugar and vitamins, containing about 2000 kcal (8.4 MJ), 15–30 g protein and 100–150 mg sodium per day, for patients suffering from congestive heart failure, cirrhosis of the liver, hypertensive disease, toxaemias of pregnancy and certain kidney disorders.
See also *salt-free diets*.

**kephalins**   Or cephalins; phosphatides similar to lecithins but composed of glycerol, fatty acids, phosphoric acid and ethanolamine (instead of choline). Found in brain and nerve tissue; part of cell structure.

**Kepler extract of malt**   Trade name for one of the earliest of the malt extracts, intended as a dietary supplement and to aid the digestion, since it was rich in diastase compared with ordinary malt extracts.

**keratin**   Insoluble protein of hair, horns, hoofs, feathers and nails. See *albuminoids*.
Not hydrolysed by digestive enzymes, therefore useless as food. Used as fertiliser, since it is slowly broken down by soil bacteria. Steamed feather meal is used to some extent as supplement for ruminants.
Those proteins not digested by proteases have been designated eukeratins, as distinct from pseudokeratins of skin and eye lens, which are digested by proteases and contain less cystine.

**Kesp** Trade name (originally Courtaulds Ltd) for a textured vegetable protein made by the spinning process.

**ketchup** (catsup or catchup) From the Chinese *koechap* or *kitsiap*, originally meaning brine of pickled fish. Now used for a spicy sauce or condiment made with juice of fruit or vegetables, vinegar and spices. Tomato ketchup is a common sauce.

**ketogenic diet** A diet poor in carbohydrate (20–30 g) and rich in fat; causes accumulation of the ketone bodies in the tissues; used to be used in the treatment of epilepsy.

**ketonaemia** Accumulation in the blood of ketone bodies, which see.

**ketone bodies** Name given to the penultimate products of fatty acid metabolism – acetoacetic acid, betahydroxybutyric acid and acetone. They can be oxidised at only a limited rate, and when their production rate is excessive, as in diabetes and starvation, they accumulate in the blood (ketonaemia), and are excreted in the urine (ketonuria).

**ketonic rancidity** Certain moulds of *Penicillium* and *Aspergillus* species attack fats containing short carbon chains and produce ketones with a characteristic odour and taste – so-called ketonic rancidity. Fats such as butter, coconut and palm kernel are most susceptible.

**Ketonil** Trade name (Merck, Sharp & Dohme, USA) for protein-rich food low in phenylalanine for feeding patients with phenylketonuria.

**ketonuria** See *ketone bodies*.

**ketosis** Clinical condition in which ketone bodies (which see) accumulate in the blood and appear in the urine.

**khatta** See *clay*.

**khuri** See *clay*.

**khushkhash** Israeli term for the bitter orange. See *orange, bitter*.

**kidney clearance test** Test of kidney function by measuring the ability to excrete injected inulin, urea or a dye, in the urine. The quantity excreted per minute divided by the amount present in 1 ml of plasma is the urinary clearance.

**kieves** Irish term for mash tuns, which see.

**kilderkin** Cask for beer (18 gallons – 80 litres) and ale (16 gallons).

**kilocalorie** See *calorie*.

**kinetic energy** See *energy*.

**kipper** Herring that has been lightly salted and smoked (see also *red herrings*), invented by John Woodger, a fish curer of Seahouses, Northumberland, 1843.

Analysis per 100 g, without bones and skin, baked: protein 23 g, fat 11 g, carbohydrate nil, kcal 200 (0.8 MJ), Ca 65 mg, Fe 1.4 mg.

**kitol** An inactive form of vitamin A found in whale liver (*kitos*, Greek for whale) which is converted into retinol by heating at 200°C.

**Kjeldahl determination** Widely used method of determining total nitrogen in a substance by digesting with sulphuric acid and a catalyst in a Kjeldahl (long-necked) flask. The nitrogen is converted to ammonia which is then measured.

In foodstuffs most of the nitrogen is protein, and the term crude protein is the total 'Kjeldahl nitrogen' multiplied by the factor 6.25.

**Klim** Trade name (Borden Co., USA) for dried milk.

**klipfish** Salted and dried cod, mainly produced in Norway. The fish is boned, stored in salt for a month, washed and dried slowly. It is known as bacalao in South America.

**Kofranyi–Michaelis spirometer** Instrument that records the volume of expired air and takes samples at intervals for subsequent analysis. It thus serves as an indirect measure of the energy expended by the subject (indirect calorimetry).

**kohlrabi** Swollen stem of *Brassica oleracea gongylodes* (turnip rooted cabbage, kale turnip (USA)); green and purple varieties.

Analysis per 100 g: water 90 g, protein 2 g, fat 0.1 g, carbohydrate 6 g, vitamin C 70 mg, 30 kcal (120 kJ).

**koji** See *miso*.

**konjac** Gum derived from tubers of *Amorphophallus konjac* C. Koch; eaten in Japan as firm jelly. Chemical structure consists of linear co-polymer of D-glucose and D-mannose in molar ratio 1:1.6.

**kosher** The selection and preparation of foods in accordance with traditional Jewish ritual and dietary laws.

The only kosher flesh foods are from animals that chew the cud and have cloven hoofs, such as cattle, sheep, goats and deer, and the hindquarters must not be eaten. The only fish permitted are those with fins and scales; birds of prey and scavengers are not kosher. Moreover, the animals must be slaughtered according to ritual before the meat can be considered kosher. From Hebrew 'Kosher', meaning 'right'. (*Deuteronomy*, Chap. 14.)

**Krebs' cycle** See *citric acid cycle*.

**Krebs' solution** Solution of inorganic salts with ionic composition similar to that of mammalian blood serum; with the addition of glucose, tissue slices continue to respire in such a solution. (Contains Na, Ca, Mg, K, Cl, $PO_4$, $SO_4$, $HCO_3$, $CO_2$.)

**Kreis test** For oxidative rancidity of fats. Fat treated with a solution of phloroglucinol in ether and hydrochloric acid – a pink colour develops in rancid fat, due to the presence of epihydrin aldehyde.

**krill**  Term that refers to many species of planktonic crustaceans but is mostly used in connection with the shrimp *Euphausia superba*. This is the main food of whales, certain types of penguins and seabirds; occurs in shoals in the Antarctic, containing up to $12\,kg/m^3$. Contains 15% protein and is collected in limited quantities for use as human food.

**kryptoxanthin**  Alternative spelling of cryptoxanthin, which see.

**kuban**  See *milks, fermented*.

**kumiss**  See *milks, fermented*.

**kümmel**  Liqueur prepared from caraway seeds, fennel and orris root.

  Alcoholic strength varies from 60 to 75% of proof spirit.

**kumquat**  A citrus fruit of the genus *Fortunella*; widely distributed in S. China; resembles citrus fruits, but very small, acid pulp, and sweet, edible skin.

**Kunitz inhibitors**  Protease inhibitors found in soyabeans together with another type called the Bowman–Birk inhibitors.

**kurrat**  Plant closely related to leek.

**kwashiorkor**  See *protein-energy malnutrition*.


# L


**l-**  Obsolete prefix indicating laevorotatory, now replaced by $(-)$. See *optical activity*.

**L-**  See D-.

**labelled substances**  To follow the progress of a substance, foodstuff or drug, through the body, it is sometimes marked or labelled so that it can readily be distinguished. Such labels may be chemical radicals that are abnormal and can therefore be distinguished, e.g. the introduction of phenyl groups into fatty acids, or, more recently, the use of radioactive substances. See *irradiation; isotopes*.

**laccase**  Enzyme in bacteria, potato and mushrooms that converts polyphenols to quinones.

**lacquer**  In reference to tinned foods, a layer of gum and gum resin coated onto the tinplate and hardened with heat. The layer of lacquer protects the tin lining from attack by acid fruit juices.

**lactalbumin**  One of the proteins of milk; casein 3%, lactalbumin 0.5%, lactoglobulin 0.25%. Not precipitated from acid solution as casein is; hence, during cheese-making the whey contains the lactalbumin and lactoglobulin. They are precipitated by heat, and a whey cheese can be made in this way.

**lactaminic acid**  See *sialic acid*.

**lactase**  Enzyme that splits milk sugar, lactose, into glucose and galactose; present in the pancreatic juice.

**lactein bread** Another name for milk loaf, i.e. loaf to which skim milk powder has been added.

**lactenin** Not a specific compound but the name given (1894) to a substance believed to be present in cow and goat milk which had antibacterial properties.

**lactic acid** The acid produced by the fermentation of milk sugar and responsible for the flavour of sour milk and precipitation of the casein curd in cottage cheese.

Also produced by fermentation in silage, pickles, sauerkraut, cocoa, tobacco – its value here is in suppressing the growth of unwanted organisms.

In mammalian muscle metabolism the first stages of breakdown of glucose end at pyruvic acid. In severe exercise this is reduced to lactic acid, which can accumulate in the muscles. Similarly formed in meat muscle from glycogen immediately after death.

Used as an acidulant (as well as citric and tartaric acids) in sugar confectionery, soft drinks, pickles and sauces.

See also *pickling*; *sarcolactic acid*.

**lactic acid, buffered** Mixture of lactic acid and sodium lactate – used in sugar confectionery to provide acid taste without inversion of the sugar which would take place at lower pH.

**lactide** Compound formed by reaction between two molecules of an alpha-hydroxy acid, with the loss of two molecules of water and the formation of a ring compound containing two oxygen atoms in the ring.

**lactitol** Alcohol derivative of lactulose – galactopyranosyl-sorbitol, ($C_{12}H_{22}O_{11}$). Less sweet than lactulose and so preferred as means of reducing pH in colon (see *lactulose*). Also called lactit, lactositol, lactobiosit.

Not digested by digestive enzymes but fermented by bacteria to short chain fatty acids and yields about 2 kcal/g – hence of potential use as low-calorie bulk sweetener; also retards crystallisation and improves moisture retention.

**Lactobacillus casei factor** See *folic acid*.

**lactobiose** Lactose.

**lactochrome** Pigment in milk.

**lactoferrin** Iron-protein complex in human milk (only a trace in cow's milk) only partly saturated with iron; has a role in inhibiting the growth of *E. coli*.

**lactoflavin** Obsolete name for vitamin $B_2$; so named because it was isolated from milk.

**lactoglobulin** See *lactalbumin*.

**lactollin** Protein found (1962) in small traces in bovine milk; of unusual composition, lacking methionine and with little alanine.

**lactometer**   Floating device used to measure the specific gravity of milk (1.027–1.035).

**lactone**   Compound formed by loss of water from a molecule of a hydroxy acid to form a ring compound or inner ester, e.g. gluconic acid forms gluconolactone.

**lac-tone**   Protein-rich baby food (26% protein) made in India from peanut flour, skim milk powder, wheat flour and barley flour with added vitamins and calcium.

**lacto-ovo-vegetarian**   One whose diet is composed of vegetables, fruit, milk and eggs, but no flesh foods.

**lactose**   Milk sugar, 4.8% of milk. A disaccharide that is hydrolysed by acid or the enzyme lactase to glucose and galactose. Fermented by micro-organisms to lactic acid; hence the souring of milk by lactobacilli.

Used pharmaceutically as tablet filler and as medium for growth of micro-organisms.

Ordinary lactose is alpha lactose (16% of the sweetness of sucrose); if crystallized above 93 °C, is changed to the beta form, which is more soluble and sweeter than the alpha form.

**lactose intolerance**   See *disaccharide intolerance*.

**lacto-serum**   Grandiloquent word for whey.

**lactostearin**   See *glyceryl lactostearate*.

**lactulose**   Disaccharide, 4-*O*-beta-galactopyranosyl-D-fructose. Does not occur naturally but formed in heated or stored milk by isomerisation of lactose. About half as sweet as sucrose.

Not hydrolysed by human digestive enzymes but fermented by intestinal bacteria to form lactic and pyruvic acids. Thought to promote the growth of *Lactobacillus bifidus* and so added to some infant formulae; in large amounts is laxative.

Used to treat portal-system encephalopathy by lowering pH in colon and so restricting resorption of ammonia.

**ladies' fingers**   See *okra*; also a short kind of banana.

**laetrile**   Name given to extract of apricot kernels – amygdalin (a glucoside of benzaldehyde and cyanide). Claimed as a cure for cancer. So-called vitamin $B_{17}$.

**laevorotatory**   See *optical activity*.

**laevulose**   Alternative name for fructose.

**lager**   See *beer*.

**lamb**   Meat from sheep younger than 12–14 months. Genuine spring lamb, 3–6 months; spring lamb up to 1 year.

Analysis per 100 g: protein 13 g, fat 7 g, kcal 200 (0.5 MJ), Fe 1.5 mg, vitamin A nil, vitamin $B_1$ 0.12 mg, vitamin $B_2$ 0.15 mg, nicotinic acid 3.8 mg, vitamin C nil.

Hoggets are 1-year-old sheep; tegs are 2 years old; shearlings 15–18 months.

**langouste**  See *lobster*.

**lanoline**  The fat from wool. Consists of a mixture of cholesterol oleate, cholesterol palmitate and cholesterol stearate, and therefore not useful as food; used in various cosmetics.

**larch gum**  Polymer of 1 part arabinose and 6 parts galactose found in the aqueous extract of the Western larch tree (*Larix occidentalis*); potential substitute for gum arabic, since it is readily dispersed in water.

**lard**  Best quality from fat surrounding stomach and kidneys of pig, but also from sheep and cattle.

Neutral Lard No. 1 – kidney and bowel fat rendered below 50°C; Neutral Lard No. 2 – back fat rendered below 50°C; Leaf Lard – residues from top two qualities rendered in autoclave; Prime Steam Lard – fat from any part of the carcass rendered in the autoclave.

**lard compounds**  Blends of animal fats, such as oleostearin or premier jus, with vegetable oils to produce products similar to lard in consistency and texture.

Vegetable shortenings made from mixtures of partially hardened vegetable fats with the consistency of lard are referred to as lard substitutes.

**lardine**  See *margarine*.

**larding**  Method of adding fat to lean meat so that it does not dry during long slow cooking. Narrow strips of bacon fat, 1–1½ inches long and ¾ inch wide, are threaded into the surface of the meat with a special larding needle. The strips are called lardoons.

Barding is the process of tying a thin sheet of bacon fat over the meat.

**lard, leaf**  Made from the residue of kidney and back fat after the preparation of neutral lard (at 50°C) by treating with water above 100°C in an autoclave. See *lard, neutral*.

**lard, neutral**  Highest-quality pig fat, prepared by agitating the minced fat with water at a temperature below 50°C. Kidney fat provides No. 1 quality; back fat provides No. 2 quality.

**lathyrism**  Spastic paralysis of the lower limbs caused by high intake of *Lathyrus sativus* (Kesari dhal, chickling pea, chickling vetch), which contains the neurotoxin β-*N*-oxalyl-amino-L-alanine (BOAA). The crop is often grown in dry districts in Asia and N. Africa together with wheat, and normally little is eaten; but when there is a drought and the wheat crop is poor, the dhal predominates and is eaten as the principal food, and lathyrism can result.

**lauric acid**  One of the long-chain fatty acids, $CH_3(CH_2)_{10}COOH$. Occurs as the triglyceride in seeds of the spice bush and to lesser extent in butter, coconut oil and palm oil.

**laver** Edible seaweed. Laver bread is made from the seaweed *Porphyra* by boiling in salted water and mincing to a gelatinous mass. It is made into a cake with oatmeal or fried. Locally known in S. Wales as Bara lawr.

**lax** (lox) Scandinavian term for salmon; term used for smoked salmon in the USA.

**laxarinic acid** See *maltol*.

**laxative** Substance that accelerates the passage of food through the intestine. If it alters peristaltic activity, it is termed a purgative; other types stimulate or depress the muscular activity of the gut.

Cellulose acts as a purgative by retaining water and increasing the volume of intestinal contents; Epsom salts function similarly through osmotic pressure. Castor oil is hydrolysed by lipase to liberate ricinoleic acid which irritates the intestinal mucosa. Drugs such as aloes, senna, cascara, rhubarb and phenolphthalein irritate the intestine.

**LC$_{50}$** Median lethal concentration; used of substances in gaseous form.

**LD$_{50}$** A measure of toxicity – the amount of the substance that kills 50% of the test population when administered as a single dose.

**LDL** Low-density lipoproteins. See *lipids, plasma*.

**lead** Of no dietary interest except that it is toxic and its effects are cumulative. May be present in food from traces naturally present in the soil, from shellfish that have absorbed it from seawater, as lead arsenate used as insecticide and from lead glazes on vessels. Traces are excreted in the urine.

**leaf lard** See *lard, leaf*.

**lean body mass** Measure of body composition excluding adipose tissue, i.e. cells, extracellular fluid and skeleton.

**Lean cuisine** Trade name (Stouffer, USA, Findus-Nestlé, Europe) for a range of frozen meals prepared to a specified energy content.

**leathers, fruit** (mango leathers, tomato leathers, etc.) Fruit purées dried in air in thin layers 4–5 mm thick then built up into thicker preparations.

**leaven** Yeast. Also used for a mixture of yeast, sugar and a small amount of flour which has already started to ferment and so is ready to add to the flour dough to make a loaf.

**leben** See *fermented milks*.

**lecithins** Fatty substances of the type called phosphatides; consist of glycerol, fatty acids, phosphoric acid and choline. Important in the body for fat transport.

Used in food technology as emulsifiers, e.g. in chocolate; help emulsification; save cocoa butter; and prevent bloom. Also used as anti-spattering agents in frying fats. Obtained commercially from soyabean, peanut and corn.

From a dietary point of view lecithins form a very small fraction of the total fat intake, and may be considered simply as fats.

**lectins**  Older name 'haemagglutinins' or 'phytoagglutinins'; toxic substances found in many legumes which cause red blood cells to agglutinate *in vitro*. Raw or undercooked beans of some varieties of *Phaseolus vulgaris* cause vomiting and diarrhoea within 2 hours of consumption due to the high level of lectins but they are rapidly destroyed by boiling.

**leek**  *Allium ampeloprasum*; a member of the onion family which has been known as a food for over 4000 years (eaten by the Israelites at the time of the Exodus from Egypt). The lower part is usually blanched by planting in trenches or earthing up, and is eaten along with the upper long green leaves.

Analysis per 100 g: 30 kcal (130 kJ), 2 g protein, 6 g carbohydrate, 300 mg K, 60 mg Ca, 1 mg Fe, 2 mg carotene in the leaves and only a trace in the blanched bulb, 20 mg vitamin C, small amounts of B vitamins.

**legumes, food**  Members of the Leguminosae family eaten by man and domestic animals. Consumed as dry mature seeds (grain legumes or pulses) or as immature green seeds in pod.

Include ground nut, *Arachis hypogaea* and soyabean, *Glycine max*, grown for their oil and protein. Also the yam bean *Pachyrrhizus erosus* and African yam bean *Sphenostylis stenocarpa*, grown for their edible tubers as well as seeds.

*Phaseolus vulgaris* – navy, Boston, pinto, string, snapbean (USA), haricot, kidney, and when unripe, French, wax bean (UK), flageolet (yellow variety).

*P. coccineus (P. multiflora)* – runner, scarlet runner, multiflora bean.

*P. acutifolius (var. latifolius)* – tepary, rice haricot bean, Texan bean (USA).

*P. lunatus (lumensis, inamoenus)* – Lima bean (USA), butter bean (UK), Madagascar butter, Rangoon, Burma, Sieva bean.

*Cajanus cajan (C. indicus)* – pigeon, Angola, non-eye pea, Congo bean or pea, red gram, yellow dhal.

*Vigna umbellata (P. calcaratus)* – rice bean, red bean, (also used for adzuki bean).

*Vigna mungo (P. mungo)* – urd bean, black gram, mash.

*V.* or *P. angularis* adzuki bean.

*Vigna unguiculata* (or *sesquipedalis* or *sinensis* – systematics confused) – cow pea, black-eyed bean or pea, China pea, cowgram, catjang, Southern pea.

*Vigna unguiculata* – subspecies *sesquipedalis* (L) – asparagus bean, pea bean, yard long bean.

*V. aconitifolia (P. aconitifolia)* – moth, mat bean, Turkish gram.

*V. radiata (P. aureus, P. radiatus)* – mung bean, green or golden gram.

*Lablab purpureus (Dolichos lablab)* – Bonavista, Dolichos, Egyptian kidney, Indian butter, lablab, tonga, hyacinth bean.

*Canavalia ensiformis* – jack, overlook, sword bean.

*Lens culinaris (esculenta)* – lentil, red dhal, masur dhal, split pea.

*Pisum sativa* – garden, green pea.

*Pisum sativum* var *macrocarpon* – sugar pea, mange tout.

*Pisum arvense* – field pea.

*Voandzeia subterranea* – Bambar(r)a groundnut, earth pea, ground bean, Kaffir pea, Madagascar groundnut.

*Cicer aretinum* – chick pea, Bengal gram.

*Cyamopsis tetragonoloba* – cluster bean.

*Lathyrus sativus* – grass, lathyrus, chickling pea, Indian vetch, khesari dhal.

*Macrotyloma uniflorum (Dolichos uniflorus)* – horse gram, horse grain, kulthi bean, Madras gram.

*Mucuna pruriens* – velvet bean.

*Psophocarpus tetragonolobus* – winged bean, asparagus bean or pea, four-cornered, Goa, Manila, Mauritius bean.

*Vicia faba* – broad bean, faba, field, horse, pigeon, trick, windsor bean.

**legumin** Globulin protein in pea, bean and lentil.

**Lehmann process** Method of treating straw to render it digestible by cattle. The straw is chopped and soaked in 1.5% sodium hydroxide, when it is delignified. The process raises the starch equivalent by a factor of 3–4.

**lemon** Fruit of *Citrus limon*; contains 40–60 mg vitamin C per 100g fruit or per 100 ml juice.

**lemon curd** Cooked mixture of sugar, butter, eggs and lemons. Legally 4% fat, 0.33% citric acid, 1% dried egg or equivalent, 0.125% oil of lemon or 0.25% oil of orange, not less than 65% soluble solids (UK regulations.)

**lemon oil** The peel oil – 0.15–0.3% of the weight of the fruit; 90% limonene, together with phellandrene, terpinene, camphene, bisabolene, cadinene, citral, etc.

**Lenhartz diet** For peptic ulcer patients (originated 1915); mainly fluid diet including raw eggs, milk, boiled rice and vegetable purées fed at frequent intervals.

**lentils** Seeds of many varieties of *Lens esculenta*; fall into the same group as peas and beans. There is a green variety and an orange-red variety that are commonly imported into Europe from Egypt and India. Frequently used as a soup thickener in the powder form. See *legumes, food*.

Analysis per 100 g: protein 24 g, fat 1.8 g, kcal 350 (1.45 MJ), Ca 60 mg, Fe 6 mg, carotene 30 μg, vitamin $B_1$ 0.5 mg, vitamin $B_2$ 0.2 mg, nicotinic acid 1.8 mg.

**lettuce** Leaves of the plant *Lactuca sativa*. Not a very valuable food: the vitamin C is only one-seventh of that of cabbage.

Analysis per 100 g: protein 0.9 g, fat 0.1 g, kcal 10 (0.04 MJ), Ca 17 mg, Fe 0.3 mg, carotene 40 μg, vitamin $B_1$ 0.03 mg, vitamin $B_2$ 0.06 mg, nicotinic acid 0.1 mg, vitamin C 5 mg.

**leucine** An essential amino acid; rarely limiting in foods. Chemically, amino isocaproic acid.

**leucocytes** White blood cells, normally 5000–9000 per cubic millimetre; includes polymorphonuclear neutrophils, lymphocytes, monocytes, polymorphonuclear eosinophils and polymorphonuclear basophils. A 'white cell count' determines the total; a 'differential cell count' estimates the numbers of each type.

Fever, haemorrhage, violent exercise cause an increase – leucocytosis; starvation and debilitating conditions cause a decrease – leucopenia.

**leucocytosis** Increase in the white cells in the blood. See *leucocytes*.

**leucopenia** Decrease in the white cells in the blood. See *leucocytes*.

**leucosin** One of the water-soluble proteins of wheat flour.

**leucovorin** Growth factor for *Leuconostoc citrovorum*, related to folic acid, which see.

**levans** Polymers of fructose (principal one is inulin) which occur in tubers and some grasses; hydrolysed to fructose.

**levitin** One of the proteins of egg yolk, about one-fifth of the total, the remainder being vitellin. Rich in sulphur and accounts for half of the sulphur in the yolk.

**Lieberkuhn, crypts of** Glands lining the small intestine which secrete intestinal juice.

**Liebermann–Burchard reaction** Test for unsaturated sterols; green colour when treated with chloroform, acetic anhydride and concentrated sulphuric acid.

**light** (or lite) As applied to foods usually indicates
(1) a lower content of fat compared with the standard product (breadspreads, sausages).

(2) Sodium chloride substitutes lower in sodium.

(3) Low-alcohol beers.

**lights**  Butchers' term for the lungs of an animal.

**lignin**  Associated with the carbohydrates of the cell wall of plants but not, itself, a carbohydrate, but a high molecular weight aromatic compound.

**lignocellulose**  Alternative name for lignin.

**lignoceric acid**  Long-chain fatty acid containing total of 24 carbon atoms (tetracosanoic acid); present in the cerebrosides and sphingomyelins.

**lime**  Fruit of *Citrus aurantifolia*, cultivated almost solely in the tropics, since it is not as hardy as other citrus fruits. Used to prevent scurvy in the British Navy (replacing, at the time, lemon juice) and so giving rise to the nickname of 'Limeys' for British sailors and for British people in general. Contains about 10–20 mg vitamin C per 100 g fruit or fresh juice.

**limit dextrin**  When a branched polysaccharide such as glycogen is hydrolysed enzymically (e.g. by phosphorylase), glucose is split off step by step until the branch point is reached. The hydrolysis then stops, leaving what is termed a limit dextrin. Further hydrolysis requires a different enzyme.

**limiting amino acid**  See *amino acid, limiting*.

**Limmisax**  Trade name (Leas Cliff) for saccharine.

**Limmits**  Trade name (Leas Cliff) for a 'slimming' preparation composed of wholemeal biscuits with a vitamin–methyl cellulose mixture as filling, containing vitamins A, $B_1$, $B_2$, nicotinamide, vitamins C and D, with iron, calcium, iodide and phosphate. Intended to replace a meal or meals with a reduced calorie diet. Six biscuits contain 1050 kcal (4.2 MJ).

**limonin**  Bitter principle in the albedo of the Valencia orange. Similarly, isolimonin is the bitter principle of the navel orange. Both are present in a non-bitter, water-soluble state, and are liberated into the juice during extraction. On standing they slowly hydrolyse and the juice becomes bitter. Not present in the ripe fruit.

**linamarin**  Cyanogenetic glucoside found in cassava (manioc) which may be a cause of neuropathies in areas where cassava is a major food. 2[β-D-glucopyranosyl oxy] isobutyro nitrite. Usually the cyanide is removed by enzymic action initiated by grating the tuber and then exposing to the air.

**linoleic acid**  Straight chain fatty acid of 18 carbon atoms with two double bonds. Chemical nomenclature numbers carbons from carboxyl group, i.e. double bonds are at carbons 9–10 and 12–13. For metabolic purposes biochemical nomenclature numbers from the terminal methyl group so linoleic is

18:2ω6-*cis*, 9-*cis* (ω indicating the first carbon with the double bond).

Cures all symptoms of essential fatty acid deficiency; is the predominant polyunsaturated fatty acid in most edible vegetable oils. See *essential fatty acids*.

**linolenic acid**   α-form, 18:3ω 3-*cis*, 6-*cis*, 9-*cis* (see *linoleic acid* for nomenclature); has some essential fatty acid properties but restores only growth in deprived animals; found in oils from seeds of evening primrose, borage and blackcurrant.

γ-linolenic, 18:3ω6, is more potent than linoleic in curing all symptoms of EFA deficiency; a minor constituent of oils except linseed, soya and rapeseed. See *essential fatty acids*.

**Lintner value**   Measure of diastatic activity using soluble starch as a substrate and measuring the effect by Fehling's solution. Applied to flour, malt extract, etc.

**liothyronine**   Alternative name for L-tri-iodo thyronine, the most potent of the hormones of the thyroid gland. Used as an aid to weight reduction by stimulating the metabolism of the body.

**lipase**   Enzyme that hydrolyses fat to glycerol and fatty acid. Has a low specificity and will attack any triglyceride or long-chain ester. Present in the intestinal juice and in many seeds and grains. Sometimes responsible for development of rancidity in stored foods.

Lipases from different sources, e.g. digestive juices or seeds, appear to be similar but attack the substrates at different rates.

**lipides**   See *lipids*.

**lipids** (lipides, lipins)   General term embracing fats, oils, waxes, complex compounds such as phosphatides and cerebrosides, sterol esters and terpenes. Their common property is insolubility in water and solubility in non-polar solvents, including chloroform, hydrocarbons and alcohols. Most include fatty acids in their structure.

**lipids, plasma**   Triglycerides, free and esterified cholesterol and phospholipids found in the blood plasma bound in specific lipoprotein complexes. The latter can be separated by electrophoresis or by density; the heaviest are the chylomicrons of triglycerides, very low-density lipoproteins (VLDL), low-density lipoproteins (LDL), and high-density lipoproteins (HDL).

**lipins**   See *lipids*.

**lipocaic**   Unidentified factor in the pancreas that prevents the deposition of fat in the liver.

**lipochromes**   Plant pigments soluble in fats and organic solvents, e.g. chlorophyll, carotenoids.

**lipofuscin**   Group of pigments that accumulate in several body tissues, particularly the myocardium, during life and are consequently associated with the aging process.

**lipoic acid** Essential growth factor for various micro-organisms; discovered in yeast and liver extracts and called by various workers acetate replacement factor, pyruvate oxidation factor, thioctic acid and protogen. Chemically, dithio-octanoic acid.

In combination with vitamin $B_1$, phosphate and coenzyme A, lipoic acid forms lipothiamide, essential for the oxidative decarboxylation in carbohydrate metabolism.

**lipolysis** The splitting of fats (to glycerol and fatty acid).

**lipolytic** Fat-splitting. Lipases are lipolytic enzymes.

**lipolytic rancidity** Some micro-organisms produce lipases, and these fat-splitting enzymes are also present in tissues. In stored foods they hydrolyse the fats to free fatty acids – so-called lipolytic rancidity. As the enzyme is destroyed by heat, this type of rancidity occurs only in uncooked foods.

**Lipomul** Trade name (USA) for a mixture of 10% glucose and 40% vegetable oil.

**lipothiamide** See *lipoic acid*.

**lipotropic substances** See *liver, fatty infiltration of*.

**lipovitellenin** A lipoprotein complex of egg comprising about one-sixth of the solids of the yolk.

**liquamen** (Garum) Ancient Roman sauce made from dried salted entrails of small fish.

**liqueurs** Distilled, flavoured and sweetened liquors from fermented sugar. For example, curaçao 30% (w/v) alcohol, 30% sugar; cherry brandy 19% alcohol, 33% sugar; advocaat 13% alcohol, 30% sugar, 0.75% nitrogen.

**liquid paraffin** See *medicinal paraffin*.

**liquefied herring** Herring reduced to liquid state by enzyme action at slightly acid pH; used as protein concentrate for animal feed.

**liquorice** Liquorice root and extract are obtained from the plant *Glycyrrhiza glabra*; stick liquorice is the crude evaporated extract of the root.

The plant has been grown in the Pontefract district of Yorkshire since the sixteenth century; hence the name of Pontefract cakes for the sugar confection of liquorice.

**lite** See *light*.

**litchi** *Litchi chinensis*, also lychee; native of China; the size of a small plum, with a translucent white jelly-like interior surrounding the seed.

Analysis per 100 g: 0.9 g protein, 0.5 g fat, 16 g carbohydrate, 70 kcal (0.28 MJ), 0.5 mg Fe, 0.04 mg vitamin $B_1$, 0.04 mg vitamin $B_2$, 0.3 mg nicotinic acid, 50 mg vitamin C.

**liver**   Liver from animals has the general composition of meat but is exceptionally rich in vitamins A, $B_1$, $B_2$, niacin and $B_{12}$. Vitamin A varies with the age and type of animal and its diet, and ranges between 3 and 50 mg per 100 g. Also contains vitamin D – 0.2–1 µg per 100 g.

Fish liver is a particularly rich source of vitamins A and D.

**liver factor 2**   Obsolete name for pantothenic acid.

**liver, fatty infiltration of**   Under the influence of liver poisons, and in the absence from the diet of substances containing methyl groups, there is a flow of fats to the liver – so-called fatty liver. This is prevented by lipotropic substances, which include choline, methionine and a pancreatic extract called lipocaic.

The affliction is aggravated on a high-fat diet and is found clinically on chronic low-protein diets.

**liver filtrate factor**   Obsolete name for panthothenic acid.

**livetin**   A water-soluble protein fraction of egg yolk.

**lobster**   Shellfish of various tribes of the suborder Macrura. True lobster (with claws), species of *Homarus*.

Norway lobster, scampi or Dublin Bay Prawn – *Nephrops norvegicus*.

Squat lobster – family Galatheidae.

Crayfish, freshwater – families Astacidae, Parastacidae and Austroastacidae.

Crawfish, spiny lobster, rock lobster or sea crayfish (without claws) – species of family Palinuridae.

Langouste – *Palinurus vulgaris*.

Analysis per 100 g: 20 g protein, 3 g fat, 120 kcal (0.5 MJ), 60 mg Ca, 0.8 mg Fe, 0.05 mg vitamin $B_2$, 1.5 mg nicotinic acid.

**Locasol**   Trade name (Trufood Ltd) for a low-calcium milk substitute.

Analysis per 100 g: protein 22.8 g, fat 19.9 g, carbohydrate 51.9 g, Ca 46 mg (dried milk Ca 960 mg), Fe 1.5 mg, kcal 474 (2.0 MJ).

**locksoy**   Fine drawn rice macaroni, Chinese.

**locoweed**   *Astralagus* spp. and *Oxytropus* spp. common in arid areas of western USA. Toxic to cattle causing neurologic damage and damage to reproduction (abortion, birth defects) – called locoism. Apparently caused by an alkaloid, swainsonine (alpha-mannosidase inhibitor), also found in mouldy hay.

**locust bean**   (1) Carob seed, which see.

(2) African locust bean, *Parkia* spp.

Analysis per 100 g: 26 g protein, 10 g fat, 47 g carbohydrate, 380 kcal (1.6 MJ), 300 mg Ca, 4 mg Fe, 0.06 mg vitamin $B_1$, 0.2 mg vitamin $B_2$, 3 mg nicotinic acid.

**Lofenalac**   Trade name (Mead Johnson) for food low in phenylalanine for treatment of phenylketonuria.

**loganberry**  Cross between the European raspberry and the Californian blackberry (named after L. H. Logan). Vitamin C content 40 mg per 100 g.

**logarithmic phase**  In reference to bacteria, means the most rapid period of growth when the numbers increase in geometric progression. Under ideal conditions bacteria can double in numbers every 20 minutes.

**Lohmann reaction**  Transfer of phosphate, with its energy, from adenosine triphosphate to creatine, to form adenosine diphosphate and creatine phosphate.

The first source of energy on muscle stimulation is adenosine triphosphate, leaving the diphosphate. This is resynthesised to the triphosphate by creatine phosphate, which thus serves as the reserve of energy. It is resynthesised during the recovery period by the Lohmann reaction.

**Lonalac**  Trade name (Mead Johnson) for a milk preparation free from sodium.

**loonzein**  Rice from which the husk has been removed; also known as brown rice, hulled rice and cargo rice.

**loquat**  *Eriobotyra japonica*, also known as Japanese medlar; small pear-shaped fruit; member of apple family.

**lotus**  *Nelumbium nuciferum*. Sacred lotus of India and China; water plant whose rhizomes and seeds are used as food. Other water plants of the same family whose seeds and rhizomes are eaten are the water-lilies, *Nymphaea*.

Analysis of rhizome per 100 g: 1.7 g protein, 11 g carbohydrate, 50 kcal (200 kJ), 1.5 mg Fe, 0.05 mg vitamin $B_1$, 20 mg vitamin C.

**Lovibond comparator**  Instrument for visual comparison of the depth of colour of a solution with a standard coloured glass slide.

A set of colour standards is usually made for each specific colour reaction, e.g. phosphate, pH determinations, etc. The comparator thus differs from the Tintometer (which see), as the latter is for general application and includes a range of colours and intensities.

**low-salt diets**  See *salt-free diets*.

**lox**  See *lax*.

**lozenges**  Shapes stamped out of mixture of icing sugar, glucose syrup and gum arabic or gelatin with flavourings, then hardened at 32–43°C.

**LSM**  US trade name for a low-sodium milk – contains 50 mg per litre; ordinary milk contains 500 mg sodium per litre.

**lucerne**  *Medicago sativa* L. Essentially a forage crop but eaten by man to a small extent.

**Lucozade**  Trade name (Beecham Foods Ltd) for a glucose beverage: 17.9% carbohydrate, 67 kcal per 100 g.

**Lugol's solution**  5% iodine in 10% potassium iodide.

**lumpfish**  Large sea fish, *Cylopterus lumpus*, pink eggs of which are salted, pressed and coloured and sold as Danish or German caviare.

**lupeose**  See *stachyose*.

**lupins**  Legumes of *Lupinus* spp. The ordinary lupin contains toxic alkaloids (quinolizidines) and tastes bitter; varieties selected for animal feed and grain crop are low in alkaloids and known as sweet lupins. 35–40% protein, 6–12% fat.

**lutein**  Alternative name for xanthophyll.

**luteol**  Alternative name for xanthophyll.

**luxus konsumption**  See *specific dynamic action*.

**Lycasin**  Trade name for hydrogenated glucose syrup. See *sweeteners, bulk*.

**lycine**  Obsolete name for betaine.

**lychee**  See *litchi*.

**lycopene**  Red pigment found in tomato, pink grapefruit and palm oil; straight-chain derivative of carotene with no vitamin A activity. The synthetic material is sometimes used as a food colour.

**lye-peeling**  Method of removing skins from vegetables by immersion in hot caustic soda followed by 'tumbling' in a washer to remove skin and chemicals.

**lymph**  The fluid intermediate between the blood and the tissues; the medium in which oxygen and nutrients are conveyed from the blood to the tissues, and waste products back to the blood.

Chemically similar to blood plasma; contains salts, serum albumin and globulins, fibrinogen, prothrombin and leucocytes (and can coagulate).

Part of the fat of the diet is absorbed without hydrolysis into the lymph, and transported to the thoracic lymph duct, whence the fat is discharged into the bloodstream. The lymph, rich in emulsified fat, is milky owing to the presence of fat droplets, called chylomicrons; the milky lymph is called chyle. Chyle and lymph differ only in their fat content.

**lymphatics**  Vessels through which the lymph flows.

**lyophilisation**  Expertise for freeze-drying, which see.

**lysergic acid**  See *ergot*.

**lysine**  An essential amino acid of special importance, since it is the limiting amino acid in many cereals. Can be synthesised on the commercial scale, and when added to bread or rice or cereal-based animal feeds, it improves the nutritive value of the protein.

Is dibasic and can be produced as the free lysine, and the mono- and dihydrochlorides. Appears to occupy a special position in amino acid metabolism, since it has a low 'turnover rate' in the body compared with other amino acids. Chemically, diaminocaproic acid.

See also **amino acid, limiting**.

**lysinoalanine** Amino acid (*N*-(DL-2-amino-2-carboxyl ethyl-L-lysine)) formed when proteins are heated or treated with alkali, by reaction between epsilon-amino group of lysine and dehydroalanine from cystine or serine. Present in many foods at levels about 1000 ppm and although high doses cause nephrocytomegaly in rats (lesions in kidney tubules) not considered a hazard to health.

**lysozyme** Enzyme that digests certain high-molecular-weight carbohydrates. Bacteria that contain these carbohydrates as part of their cell wall structure disintegrate or lyse under attack by lysozyme. Widely distributed, but particularly in egg-white, of which it comprises 2.5% of the total solids.

**lyxoflavin** Substance isolated from human heart muscle, similar to riboflavin but containing the sugar lyxose; function unknown.

**lyxose** Pentose sugar differing from xylose only in the position of the OH group on C2.

**lyxulose** Xylulose.

# M

**MA** Modified atmosphere, see **gas storage, controlled**.

**macaroni** See **alimentary pastes**.

**macassar gum** See **agar**.

**maccaroncelli** See **alimentary pastes**.

**mace** See **nutmeg**.

**macedoine** Mixture of fruits or vegetables, diced, or cut into even-shaped pieces.

**macerases** A group of enzymes (usually extracted from the mould *Aspergillus*) used to break down pectin in fruits to facilitate maximum extraction of the juice (breaks down the rhamnogalacturonan backbone of the pectin).

**mackerel** See **fish, fatty**.

**macon** Bacon made from mutton.

**maconochie** A tinned, meat stew much used in the First World War; made by Maconochie Brothers.

**macrobiotic diet** A system of eating associated with Zen Buddhism; consists of several stages finally reaching Diet 7 which is restricted to cereals. Cases of severe malnutrition have been reported on this 'diet'.

Includes the concept of 'yin' and 'yang' whereby foods, even different vitamins (and everything in life) are one or the other and must be balanced.

**macrocytes** Large red cells found in the blood in pernicious anaemia, due to disturbed development of the red blood cell. Hence macrocytic anaemia.

**magma** Mixture of sugar syrup and sugar crystals produced during sugar refining.

**magnesium** A dietary essential; present in all human tissues, especially bone. Involved in the utilisation and metabolism of ATP.

Present in chlorophyll and so in all green plant foods, and is generally plentiful in the diet. Deficiency in human beings gives rise to disturbances of muscle and nervous system; in cattle gives rise to grass tetany; in plants causes yellowing or 'chlorosis'.

**Maillard reaction** Two processes in foods can produce a brown colour. One is the enzymatic oxidation of phenolic substances, such as occurs at the cut surface of an apple. The other is a reaction between proteins or amino acids and sugars, and is variously known as the Maillard reaction, the browning reaction and non-enzymic browning. It takes place on heating or on prolonged storage and is one of the deteriorative processes that take place in stored foods. It is accompanied by a loss in nutritive value, since the part of the protein that reacts with the sugar is the free amino part of the lysine. This complex is not digested and there is thus a reduction in the biologically available lysine.

**maize** Grain of *Zea mays*, also called Indian corn. Staple food in many countries, made into tortillas in Latin America, made into polenta in Italy, and flaked as corn flakes commonly eaten as a breakfast cereal; various preparations in the southern states of the USA are known as hominy, samp and cerealine.

Two varieties of major commercial importance are flint corn (*Zea indurata*), which is very hard, and dent corn (*Zea dentata*); there is also sweet corn *Z. saccharata*, and a variety that expands on heating (popcorn).

The starch prepared from maize *Z. dentata* is termed corn flour; the ground maize is termed maize meal.

Analysis of sweetcorn, corn on the cob, per 100g: protein 4g, carbohydrate 24g, fat 2.5g, Fe 1mg, niacin 1.8mg, (not fully available), carotene 250µg.

Analysis of dent corn per 100g: 10g protein, 4g fat, 70g carbohydrate.

There is a white variety without any carotene; the yellow colour is partly due to cryptoxanthin (a vitamin A precursor).

The protein is low in both lysine and tryptophan, although there are high-lysine hybrid varieties.

**maize, flaked**  Partly gelatinised maize used for animal feed. The grain is cracked to small pieces, moistened, cooked and flaked between rollers.

**maize flour**  Highly refined and very finely ground maize meal from which all bran and germ has been removed.

**maize rice**  Finely cut maize with bran and germ partly removed; also called mealie rice.

**maize starches, waxy**  Starch obtained from hybrids of maize consisting wholly or largely (99%) of amylopectin compared with ordinary maize starch with 26% amylose and 74% amylopectin. The paste is semi-translucent, cohesive and does not form a gel.

**malabsorption syndrome**  Defect of absorption of one or more nutrients; signs include diarrhoea, steatorrhoea, abdominal distension, weight loss and specific signs of the nutrient deficiency.

**malic acid**  Organic acid occurring in many fruits, particularly in apples, tomatoes and plums. Molecular formula, $COOHCH(OH)CH_2COOH$ (i.e. hydroxysuccinic acid).

**mallorising**  Application of high temperature to pasteurising process – up to 265°F (129°C); named after inventor.

**malnutrition**  Disturbance of form or function arising from a deficiency or excess of one or more nutrients.

**Malpighia**  See *cherry, West Indian*.

**malt, malt extract**  Mixture of starch breakdown products containing mainly maltose (malt sugar), prepared from barley or wheat.

   The grain is allowed to sprout, when the enzyme diastase (or amylase) develops and hydrolyses the starch to maltose. The mixture is then extracted with hot water, and this malt extract contains a solution of starch breakdown products together with diastase. Malt extract may be the concentrated solution or evaporated to dryness.

   For brewing, a barley low in protein and rich in diastase is used and mixed with extra unmalted barley to provide more starch for the yeast fermentation.

   See also *diastatic activity*; *maltose*.

**maltase**  Enzyme that splits maltose (malt sugar) into two molecules of glucose; present in the pancreatic juice and intestinal juice.

**malted barley**  See *malt; malt extract*.

**malt flour**  Germinated barley or wheat, in dried form. As well as dextrins, glucose, proteins and salts derived from the cereal, it is rich in diastase and is added to wheat flour of low diastatic content for breadmaking; used as an ingredient of 'malt' loaf.

**Malthus**   Author of an essay in 1798 postulating that any temporary or local improvement in living conditions will increase population faster than the food supply, and that disasters such as war and pestilence, which check population growth, are inescapable features of human society.

**malting**   See *beer*.

**maltitol**   A polyol sweetener, 4-$O$-α-D-glucopyranosyl-D-sorbitol, produced by hydrogenation of maltose. Slowly hydrolysed in the digestive tract to glucose and sorbitol and fairly completely utilised, providing 4 kcal per gram; 90% as sweet as sucrose; (sweeter than maltose).

**maltol**   Also termed laxarinic acid, palatone, veltol; 3-hydroxy-2-methyl-γ-pyrone. Found in the bark of young larch trees, pine needles, chicory and roasted malt; synthesised for use as a fragrant, caramel-like flavour for addition to foods; imparts a 'freshly baked' flavour to bread and cakes.

**maltose**   Malt sugar, maltobiose; 4-$O$-α-D-glucopyranosyl-D-glucopyranose. Double molecule of glucose which is hydrolysed during digestion to glucose. Does not occur in foods (unless specifically added as malt) but is formed as an intermediate during acid or enzymic digestion of starch. 33% as sweet as sucrose; a reducing sugar.

**maltose figure**   See *diastatic activity*.

**maltose intolerance**   See *disaccharide intolerance*.

**manganese**   Constituent of at least three mammalian enzymes and therefore a dietary essential, although dietary deficiencies have not been reported.

Toxicity has been found among manganese miners. Deficiency in animals leads to defects in the synthesis of mucopolysaccharides.

**mangelwurzel, mangoldwurzel**   *Beta vulgaris rapa*. Cross between red and white beetroot, used as cattle food.

Analysis: water 75.4–94.3%, nitrogenous substances 0.47–3.65%, fat 0.02–0.45%, N-free extract 5.75–10.0%, fibre 0.39–2.14%, ash 0.59–2.77%, sucrose 3.5–8.7%.

**mange tout**   Immature pods and embryo seeds of *Pisum sativum* var *macrocarpum (macrocarpon)* eaten wholly; sometimes immature French beans, *P. vulgaris*.

**mango**   *Mangifera indica*. Fruit of Indo-Burmese origin extensively grown throughout the tropics; 3–6 inches diameter; orange-coloured edible flesh surrounding central stone. The depth of colour is an index of vitamin A activity, which can be up to 700 μg per 100 g.

Analysis per 100 g: 0.5 g protein, 15 g carbohydrate, 60 kcal (0.25 MJ), 0.5 mg Fe, 200 μg carotene, 0.03 mg vitamin $B_1$, 0.04 mg vitamin $B_2$, 0.3 mg nicotinic acid, 30 mg vitamin C.

**mangosteen**   Fruit of Indian origin, the size of an orange with thick purple rind and sweet white pulp in segments (*Garcinea mangostana*). Vitamin C content 9 mg per 100 g.

**manihot starch**   See *cassava*.

**manioc**   See *cassava*.

**manna**   Dried exudate from the manna-ash tamarisk tree (*Fraxinus ornus*). Abundant in Sicily and used as a mild laxative for children.

Analysis 40–60% mannitol, 10–16% mannotetrose, 6–16% mannotriose, plus glucose, mucilage and fraxin.

This is thought to be the food eaten by the children of Israel in the wilderness.

**manna loaf**   A cake-like product made from crushed sprouted wheat made into a dough (no yeast) and baked. Analysis per 100 g: 215 kcal (720 kJ), 7 g protein, 47 g carbohydrate, 1 g fat, 3 mg sodium, 350 mg potassium.

**mannitol**   Mannite, or manna sugar. Formed by hydrogenation of the hexose sugar mannose, when the terminal −CHO group is reduced to −$CH_2OH$. Also extracted commercially from seaweed (*Laminaria*).

**mannose**   Also termed seminose and carubinose. Hexose sugar found in small amounts as polysaccharide complexes (mannosans) in legumes, in manna (exudate of the tamarisk) and in some gums. Chemical structure similar to that of glucose, except that the hydroxyl group on C2 is on the 'left'.

**mannotetrose**   See *stachyose*.

**Manucol**   Trade name (Kelco/AIL International) for sodium alginate.

**maple syrup**   Sap of certain varieties of the maple tree, *Acer saccharum* (USA and Canada). Evaporated either to syrup or finally to sugar.

Maple syrup, 63% sucrose, 1.5% invert sugar.

**maple syrup urine disease**   An inborn error of metabolism in which unusually large amounts of the three amino acids leucine, isoleucine and valine are excreted in the urine; the urine smells like maple syrup. There is progressive cerebro-degeneration leading to early death.

**marasmus**   See *protein-energy malnutrition*.

**margarine**   Also termed butterine, lardine and oleomargarine. An emulsion of fat from any of a variety of vegetable, animal or marine oils, with about 16% water, flavoured, and coloured.

So-called 'soft' margarines are usually (not necessarily) relatively rich in the polyunsaturated fatty acids (up to 60% of the total fat), compared with ordinary margarines, which may contain 10% polyunsaturated fatty acids.

In most countries margarine is fortified with vitamin A (4.5–9 mg per kg) and vitamin D (15–100 µg per kg).

**margarine, kosher**  Made only from vegetable fats, since ordinary margarine can include animal fats that may not be kosher (see *kosher*); also, the margarine is fortified with carotene (which is derived from vegetable sources) instead of retinol (which can be obtained from non-kosher sources).

**marinade**  Preparation of wine or vinegar with olive oil, lemon juice and herbs and spices, used to soak meat or fish both to give flavour and to tenderise. Anchovy and Bismarck herrings are marinated before cooking.

**marinate**  The verb from marinade.

**marine biotoxins**  Toxins in shellfish and marine fish either produced naturally or accumulated by the fish from their diet (includes ciguatera and paralytic shellfish poisoning).

**marjoram**  Dried leaves of a number of aromatic plants of different species. The most widely accepted marjoram herb is *Origanum majorana* (perennial bush) and a sweet marjoram *majorana hortensis* (annual). Spanish wild marjoram is *Thymus mastichina*. The volatile oils contain terpenes and terpene alcohols. Used as seasoning for poultry and meats.

**marmalade**  Originally a jam made from the Portuguese marmelo or quince. Now the name given to jam made from citrus fruits such as orange, lime, lemon, grapefruit.

**marmite**  (1) The original form of pressure cooker used by Papin in 1681; it was an iron pot with a sealing lid.

(2) Cookery term for a stock.

**Marmite**  Trade name (Beecham's) for an extract of yeast flavoured with vegetable extract and used as a bread spread, beverage and flavouring agent.

Analysis per 100 g: Ca 123 mg, Fe 7 mg, vitamin $B_2$ 5.2 mg, nicotinic acid 59 mg.

**marrow**  See *gourds*.

**marshmallow**  Soft sweetmeat made from an aerated mixture of gelatin or egg albumin with sugar or starch syrup. Differs from nougat in containing less glucose and more water.

Originally made from the root of the marshmallow plant (*Althaea*), which provides a mucilaginous substance as well as starch and sugar.

**marumillon 50**  Trade name (Japan) for mixture of the sweet glycosides extracted from stevia leaves. See also *stevioside; rebaudoside*.

**marzipan**  Sweetmeat or cake decoration composed of 25% ground almond paste and 75% sugar; also called almond paste.

**mashing**  In the brewing of beer (see *beer*) the malted barley is heated with water both to extract the soluble sugars and to continue enzymic reactions started during malting.

**mash tun**  Vessel used in brewing in which the malt is extracted from the sprouted barley with hot water.

**maslin, mashlum**  (1) Old term still used in Scotland, for mixed crop of beans and oats used as cattle food.

(2) In Yorkshire and north of England it means a mixed crop of 2–3 parts of wheat and 1 part of rye, which is used for bread.

**Mason jar**  Screw-topped glass jar for home bottling; patented 1858.

**massecuite**  The mixture of sugar crystals and syrup mother liquor obtained during the crystallisation stage of sugar refining.

**mast**  See *milks, fermented*.

**maté**  Also yerba maté, or Paraguay or Brazilian tea. Made from the dried leaves of *Ilex paraguayensis*. Contains caffeine and tannin.

**matoké**  Cooked (steamed) green banana.

**maturation factor**  Substance in the liver which aids maturation of red blood cells. May be vitamin $B_{12}$ or combination of $B_{12}$ with the intrinsic factor produced by the stomach.

**Matzka process**  Sterilisation by combined use of silver ions (oligodynamic process) and limited heat – katadyn process employs silver ions alone. In the presence of the silver the pasteurisation temperature is only 8–11°C (15–20°F). Applied to fruit juices.

**matzo, motza**  (matzoth is the plural.) Unleavened bread or Passover bread made as thin, flat, round or square water biscuits, and, according to the injunction in Exodus, eaten by Jews during the eight days of Passover in place of leavened bread.

**maw**  Fourth stomach of the ruminant.

**mawseed**  Poppyseed.

**MaxEPA**  Trade name (Duncan Flockhart) for standardised mixture of eicosapentaenoic and docosohexaenoic acids (EPA and DHA) long chain marine fatty acids.

**mayonnaise**  See *salad cream*.

**maysin**  Coagulable globulin protein of maize.

**mazun**  See *milks, fermented*.

**mazzard**  See *gean*.

**mealie(s)**  Maize.

**mealie rice**  See *maize rice*.

**meat**  Generally refers to the muscle tissue of any animal – beef, lamb, veal, mutton, pork or poultry. 'Organ meats' or 'offal' is the term used for non-muscle tissue such as liver, kidneys, etc. Most muscle meat is about 20% protein, 10–30% fat, and the remainder water.

**meat bar**   Dehydrated cooked meat and fat; a modern form of pemmican.

Analysis per 100 g: 7.5 g water, 49 g protein, 570 kcal (2.4 MJ).

**meat conditioning**   After an animal has been slaughtered, muscle glycogen breaks down to lactic acid, which tends to improve the texture and keeping qualities of the meat. Meat that has been left until these changes have occurred is 'conditioned'. See also *rigor mortis*.

**meat, curing**   Pickling with the aid of sodium chloride, sodium nitrate and some sodium nitrite, which permits the growth of only salt-tolerant bacteria and inhibits the growth of *Clostridium botulinum*. The nitrite is the effective preserving agent and the nitrate is converted into nitrite during the process. The red colour is due to the formation of nitrosomyoglobin from the myoglobin and nitric oxide.

**meat extract**   The water-soluble part of meat that is mainly responsible for flavour. Commercially is made during the manufacture of corned beaf; minced meat is immersed in boiling water, when the water-soluble extractives are partially leached out. This 'soup' is concentrated and produces the meat extract (so-called No. 1 extract) of commerce. (Exhaustive extraction of the meat produces 'Direct Extract', containing more gelatin.)

Rich in the B vitamins (particularly $B_2$, nicotinic acid and $B_{12}$), meat bases and potassium. Shown by Pavlov that meat extract is the most powerful oral stimulant of gastric acid secretion.

**meat factor**   Factor used to determine the fat-free meat content of sausages and similar meat products from a nitrogen estimation: $100 \times N/3.4$; applies to both pork and beef.

**meat speciation**   Identification of species of animal from which the meat originated. After processing it becomes less recognisable and serological testing becomes necessary.

See also *nitrate*.

**meat sugar**   Obsolete name for inositol.

**medicinal paraffin**   A mineral oil of no nutritive value since it is not affected by digestive enzymes and passes through the intestine unchanged.

Used as a mild laxative because of its lubricant properties; if taken at the same time as the fat-soluble vitamins, these go into solution in the oil and pass through the digestive tract unabsorbed.

**medlar** *Mespilus germanica*. Can be eaten fresh from tree in Mediterranean areas but in colder climates, as Great Britain, does not become palatable until it is half rotten (bletted).

**Meeh formula** See *surface area*.

**melampyrin** Dulcitol, which see.

**melangeur** Mixing vessel consisting of rollers riding on a rotating horizontal bed. Used to mix substances of pasty consistency (hence melangeuring).

**melangolo** Italian term for the bitter orange. See *orange, bitter*.

**melezitose** Trisaccharide composed of two glucose and one fructose; hydrolysed to glucose plus the disaccharide turanose (3-$\alpha$-D-glucosido-D-fructose).

**melibiose** Disaccharide, 6($\alpha$-D galactoside)-D-glucose.

**melitose** See *raffinose*.

**melitriose** See *raffinose*.

**mellorine** US term for ice-cream made from non-butter fat.

**melon** See *gourds*.

**melting point** Often characteristic of a particular chemical and used as a means of identification. Particularly valuable as an index of purity, as impurities lower the melting point.

**membrane, semi-permeable** One that allows the passage of small but not large molecules: e.g. pig's bladder is permeable to water but not salt; collodion is permeable to salt but not protein molecules.

The exchange of water and salts between tissues of the body and red blood cells is possible because of the semi-permeable nature of the walls.

See *isotonic*; *osmotic pressure*.

**menadione** Obsolete term for vitamin $K_3$, 2-methyl-1,4-naphthoquinone. See *vitamin K*.

**menaquinone** 2-methyl-1,4-naphthoquinone, generic descriptor of substances with vitamin K activity; formerly called menadione.

**mercapturic acid** Complex of cysteine with naphthalene or various halogenated aromatic hydrocarbons (such as bromobenzene) whereby the latter compounds are detoxicated and excreted in the urine.

**meringues** Confections made by beating together a mixture of sugar and white of eggs.

**Meritene** Trade name (Doyle Pharmaceutical Co., USA) for a food concentrate based on skim milk powder.

Analysis per 100 g: protein 33 g, fat 0.2 g, carbohydrate 58.4 g, Ca 1 g, Fe 15 mg, kcal 365 (1.5 MJ), vitamin A 2 mg, vitamin $B_1$ 2.4 mg, vitamin $B_2$ 4.3 mg, nicotinic acid 22 mg, vitamin C 80 mg, D 14 µg.

**mescal**   See *tequila*.

**mesocarp**   See *albedo*.

**mesomorph**   Description given to a well-covered individual with well-developed muscles. See also *ectomorph*; *endomorph*.

**mesophiles**   Micro-organisms that grow best at temperatures between 25 and 40°C; usually will not grow at temperatures below 5°C.

**metabolic rate**   Rate of utilisation of energy. See also *basal metabolic rate*.

**metabolic water**   Produced in the body by the oxidation of foods.
  100 g of fat produces 107.1 g of water.
  100 g of starch produces 55.1 g of water.
  100 g of protein produces 41.3 g of water.

**metabolism**   The process of chemical change that goes on in living cells: growth of new tissues, breakdown of old tissue, production of energy. Anabolism is building up and catabolism is breaking down.

  Intermediary metabolism describes the biochemical stages in the change of, for example, glucose to carbon dioxide and water. See *glucose metabolism*.

**metabolism, inborn errors of**   See *genetic disease*.

**metalloproteins**   Proteins linked to a metal, such as haemoglobin, cytochrome, peroxidase, ferritin, siderophilin, all of which contain iron, and chlorocruorin, which contains copper.

**metaproteins**   Products of the action on proteins of dilute acids or alkalies; they are no longer soluble at their isoelectric points but are soluble in weak acid or alkali.

**Metercal**   (US product spelled Metrecal)   Trade name (Mead Johnson) for a 'slimming' preparation comprising all the dietary essentials limited to 900 kcal (3.8 MJ), per day intake (in ½ lb) – in powder, liquid and biscuit form. Based on skimmed milk with added protein and full range of vitamins.

**methaemoglobin**   Oxidised form of haemoglobin (unlike oxyhaemoglobin, which is a loose and reversible combination with oxygen) which cannot transport oxygen to the tissues. Present in small quantities in normal blood, increased after certain drugs and after smoking; found rarely as a congenital abnormality.

  Can be formed in blood of babies after consumption of the small amounts of nitrate found naturally in vegetables grown in certain areas and in some drinking water, since the lack of acidity in the stomach permits reduction of nitrate to nitrite. See also *nitrate*.

**methionine**   An essential amino acid; one of the three containing sulphur – cystine, cysteine and methionine.

  Cystine is non-essential but can replace part of the methionine of the diet; hence, the sulphur amino acids are always considered together. They occupy an outstanding position in protein nutrition, since not only are the sulphur amino acids the limiting factor in many proteins, but also they are limiting in the total diet of most peoples that have been examined. In other words, the protein nutritive value of these diets can be improved by adding either more protein or more methionine (or cystine) but no other amino acid.

Methionine is available on the commercial scale and is added to animal feeds, where it is often, but not always, the limiting amino acid.

Chemically, aminomethylthiol butyric acid.

See also *amino acid, limiting*.

**methionine sulphoximine** Substance formed by reaction between nitrogen trichloride ('agene') and the amino acid methionine when flour is treated with agene as a bleaching agent. Causes running fits in dogs, and although it has never been shown to be toxic to man, the use of agene as a bread improver was abandoned in Great Britain in 1955.

**Methocel** Trade name (Dow Chemical Co.) for methyl cellulose.

**Methofas** Trade name (Imperial Chemical Industries) for methyl hydroxypropyl cellulose.

**methyl alcohol** The first member of the alcohol series. It is a highly toxic substance and leads to mental disturbance, blindness and death when consumed over a period. It is present in methylated spirits, to which it is added to denature the ethyl alcohol and render it undrinkable. Since methylated spirits is duty-free, alcoholic addicts often drink this despite the presence of the toxic methyl alcohol.

**methylated spirits** Ethyl alcohol containing methyl alcohol, coloured with a dye and given a repulsive smell by the addition of pyridine. Its toxicity is due to the presence of the methyl alcohol.

**methyl cellulose** See *carboxymethylcellulose*.

**methylene blue** Blue dye that becomes colourless when reduced, the so-called leuco- form. Used in cell respiration experiments to indicate when oxygen is being consumed. See also *methylene blue dye-reduction test*.

**methylene blue dye-reduction test** When methylene blue or resazurin is added to milk, the bacteria present take up oxygen and change the colour of the dye. Methylene blue goes colourless; resazurin changes blue-purple–pink–white.

The speed of the change indicates the bacterial content. Pasteurised milk must not reduce dye in half an hour.

**3-methyl-histidine**  Derivative of the amino acid, histidine, found only in the contractile proteins of muscle (myosin and actin). Useful among other purposes, as an index of lean meat content since it is not present in collagen or added materials.

Urinary excretion reflects amount of muscle tissue.

**metmyoglobin**  See *nitrosomyoglobin*.

**Meulengracht diet**  For peptic ulcer patients; sieved foods such as meat, chicken, vegetables, at 2-hourly intervals. Differs from Sippy and Lenhartz diets (which see) in being much richer in protein.

The intention is to neutralise the acid in the stomach by the buffering effect of the protein.

**mevalonic acid**  Chemically, $\beta,\delta$-dihydroxy-$\beta$-methylvaleric acid; a growth-promoting factor for *Lactobacillus acidophilus* distinct from lipoic acid; can replace acetate, which is an essential factor for this organism.

It is an intermediate stage in the biosynthesis of sterols and terpenes (including possibly carotene). Isolated 1956 from distillers' dried solubles.

**Michaelis constant**  Measure of the kinetics of enzyme reaction. Defined as the substrate concentration at which half the limiting velocity of the reaction is reached.

It is a characteristic of the enzyme and is useful as a means of following the stages of purification of an enzyme.

**micro-aerophiles**  Micro-organisms that can grow in low concentrations of oxygen and so lead to spoilage of foodstuffs unless all oxygen is excluded.

**microbiological assay**  Biological assay using micro-organisms; used for vitamins and amino acids in particular.

The principle is that the organism is inoculated into a medium containing all the needed growth factors except the one under examination; the rate of growth is then proportional to the amount of this particular factor added in the test substance. Rate of growth determined by turbidity or by titrating the acid produced after 2–3 days incubation.

**microencapsulation**  Preparation of small particles of solids or droplets of liquids inside thin polymeric coatings (ranging from beeswax and starch to gelatin and polyacrylic acid). The microcapsules range from tenths to thousandths of micrometres in size and are used to prepare liquids as free-flowing powders or compressed solids, to separate reactive materials, reduce toxicity, protect against oxidation and control rate of release; used for enzymes, flavours, nutrients, etc.

**microfiltration**  Filtration under pressure through membrane of small pore size, 0.1–10 μm, larger size than ultrafiltration; used for clarification of beverages and to sterilise liquids by filtering off organisms.

**microgram**   One-thousandth part of a milligram; symbol µg.

**micrometre**   One-thousandth of a millimetre; symbol µm. Unit of measurement of bacterial size.

**micronisation**   Extremely rapid heating with infrared radiation produced by heating propane on a ceramic tile or with nichrome wire elements. Suggested as an alternative to steam heating or toasting where the shorter heating time is less damaging to the foodstuff.

**micronutrients**   Vitamins and minerals as distinct from fats, carbohydrates and proteins which are needed in vastly greater amounts (macronutrients).

**micro-organisms**   Generally refers to bacteria, moulds and yeasts; of interest in food spoilage, as causes of diseases, of value in food preservation and processing and as foodstuffs themselves (termed single cell protein).

**microwave heating**   See *irradiation*.

**middlings**   See *wheatfeed*.

**milk**   The secretion of the mammary gland of animals including cow, buffalo, goat, ass, mare, ewe and camel.

Cow's milk is particularly rich in calcium (1.2 g per litre), and riboflavin (2 mg per litre) and contains per litre 47 g lactose, 33 g protein, 38 g fat, 500 µg vitamin A (as both retinol and carotene), 0.4 mg thiamin, 0.8 mg niacin, 50 µg folate, 0.3 µg vitamin D, about 15 mg vitamin C, and small amounts of other B vitamins and minerals. Jersey, Guernsey, South Devon and Channel Islands milk contain about 48 g fat.

Buffalo milk – 75 g fat, 43 g protein and 45 g carbohydrate per litre.

**milk, accredited**   Term not used after October 1954. Referred to milk untreated by heat, from cows examined at specific intervals for freedom from disease.

**milk, acidophilus**   A preparation similar to cultured buttermilk but soured by *Lactobacillus* instead of acid-producing streptococci.

**milk–alkali syndrome**   Weakness and lethargy caused by prolonged adherence to a diet rich in milk (more than 2 pints) per day and alkalies.

**milk, Buddeised**   Milk preserved by the addition of hydrogen peroxide. Not legally permitted. See also *hydrogen peroxide*.

**milk, citrated**   Milk to which sodium citrate has been added to combine with the calcium and inhibit the curdling of caseinogen which would normally occur in the stomach. Claimed, with little evidence, to be of value in feeding infants and invalids.

**milk, designated**  Legally milk may be designated pasteurised or sterilised and also tuberculin tested.

The special designation 'accredited' has been abolished.

**milk, dried**  Milk that has been evaporated to dryness, usually by spray or roller-drying. May be whole or full-cream milk (26% fat), three-quarter cream (not less than 20% fat), half-cream (not less than 14% fat), quarter-cream (not less than 8% fat) or skim milk (1% fat).

**milk, dye-reduction test**  See *methylene blue dye-reduction test.*

**milk, evaporated**  Concentrated to about 45% of its original volume by evaporation. Also called unsweetened, condensed milk.

Legally must contain not less than 7.8% fat and 25.5% total solids. First produced in 1883 by Meyenberg.

**milk fat test**  See *Gerber test.*

**milk, filled**  Milk from which the natural fat has been removed and replaced with fat from another source. The reason may be economic, if the butter-fat can be replaced by a cheaper one, or, more recently, to replace a fat poor in the polyunsaturated fatty acids with a vegetable fat rich in these factors.

**milk, freezing-point test**  The sample of milk is cooled below its freezing point and seeded with a crystal of ice. The temperature rises to the freezing point (FP) of milk as the whole freezes – normally −0.530 to −0.560°C.

When milk has been adulterated the FP rises nearer to that of water. FPs above −0.530°C are indicative of adulteration.

**milk, frozen or fresh frozen**  Milk is pasteurised, treated with an ultrasonic vibrator at 5 million cycles per second for 5 minutes and frozen to 10°F. It will keep for a year, and when thawed is indistinguishable from the original milk.

**milk, half-cream**  Often refers to dried milk powder in which the fat content is reduced to half for infant feeding, particularly for premature infants.

**milk, homogenised**  Mechanical treatment breaks up and redistributes the fat globules throughout the milk to prevent the cream rising to the surface.

**milk, humanised**  Cow's milk that has had its composition modified to resemble human milk. The main change is a reduction in protein content often achieved by dilution with carbohydrate and restoration of the fat content.

**milk, irradiated**  Milk that has been subjected to ultraviolet light, when the 7-dehydrocholesterol present naturally is partly converted into vitamin D.

**milk, lactose-hydrolysed**  Milk in which the lactose has been hydrolysed to glucose and galactose by treatment with the enzyme lactase, intended for infants who are lactase-deficient.

**milk, long**  A Scandinavian soured milk which is viscous because of 'ropiness' caused by bacteria.

**milk, Long-life**  Trade name (Express Dairy Co. Ltd) for milk sterilised for a very short time (2 seconds) at ultra-high temperature (137°C) – also called UHT milk.

**milk, malted**  A preparation of milk and the liquid separated from a mash of barley malt and wheat flour, evaporated to dryness.

**milk, methylene blue test**  See *methylene blue dye-reduction test*.

**milk, pasteurised**  See *methylene blue dye-reduction test*; *pasteurisation*; *phosphatase test*.

**milk, protein**  See *protein milk*.

**milk, ropy**  See *rope*.

**milks, fermented**  In various countries milk, from the ass, mare, cow, goat and buffalo, is fermented with a mixture of bacteria and yeasts, when the lactose is converted to lactic acid and, in some drinks, to alcohol. These fermented milks include busa (Turkestan), cieddu (Italy), dadhi (India), kefir (Balkans), kumiss (Steppes), laban Zabadi (Egypt), mazun (Armenia), taette (N. Europe), skyr (Iceland), mast (Iran), crowdies (Scotland), kuban and yoghurt.

**milk-stone**  Deposit of calcium and magnesium phosphates, protein, etc., produced when milk is heated to temperatures above 60°C.

**milk, sweetened, condensed**  Evaporated to less than one-third volume and sugar added as preservative; may be full cream or skimmed. First patented in the USA and the UK by Borden, 1856.

**milk, toned**  Dried, skim milk added to a high-fat milk such as buffalo milk, to reduce the fat content but maintain the total solids. If the fat were diluted simply by adding water, the milk would not be 'toned up'.

**milk, TT**  Tuberculin tested. Applied to milk from herd that has been attested free from tubercle by a veterinary inspector.

**milk, turbidity test**  To distinguish sterilised milk from pasteurised. During sterilisation, the milk is held at 104–116°C for 20–40 minutes, when all the albumin is precipitated. In the test the filtrate from an ammonium sulphate precipitation should remain clear on heating, indicating that no albumin was present in solution and the milk had therefore been sterilised.

**milk, witches'**  See *witches' milk*.

**millerator**  Wheat-cleaning machine consisting of two sieves, the upper one retaining particles larger than wheat, the lower one rejecting particles smaller than wheat.

**miller's offal**  See *wheatfeed*.

**millet** Cereal of a number of species of Gramineae smaller than wheat and rice and high in fibre content.

Common millet (*Panicum* and *Setaria* species) also known as China, Italian, Indian, French hog, proso, panicled and broom corn millet, foxtail millet (*Setaria italica*); grows very rapidly, 2–2½ months from sowing to harvest.

Protein 10%, fat 2.5%, carbohydrate 73%.

Red, finger, South India millet, coracan or ragi is *Eleusine coracana*. Protein 6%, fat 1.5%, carbohydrate 75%.

Bulrush millet, pearl millet, bajoa or Kaffir manna corn is *Pennisetum typhoideum* or *P. americanum*; the staple food in poor parts of India. Protein 11%, fat 5%, carbohydrate 69%.

Other species are Kodo or haraka millet (*Paspalum scrobiculatum*) and Teff (*Eragrostis tef* or *E. abyssinica*) and jajeo millet (*Acroceras amplectens*).

**milling** The term usually refers to the conversion of cereal grain into its derivative – e.g. wheat into flour, brown rice to white rice.

Flour milling involves two types of rollers: (1) break rolls are corrugated and exert shear pressure and forces which break up the wheat grain and permit sieving into fractions containing varying proportions of germ, bran and endosperm; (2) reducing rolls that are smooth and subdivide the endosperm to fine particles.

**Millon's test** For proteins; actually a test for the hydroxyphenyl group and therefore for tyrosine, but since every protein contains some tyrosine, it is used as a general protein test.

The reagent consists of mercury in nitric acid and gives a white precipitate with proteins which turns red on heating.

**mills** See *ball mill*; *disc mill*; *hammer mill*; *querns*; *roller mill*.

**milt** The soft roe of the male fish. Also the name given to the spleen of animals.

**miltone** A toned milk developed in India in which peanut protein is added to buffalo or cow's milk to extend supplies.

**Minafen** Trade name (Trufood Ltd) for food low in phenylalanine for treatment of phenylketonuria.

**Minamata disease** Poisoning from organic (methyl) mercury, named after Minamata Bay in Japan where fish contained this poisonous organic form of mercury after waste water from mercury processing was passed into the estuary.

**minarine** Name sometimes given to low-fat spreads with less than the statutory amount of fat in a margarine.

**mincemeat** A traditional product made from apple, sugar, vine fruits and citrus peel with suet, spices and acetic acid, coloured with caramel. Preserved by the sugar content and acid.

In some countries called fruit mince. Originally a meat product; in USA a spiced mixture of chopped meat, apples and raisins.

**mineralocorticoids** Obsolescent term for the steroid hormones of the adrenal cortex which control the excretion of salt and water by the kidney. See *adrenal glands*; *aldosterone*.

**mineral salts** The inorganic salts, including sodium, potassium, calcium, chloride, phosphate, sulphate, etc.

**mineral waters** Natural, untreated, spring waters, some of which are naturally carbonated, may be slightly alkaline or salty. Numerous health claims have been made for the benefits arising from the traces of a large number of minerals found in solution. Examples are Evian, Malvern, Apollinaris, Vichy, Vittel.

The term is also applied to artificially carbonated water, 'soda water' or club soda.

**miners' cramp** Cramp due to loss of salt from the body caused by excessive sweating; occurs in tropical climates and with severe exercise – mining often combines the two. Prevented by consuming salt, e.g. salt tablets in the tropics and for athletes.

**minifoods** Name given to single cell proteins, which see.

**mint** Many varieties of the species *Mentha* – spearmint, *M. spicata*; peppermint, *M. piperita*. Used to flavour meat, fish, tobacco, etc.

Oil of peppermint is distilled from stem and leaves of *M. piperita*, and used both pharmaceutically and as a flavour.

**miotin** Unidentified urinary excretion product of biotin, together with triotin and rhiotin.

**miracle berry** *Richardella dulcifica* (also known as *Synsepalum dulcificum*); tropical fruit from W. Africa containing a taste-modifying substance that causes sour foods to taste sweet. Hence the name miracle berry, and miraculin for the active principle, a glycoprotein.

**miraculin** See *miracle berry*.

**mirepoix** Bed of vegetables used to give flavour to braised meats and also soups and sauces.

**miso** Autoclaved soyabeans mixed with cooked rice and partly fermented with *Aspergillus oryzae and A. sojae* to form koji. Salt added to stop further mould growth, bacterial fermentation continues with addition of *Lactobacillus* (1–2 months). Barley miso is an alternative to soyabeans alone.

**mithi** See *clay*.

**mixed function oxidases** See *cytochrome P450*.

**mixiria** Process of preserving meat and fish by roasting in their own fat and preserving in jars covered with a layer of fat.

**mixograph** American instrument for measuring the physical properties of a dough, similar in principle to the farinograph, which see.

**mocca** Mixture of coffee and cocoa used in bakery and confectionery products. (Mocha is a variety of coffee from Mocha, Arabia.)

**modified atmosphere** See under *gas storage, controlled*.

**molasses** Residue left after repeated crystallisation of sugar; contains sucrose, glucose and fructose and (if from beet) raffinose and small quantities of dextrans; will not crystallise; 67% sucrose, 260 kcal (1.1 MJ) per 100 g: contains more than 500 mg iron per 100 g, with traces of other minerals.

**Molisch reaction** Test for carbohydrates. The reagent is a 5% solution of alpha-naphthol in alcohol; two drops added to the test solution and concentrated sulphuric acid poured down the side of the tube to form a lower layer. Violet zone appears at the junction.

**molluscicides** Chemicals used to kill molluscs – usually slugs and snails.

**molluscs** Edible marine molluscs include cockles, mussels, oysters, scallops, whelks, winkles (periwinkles).

**molybdenum** Constituent of at least two mammalian enzymes – namely xanthine oxidase and aldehyde dehydrogenase – and therefore it is a dietary essential for man, although dietary deficiencies are never encountered. Excess is toxic.

**monellin** The active sweet principle, a protein, from the serendipity berry, *Dioscoreophyllum cumminsii*. 1500–3000 times as sweet as sucrose.

**monethanolamine** See *ethanolamine*.

**monocalcium phosphate** See *calcium acid phosphate*.

**monoglycerides** See *superglycerinated fats*.

**monophagia** Desire for one type of food.

**monosaccharides** Group name of the simplest sugars, including those composed of 3 carbon atoms (trioses), 4 (tetroses), 5 (pentoses), 6 (hexoses) and 7 (heptoses). Also known as monoses or monosaccharoses.

**monosaccharose** See *monosaccharides*.

**monose** See *monosaccharides*.

**monosodium glutamate** See *glutamic acid*.

**montmorillonite** See *Fuller's earth*.

**Moreton Bay bug** Or Bay lobster, a variety of sand lobster found in Australia.

**mortadella** See *sausage*.

**moss, Irish** See *carrageenan*.

**mother of vinegar** See *vinegar*.

**mottled teeth**   In areas where the drinking water contains fluoride at a level of several parts per million, dull, chalky patches occur on the teeth known as mottling. These teeth are relatively free from decay, and lower levels of fluoride, about 1 ppm, reduce decay without causing mottling.

**mould bran**   A fungal amylase preparation produced by growing mould on moist wheat bran; used as source of starch-splitting enzymes.

**mould inhibitors**   See *antimycotics*.

**moulds**.  Fungi characterised by their branched filamentous structure of mycelium. (1) They can cause food spoilage very rapidly – white *Mucor*, grey-green *Penicillium*, black *Aspergillus* – and produce mycotoxins. (2) Used for large-scale production of citric acid (*Aspergillus niger*), ripening of cheese (species of *Penicillium*) and as source of enzymes for use in the food industry. (3) Mushrooms belong to this family of fungi. (4) A number of foods are fermented with moulds, e.g. idli, miso and tempeh. (5) The mycelium of *Fusarium* species is used as a manufactured food product. (6) Most of the antibiotics are mould products.

**MPD**   See *polydextrose, modified*.

**MSG**   See *glutamic acid*.

**MUAC**   Mid-upper-arm-circumference. Rough method of rapid screening of large groups of children for undernutrition.

**mucin**   Naturally occurring complexes of protein and carbohydrates; highly viscous.

**mucopolysaccharides**   Group of polysaccharides containing an amino sugar and uronic acid; constituent of mucoproteins of cartilage, tendons, connective tissue, cornea, heparin and blood group substances.

**mucoproteins**   Members of the group of glycoproteins containing a sugar, usually chondroitin sulphate, combined with amino acids or peptides; occur in mucin secreted in the stomach, saliva and various glands.

**mucor**   See *moulds*.

**mucosa**   Name given to the moist tissue lining, for example, the mouth (buccal mucosa), intestines and respiratory tract.

The intestinal wall has two sides, the inner, or mucosal, side, and the outer, or serosal, side.

**muffins**   See *dough cakes*.

**mulberry**   *Morus nigra* (also white mulberry, *M. alba*). Of little commercial importance.

Analysis per 100 g: 14 g carbohydrate, 1.5 g protein, 60 kcal (0.24 MJ), 10 mg vitamin C.

**multipurpose food** Indian multipurpose food is made from peanut flour and chickpea flour with calcium carbonate, and vitamins A, $B_1$ and $B_2$, and contains 40% protein.

American multipurpose food is based on soya.

**muscarine** Quaternary trimethylammonium salt of 2-methyl-3-hydroxy-5-(aminomethyl)-tetrahydrofuran; toxic material in red variety of the mushroom *Amanita muscaria*, the fly fungus and other fungi.

**muscatels** Made by drying the large seed-containing grapes grown almost exclusively in Malaga (Spain). They are partially dried in the sun and drying is completed indoors; they are left on the stalk and pressed flat for sale.

Muscatel is the name given to a sweet wine made from the same grape.

For analysis see *fruit, dried*. See also *currants*; *raisins*; *sultanas*.

**muscle** The contractile cellular unit of skeletal muscle is the fibre. This is a long cylinder in shape and composed of many myofilbrils. Chemically, the muscle fibre is composed of three proteins: myosin, actin and tropomyosin.

The muscle fibre is surrounded by a thin membrane, the sarcolemma. Within the muscle fibre surrounding the myofibrils is the sarcoplasm or cytoplasm. Individual fibres are separated by a thin network of connective tissue, the endomysium, and bound together in bundles by larger sheets of connective tissue, the perimysium.

Muscle tissue also contains structural elements, collagen, reticulin and elastin.

**muscle adenylic acid** Adenosine-5-phosphoric acid; yeast adenylic acid is adenosine-3-phosphoric acid.

**Muscovado sugar** See *sugar*.

**mushroom** *Agaricus campestris*.

Analysis per 100 g, raw: water 91.5 g, protein 1.8 g, fat trace, carbohydrate nil, kcal 7 (30 kJ), Fe 1 mg, vitamin $B_1$ 0.1 mg, vitamin $B_2$ 0.4 mg, nicotinic acid 4 mg, vitamin C 3 mg.

**mushroom alcohol** (champignol) 1-octo-3-ol.

**mushroom sugar** Trehalose, which see.

**mussel** *Mytilus edulis*. Bivalve, cultivated at 25–50 tons per acre, yield 6–10 tons wet weight of meat per acre; take 4 years to reach marketable size – 5 cm; 20% of weight is meat.

Analysis per 100 g boiled: water 79 g, protein 16.8 g, fat 2 g, carbohydrate trace only, kcal 90 (0.36 MJ), Ca 200 mg, Fe 13 mg.

**mustard**  Powdered seeds of black or brown mustard (*Brassica nigra* or *B.juncea*) mixed with yellow or white (*Sinapsis alba*). Active principles are glycosides – sinigrin in black, sinalbin in white. When moistened the enzyme myrosinase liberates the characteristically flavoured oil (allyl isothiocyanate).

'English mustard' contains not more than 10% wheat flour; still referred to in parts of England as Durham mustard, after Mrs Clements of Durham, who made the first commercial preparations of ground mustard seed, wheat flour and turmeric, 1711; based on white and brown mustard which produces more pungent product.

Dijon mustard – made from *B. nigra* or *B. juncea* with vinegar, grape juice or wine and not coloured.

French mustard – brown mustard, vinegar, salt, turmeric, cayenne pepper, cloves, pimento – mild.

Violet mustard – coloured with grape juice.

**mustard and cress**  Salad herb mixture of leaves of mustard (*Brassica alba*) and garden cress (*Lepidium sativum*). Often mustard is replaced with rape (*Brassica napus var. oleifera Del*) – a different strain from that used for rape seed oil – it has a larger leaf and grows faster than mustard. Analysis per 100 g mixture: 1.6 g protein, 0.9 g carbohydrate, 10 kcal (40 kJ), 70 mg calcium, 4.5 mg iron, 80 µg carotene, 80 mg vitamin C, 4 g fibre.

**mustard oil**  Used as cooking fat in Bengal and Bihar. The seeds are often contaminated with seeds of *Argemone mexicana*, which contains an alkaloid, argemone oil. The contaminated mustard oil is the cause of epidemic dropsy, as the sanguinarine inhibits the oxidation of pyruvic acid which accumulates in the blood.

**mutachrome**  See *citroxanthin*.

**mutagen**  Substance able to produce genetic damage by affecting spermatozoa or ova.

**mutton**  Meat of sheep older than 1 year.

Analysis per 100 g: protein 12 g, fat 20 g, kcal 240 (1.0 MJ), Fe 1.4 mg, vitamin $B_1$ 0.1 mg, vitamin $B_2$ 0.14 mg, nicotinic acid 3.6 mg.

**mycelia**  See *moulds*.

**mycelial protein**  Name given to mould mycelium prepared as foodstuff. *Fusarium* species and *Neurospora* species grown on carbohydrate have been used.

***Mycoderma aceti***  See *Acetobacter*.

**mycoprotein**  Name given to mould mycelium used as a food ingredient. Analysis per 100 g; 12 g protein, 4 g fat, 7 g dietary fibre, 70 g water. See *Quorn*.

**mycotoxins** Toxins formed by fungi (moulds) especially *Aspergillus flavus* under tropical conditions and *Pencillium* and *Fusarium* species under temperate conditions. The problem is created by the storage of food under damp conditions which favour the growth of the moulds.

They include aflatoxin (on nuts and cereals), ochratoxin (on meat products and pulses), patulin (on fruit products), zearalenone and sterigmatocystin.

See also *aflatoxin*.

**Myoacets** Trade name (Distillation Products, USA) for a range of distilled monoglycerides. See *superglycerinated fats*.

**myocardial infarction** Damage to heart muscle due to failure of the blood supply to the muscle (ischaemia).

**myofibril** See *muscle*.

**myogen** Protein of muscle, about 20% of the total; an albumin, not present in the muscle fibrils but only in the sarcoplasm in which the fibrils are embedded.

**myoglobin** A complex protein in muscle, similar to the haemoglobin of the blood (but one-fourth of its molecular weight), composed of the iron-containing pigment haem and the protein globin. It serves as a storage mechanism for oxygen for the cells, as it can reversibly add oxygen to form oxymyoglobin.

The globin is denatured by heat to a brown pigment; hence the change from the red colour of raw meat to brown on cooking.

When meat is cured with nitrite, the myoglobin is converted into bright red nitric oxide-myoglobin or nitrosomyoglobin.

**myosin** Major fraction, about two-fifths, of muscle protein. A globulin, insoluble in water but soluble in salt solution. Combines with the protein actin to form actomyosin; the complex dissociates in the presence of ATP.

**myristic acid** One of the long-chain saturated fatty acids, $CH_3(CH_2)_{12}COOH$. Occurs as triglyceride in nutmeg butter, coconut butter, lard, spermaceti and wool wax.

**myrosinase** Glycosidase enzyme in mustard seed that hydrolyses myrosin or sinigrin to glucose and allyl isothiocyanate (mustard oil). See also *horse radish*; *mustard*.

**Mysore flour** Blend of 75% tapioca flour and 25% peanut flour, used as a partial substitute for cereals in large-scale feeding trials in Madras State, India.

**myxoedema** Severe hypothyroidism in the adult (name derived from puffiness of hands and face due to thickening of skin).

**myxoxanthin** Carotenoid pigment in algae with vitamin A activity.

# N

**NACNE** National Advisory Committee on Nutrition Education (UK). An ad hoc working party that published a discussion paper on nutritional guidelines in 1983.

**NAD, NADP** See *nicotinamide adenine dinucleotide*; *nicotinamide adenine dinucleotide phosphate*.

**naphthoquinone** Basic part of the molecule of vitamin K; the various forms of vitamin K are referred to as substituted naphthoquinones.

**naringin** Trihydroxyflavonone rhamnoglucoside, found in grapefruit, especially in the immature fruit; extremely bitter and dilutions of 1 part in 10000 parts of water can be detected. Sometimes found in canned grapefruit segments as tiny, white beads.

Hydrolysed to the aglucone, trihydroxyflavonone (naringenin), which is not bitter.

**national flour** See *wheatmeal, national*.

**natto** Fermented soya bean (Japan) using *Bacillus natto*.

**natural waters** See *mineral waters*.

**nature-identical** Term applied to food additives that are synthesised in the laboratory and are identical with those that occur in Nature.

**N conversion factor** See *nitrogen conversion factor*.

**NDGA** See *nordihydroguaiaretic acid*.

**NDpCal** See *net dietary protein energy ratio*.

**neat's foot** Ox or calf's foot used for making soups and jellies. Now called cow's heels.

**neat's-foot oil** Oil obtained from the knuckle bones of cattle; used in leather working and for canning sardines.

**NEFA** See *non-esterified fatty acids*.

**negus** Drink of port or sherry with spices, sugar and hot water.

**NEO-DHC** Neohesperidin dihydrochalcone (which see); non-nutritive sweetener.

**neohesperidin dihydrochalcone** 1000 times as sweet as sucrose; formed by hydrogenation of naturally occurring flavonoid neohesperidin.

**neomycin** Antibiotic isolated 1949 from *Streptomyces fradii*, used to some extent in controlling infections in food processing.

**neroli oil** Prepared from blossoms of the bitter orange by steam distillation (S. France, Spain, Italy, South America). Yellowish oil with intense odour of orange blossom.

**Nescafé** Trade name (Nestlé Ltd) for a dried, instant coffee. Contains more potassium than any other food – 5.5%.

**Nessler reagent** Alkaline solution of the double iodide of mercury and potassium. Gives an orange-brown with ammonia and used for quantitative estimation.

**net dietary protein calories**   See *net dietary protein energy ratio*.

**net dietary protein energy ratio**   The protein content of a diet or food expressed as protein energy multiplied by net protein utilisation (which see) divided by total energy.

Before the change from calories to joules this was termed net dietary protein calories per cent, NDpCal%.

**net protein ratio**   See *protein quality*.

**net protein utilisation**   Measure of quality of protein in terms of the amount of dietary protein retained in the body under specified experimental conditions. Previously expressed as a percentage, i.e. egg protein and human milk had NPU 100; wheat protein 50. Now expressed as ratio, 1.0 and 0.5, respectively.

By convention measured at 10% dietary protein level, $NPU_{10}$, at which level the protein synthetic mechanism in the growing animal can utilise all the protein so long as the balance of amino acids is correct. When fed at 4% dietary protein level, said to be that level at which the NPU is maximum, the value is termed NPU standardised. If the food or diet is fed as it is, i.e. not incorporated into a diet with other ingredients, the value is NPU operative ($NPU_{op}$).

**net protein value**   Product of net protein utilisation and protein content per cent.

**Neuberg ester**   Name given to fructose-6-phosphate, one of the intermediates in glucose metabolism, which see.

**neuraminic acid**   Sialic acid.

**neurine**   Trimethylvinylammonium hydroxide, formed during putrefaction by dehydration of choline and also found in egg yolk, brain and bile; toxic.

**New Zealand process**   Drying process applied to meat. It is immersed in hot oil under vacuum, when it dries to 3% moisture in about 4 hours. The fat is removed from the dry meat in a hydro-extractor.

**NFE**   Nitrogen-free extract. In the analysis of foods and animal feedingstuffs this fraction contains the sugars and starches plus small amounts of other materials.

**niacin**   Generic descriptor for pyridine-3-carboxylic acid and derivatives exhibiting qualitatively the biological activity of nicotinamide. The term nicotinic acid refers specifically to pyridine-3-carboxylic acid; its amide is nicotinamide.

In the old, obsolete nomenclature niacin was synonymous with nicotinic acid and niacinamide with nicotinamide. Earlier designation was PP-factor, pellagra-preventative.

See *nicotinic acid*.

**niacinamide**   Obsolete term for nicotinamide. See *nicotinic acid*.

**niacinogens**   Name given to protein–niacin complexes found in cereals. See *niacytin*.

**niacytin**   The bound forms of the vitamin niacin, found in some foods, particularly cereals. Complexes of niacin with polysaccharides of cellulose type and peptide or glycopeptide; not hydrolysed by intestinal enzymes, so biologically unavailable, but can be liberated by acid or alkaline hydrolysis or by baking the cereal, especially with an alkaline baking powder.

**nib**   See *chocolate*.

**niceritol**   Derivative of the vitamin, niacin (penta erythritol tetranicotinate) used in large doses (several grams) to reduce plasma cholesterol levels.

**nickel**   Present in foods and in animal and human tissues. Not shown to be essential for plants or animals but improves growth of many plants.

Metallic nickel used as catalyst in hydrogenation of fats.

**Nicol prism**   See *polarimeter*.

**nicotinamide**   See *nicotinic acid*.

**nicotinamide adenine dinucleotide** (NAD)   Complex of nicotinamide with adenine, two molecules of ribose and two molecules of phosphate. Also known as Coenzyme I, diphosphopyridine nucleotide (DPN) cozymase and as Euler's yeast coenzyme.

Essential part of the mechanism of oxidation in the tissues.

**nicotinamide adenine dinucleotide phosphate** (NADP)   Complex of nicotinamide with two molecules of ribose, adenine and three molecules of phosphate. Also known as triphosphopyridine nucleotide (TPN), Coenzyme II and Warburg and Christian's coenzyme.

Essential part, along with NAD, of the mechanism of oxidation in the tissues.

**nicotinamide nucleotides**   Nicotinamide adenine dinucleotide (NAD) and nicotinamide adenine dinucleotide phosphate (NADP) are common carriers of hydrogen and electrons in oxidation and reduction reactions.

**nicotinate, sodium**   Sodium salt of nicotinic acid; used, among other purposes, to preserve the red colour in fresh and processed meats.

**nicotinic acid**   Vitamin of the B complex with no numerical designation; sometimes called vitamin PP (pellagra preventative). The amide, nicotinamide, has the same biological function and both are known according to internationally agreed nomenclature as niacin. (In the USA the old designations niacin and niacinamide for nicotinic acid and its amide are still used.)

Functions as a coenzyme in the oxidation of carbohydrates as nicotinamide adenine dinucleotide. Deficiency leads to pellagra

– mental disorder, intestinal disorders and dermatitis. Can be formed in the body from the amino acid tryptophan at the rate of 1 mg from 60 mg tryptophan; hence, niacin content of foods often recorded as niacin equivalents, being the sum of pre-formed niacin plus one-sixtieth of the tryptophan.

Pellagra occurs particularly in maize-eating areas, because the niacin in maize is not available and maize protein is low in tryptophan.

Recommended daily intake 10 mg; found in meat, liver and yeast; that present in cereals often largely unavailable; added to flour in many countries.

See also *pellagra*.

**nicotinic acid, bound form**   See *niacytin*.

**nigerseed**   *Guizotia abyssinica*, or nug; grown in India and Ethiopia as food crop, 17% protein, 17% fat, 37% carbohydrate.

**night blindness**   Nyctalopia. Inability to see in dim light through deficiency of vitamin A. Dark-adaptation test is used as an index of vitamin A deficiency, as night blindness is the first symptom. See *dark adaptation*.

**ninhydrin test**   For proteins and amino acids (actually for the amino group). Pink, purple or blue colour is developed on reacting the amino acid or peptide with ninhydrin (triketohydrindene hydrate).

**nioigome**   Perfumed rice.

**NIRS**   Near infra-red spectroscopy.

**nisin**   Antibiotic isolated 1944 from lactic streptococci group N. Non-toxic, polypeptide, inhibits some but not all clostridia; not used medically.

The only antibiotic permitted in Great Britain in food preservation (in certain foods). It is naturally present in cheese, being produced by a number of strains of cheese starter organisms. Useful to prolong storage life of cheese, milk, cream, soups, canned fruits and vegetables, canned fish and milk puddings. Used at 2–4 µg per g of processed cheese and 1–5 µg per g of canned peas. It also lowers the resistance of many thermophilic bacteria to heat and so permits a reduction in the time and/or temperature of heating in the processing of canned vegetables.

**nitrate**   Natural constituent of plants; beets, rhubarb, cabbage, broccoli, cauliflower can contain up to 1 g/kg. Within one or two days after harvesting, some of the nitrate is converted into nitrite.

Used together with nitrite in pickling of meats and is converted into nitrite in the process. Nitrites can react with haemoglobin to form methaemoglobin (which see), especially in young infants, and an upper limit of 45–50 mg nitrate per litre drinking water has been recommended for infants.

**nitrites**  Found in many plant foods, since they are rapidly formed by the reduction of naturally occurring nitrate. Nitrite is the essential agent in preserving meat by pickling, since it inhibits the growth of clostridia; it also combines with the myoglobin of meat to form the characteristic red nitrosomyoglobin.

**nitrogen**  This is, of course, a gas, comprising about 80% of the atmosphere, but in nutrition the term 'nitrogen' is used to refer to ammonium salts and nitrates as plant fertilisers, to proteins and amino acids as animal nutrients, and to urea and ammonium salts as excretory products. In other words, all nitrogen-containing substances are loosely referred to as 'nitrogen'.

**nitrogen balance**  The difference between the dietary intake of nitrogen (as protein) and its excretion (as urea and other waste products).

During growth and tissue repair (convalescence) the body is in positive N balance, i.e. ingestion is greater than loss. In fevers, fasting and wasting diseases the loss is greater than the intake, and the individual is in negative balance.

Healthy adults are excreting the same amount as is being ingested and so are in N equilibrium.

**nitrogen conversion factor**  Factor by which total N in a material is multiplied to determine the protein; depends on the amino acid composition of the protein of the food. Wheat and most cereals 5.8, rice 5.95, soya 5.7, most legumes 5.3, most nuts 5.3, milk 6.38, other foods 6.25. Errors arise if part of the nitrogen is present as non-protein nitrogen. In mixtures of proteins, as in dishes and diets, the factor of 6.25 is used. 'Crude protein' is defined as N × 6.25.

**nitrogen equilibrium**  See *nitrogen balance*.

**nitrogen, metabolic**  Nitrogen of the faeces derived from internal or endogenous sources, as distinct from nitrogen residue from dietary sources (exogenous nitrogen). This nitrogen consists of unabsorbed digestive juices, the shed lining of the gastrointestinal tract and bacteria from the intestine, and continues to be excreted on a protein-free diet.

**nitrogen trichloride**  As bread 'improver', see *agene*.

**nitrosamines**  Group of compounds bearing the nitroso group on the N of the corresponding amines – *N*-nitrosodimethylamine, *N*-nitrosodiethylamine; found in amounts of a few micrograms per kg in mushrooms, fermented fish meal and smoked fish, and in pickled foods by reaction between nitrite and secondary amines. Causes cancer in all species of animals examined, but not clear whether these amounts affect human beings, especially since it has also been found in human gastric juice (possibly by reaction between amines and nitrites or nitrates from the diet).

**nitrosomyoglobin**  The red colour of cured meat. It is formed by the reaction of nitric oxide from the pickling salts (saltpetre) with the muscle pigment, myoglobin.

Fades in light to yellow-brown metmyoglobin.

**nitrous oxide**  A gas used as a propellant in pressurised containers, e.g. to eject cream or salad dressing from containers.

**NOAE**  With respect to food additives – No Adverse Effect Level – equivalent to No Effect Level.

**No Effect Level (NEL)**  With respect to food additives, the maximum dose of an additive that has no adverse effects.

**noggin**  Used as a measure of liquor = ¼ pint; also known as a quartern.

**N-oil**  Trade name (National Starch and Chemical, UK) for modified tapioca which forms fat-like gel when heated in aqueous solution; mixes well with fats to give a creamy texture.

**non-enzymic browning**  See *Maillard reaction*.

**non-essential amino acids**  See *amino acid*.

**non-esterified fatty acids**  Free fatty acids in the blood, about 10% of the total blood fatty acids, usually 0.5–1.0 micromole per litre.

They have a rapid turnover rate and may be the primary fuel of working muscles. The fuel for sudden bursts of hard exercise is glycogen, but for long-continued work the free fatty acids are said to be the source of energy. Also known as unesterified fatty acids, or UFA or NEFA.

**non-pareils**  The silver beads used to decorate confectionery, made from sugar coated with silver foil or aluminium–copper alloy.

**non-saponifiable fraction**  See *saponification*.

**noodles**  See *alimentary pastes*.

**nor-**  Chemical prefix to the name of a compound indicating one methyl group less, e.g. noradrenalin contains a methyl less than adrenalin, similarly norleucine, norvaline.

**noradrenaline**  Hormone secreted by the adrenal medulla together with adrenaline (which see); also known as nor-epinephrine. Physiological effects similar to those of adrenaline; chemically differs only by the loss of a methyl group.

The nerve endings in certain parts of the nervous system liberate noradrenaline as a chemical stimulator of the muscles.

**norconidendrin**  See *conidendrin*.

**nordihydroguaiaretic acid** (NDGA)  Substance of plant origin (the creosote bush) used as an antioxidant for fats.

**norepinephrine**   See *noradrenaline*.

**norite**   Activated carbon used to decolorise solutions.

**norite eluate factor**   Early name given to folic acid.

**normocytes**   Red blood cells.

**notatin**   See *glucose oxidase*.

**nougat**   Sweetmeat made from a mixture of gelatin or egg albumin with sugar and starch syrup, and the whole thoroughly aerated.

**Novadelox**   Trade name for benzoyl peroxide used for treating flour. See *aging*.

**novain**   Old name for carnitine.

**NPR**   Net protein ratio. See *protein quality*.

**NPU**   Net protein utilisation.

**NPV**   Net protein value.

**nubbing**   Term used in the canning industry for 'topping and tailing' of gooseberries.

**nucellar layer**   Of wheat, the layer of cells that surrounds the endosperm and protects it from the entry of moisture.

**nucleic acids**   Combined with proteins they form the nucleoproteins of cell nuclei.

There are two main types of nucleic acid: ribonucleic acid (RNA), consisting of phosphoric acid, two purines (adenine and guanine), two pyrimidines (cytosine and uracil) and the sugar ribose; and desoxyribonucleic acid (DNA), which differs in containing desoxyribose as the sugar, and thymine in place of uracil.

RNA and DNA are believed to play a key role in the synthesis of proteins in the body and in the transmission of hereditary characteristics.

Nucleoproteins are present in some foods such as fish roe, and are useful as a source of protein, but they are not essential to the diet and the nucleic acids are readily synthesised in the body.

**nucleo-albuminate, iron**   A preparation of iron and casein, also called iron caseinate.

**nucleoproteins**   Specific type of proteins found in cell nuclei of both plants and animals. See *nucleic acids*.

**nucleosides**   Compound of purine or pyrimidine base with a sugar. For example, adenine plus ribose forms adenosine – the nucleoside. With the addition of phosphoric acid a nucleotide is formed.

**nucleotides**   Compound of purine or pyrimidine base with sugar and phosphoric acid.

**nug**   See *nigerseed*.

**nuoc mam**   Fermented fish sauce from Vietnam and Cambodia. The fish is digested by autolytic enzymes in the presence of added salt to inhibit bacteria.

**nutmeg**  Dried ripe seed of *Myristica fragrans*; mace is the seed coat (arillus) of the same species. Both contain fixed oils and their volatile oils are similar but not identical. Both mace and nutmeg are used as flavourings in meat products and bakery goods.

**Nutrasweet**  Trade name (Nutrasweet Co.) for aspartame.

**nutrient enemata**  Rectal feeding can be carried out with nutrient solutions as the colon can absorb 1–2 litres of solution per day; maximum daily amount of glucose that can be given is 75 g, and of nitrogen, in the form of hydrolysed protein, 1 g.

**nutrients**  Essential dietary factors such as vitamins, minerals, amino acids and fats. Sources of energy are not termed nutrients so that a commonly used phrase is 'energy and nutrients' (calories and nutrients).

**nutrification**  Term used of the addition of nutrients to foods at such a level as to make a major contribution to the diet.

**nutrition**  Study of foods in relation to the needs of living organisms.

**nutritionist**  According to the United States Department of Labour, Dictionary of Occupational Titles – one who applies the science of nutrition to the promotion of health and control of disease; instructs auxiliary medical personnel; participates in surveys. See also *dietitian*.

**nutritive ratio**  Measure of the value of a feeding ration for growth (or milk production) compared with its fattening value. It is the sum of the digestible carbohydrate, protein and 2.3 × fat, divided by digestible protein. (Calorie value of fat is 2.3 times carbohydrate and protein.) Ratio 4–5 for growth, 7–8 for fattening.

**nutritive value index**  Term used in animal feeding; intake of digestible energy expressed as energy digestibility multiplied by voluntary intake of dry matter of a particular feed divided by metabolic weight (weight to the power of 0.75), compared with standard feed.

**nutro-biscuit**  Biscuit baked from a mixture of 60% wheat flour and 40% peanut flour – contains 16–17% protein; developed in India.

**nutro-macaroni**  Mixture of 80 parts wheat flour, 20 parts defatted peanut meal (total 19% protein); developed in India.

**nuts**  Hard-shelled fruit of a wide variety of trees, e.g. almonds (*Prunus amygdalis*), Brazil nut (*Bertholletsia excelsa*), cashew nuts (*Anacardium occidentale*), walnut (*Juglans regia*) – all have high fat content, 45–60%; high protein content, 15–20%; 15–20% carbohydrate, much of which is in the form of pentosans and other indigestible forms.

The chestnut (*Castanea sativa*) is something of an exception, with 3% fat and 3% protein, being largely carbohydrate, 37%.

A number of nuts are grown specially for their fat content, such as groundnut, coconut, and palm, which see.

**nyctalopia**   See *night blindness*.


# O


**oats**   Grain from species of *Avena*, the three best-known being *A. sativa*, *A. steritis* and *A. strigosa*.

Analysis per 100 g: protein 13 g, fat 7.5 g, carbohydrate 73 g, kcal 380 (1.6 MJ), calcium 60 mg, iron 4 mg, vitamin $B_1$ 0.6 mg, vitamin $B_2$ 0.1 mg, nicotinic acid 0.9 mg.

Contains large amounts of phytic acid, which can prevent the absorption of calcium from the diet and so induce rickets unless extra calcium and vitamin D are consumed.

Oatmeal – ground oats; oatflour – ground, and bran removed; groats – husked oats; Embden groats – crushed groats; Scotch oats – groats cut into granules of various sizes; Sussex ground oats – very finely ground oats; rolled oats – crushed by rollers and partially precooked.

**obesity drugs**   See *anorectic drugs*.

**octave**   A cask for wine containing 1/8 of a pipe, about 13 imperial gallons (59 litres).

**odoratism**   Disease experimentally produced by feeding sweet-pea seeds, *Lathyrus odoratus*, to rats. Damage to the spine and aorta, caused by the presence of a toxic substance, BAPN (beta-amino propion nitrile). This is present in both the sweet pea and the Singletary pea (*L. pusillus*), but not in the chick pea, *L. sativus*, which causes lathyrism in man. See also *lathyrism*.

**oedema**   Excess fluid in the body indicated by pitting of the subcutaneous tissues when pressure is applied with the finger. May be caused by cardiac, renal or hepatic failure and by starvation (famine oedema).

**oenin**   An anthocyanidin from the skin of purple grapes.

**oestradiol**   See *oestrogens*.

**oestriol**   Urinary excretion product of the female hormones oestrone and oestradiol. See *oestrogens*.

**oestrogens**   Female sex hormones. There are two groups, oestrone and oestradiol, which stimulate the ovaries, and progesterone, produced by the corpus luteum, which stimulates the uterus.

Synthetic hormones include ethinyl oestradiol, stilboestrol

and hexoestrol. The latter two are used in chemical caponisation of cockerels, by implantation under the skin, and to increase the growth rate of cattle, by implantation during the last 3 months before slaughter.

Oestrogenic substances are also found in spring grass.

**oestrone** One of the female sex hormones. See *oestrogens*.

**offal** Corruption of 'off-fall'. With reference to meat, the term includes all parts that are cut away when the carcass is dressed, including liver, kidneys, brain, spleen, pancreas, thymus, tripe and tongue. In the USA the term used is 'organ meats'.

With reference to cereals, offals are the bran and germ discarded when milling to a white flour.

**ohmic heating** Sterilisation by heat generated in fluid passing through a tube while voltage is applied between a series of electrodes. Applied to food products containing particles and liquid, such as meat and vegetables in liquid medium.

**oilseed** A wide variety of seeds are grown as a source of oils, e.g. cottonseed, sesame, groundnut, sunflower, soya, palm, etc. After extraction of the oil the residue is a valuable source of protein, the so-called seed cake.

**oils, essential** See *essential oils*.

**oils, fixed** Refers to the triglycerides, the edible oils, as distinct from the volatile or essential oils, which see.

**okra** Also known as gumbo, bamya, bamies and ladies' fingers (*Hibiscus esculentus*). Small ridged mucilaginous pods resembling a small cucumber, grown in South America, West Indies and India; used in soups and stews.

Analysis per 100 g: carbohydrate 6 g, protein 2 g, Fe 1 mg, carotene 250 μg, vitamin $B_1$ 0.1 mg, vitamin $B_2$ 0.1 mg, nicotinic acid 0.8 mg, vitamin C 25 mg.

**oleandomycin** Antibiotic sometimes used as additive to chicken feed.

**oleic acid** Long-chain fatty acid with total of 18 carbon atoms; unsaturated with one double bond, 9-octadecenoic acid; found in most fats; high percentage in human fat, and butter. By far the most abundant of the unsaturated acids.

**oleomargarine** See *margarine*.

**oleo oils** See *premier jus*; *tallow, rendered*.

**oleoresins** In the preparation of some spices such as pepper, ginger and capsicum, the aromatic material is extracted with solvents which are evaporated off, leaving behind thick oily products known as oleoresins.

**oleostearin** See *premier jus*; *tallow, rendered*.

**Olestra** Trade name (Procter and Gamble) for sucrose polyesters, which see.

**oligoallergenic diet**   Comprised of very few foods or an elemental diet used to diagnose whether particular symptoms are the result of allergic response to food.

**oligodynamic**   Sterilising effect of traces of certain metals. For example, silver in concentration of 1 in 5 million will kill *Escherichia coli* and staphylococci in 3 hours.

Electrolytic method of getting silver into water is katadyn process. Suggestions have been made for its use for the treatment of water, fruit juices and various foods.

**oligosaccharides**   Carbohydrates composed of 3–10 monosaccharide units (with more than 10 units they are termed polysaccharides).

**olive**   Fruit of evergreen tree, *Oleo europea*; picked unripe when green or ripe when they have turned dark blue or purplish, and usually pickled in brine. Olives have been known since ancient times; tree continues to fruit for many years and there are claims that trees are still fruiting after 1000 years.

Analysis per 100 g: 0.9 g protein, 11 g fat, trace carbohydrate, 100 kcal (0.45 MJ), 2 g Na, 60 mg Ca, 1 mg iron. Little or no vitamins when pickled.

Olive oil, obtained by pressing the ripe fruits, is used in cooking, as salad oil and for canning sardines. It is one of the few vegetable oils to contain only small amounts of polyunsaturated fatty acids but 70% oleic acid (monounsaturated).

**omasum**   See *rumen*.

**omega-3 marine triglycerides**   A mixture of eicosapentaenoic acid (20 carbons, 5 double bonds) and docosohexaenoic (22 C,6 double bonds) both of the omega-3 series of polyunsaturated fatty acids.

**omega (3, 6 or 9) fatty acids**   Three series of long chain fatty acids derived respectively from linolenic, linoleic and oleic acids. Omega (ω) or n being the position of the first double bond counting from the terminal methyl group (a procedure more useful to the biochemist than the more correct method of numbering from the opposite end, i.e. the COOH group).

**omophagia**   Eating of raw or uncooked food.

**oncotic pressure**   The osmotic pressure of colloids. Blood plasma has an oncotic pressure of 28 mm of mercury.

**onion**   Bulb of *Allium cepa*.

Analysis of mature bulb per 100 g: 93 g water, 5 g sugars, 1 g protein, 25 kcal (100 kJ), 3–15 mg vitamin C.

Spring onion per 100 g: 87 g water, 9 g sugar, 3 g dietary fibre, 1 g protein, 140 mg Ca, 1 mg Fe, 35 kcal (150 kJ), 20–30 mg vitamin C.

**onion, Welsh**   Perennial onion, *Allium cepa perutile*, cropped by breaking off leaves and leaving plant to grow. Similar to but smaller than the Japanese bunching onion, *Allium fistulosum*.

**Oolong tea** See *tea*.

**ophthalamin** Obsolete name for vitamin A.

**opsomania** Craving for special food.

**optical activity** The ability of certain substances such as sugars and acids to rotate the plane of polarised light. This depends on the molecule being asymmetrical. If the plane of light is rotated to the right, the substance is dextrorotatory and is designated by the prefix ($+$); if laevorotatory, the prefix is ($-$). A mixture of the two forms is optically inactive and is termed racemic.

The degree of rotation measured in the polarimeter under standard conditions serves as a measure of purity and concentration of the substance.

Sucrose is dextrorotatory but is hydrolysed to glucose (dextrorotatory) and fructose, which is more strongly laevorotatory, so hydrolysis changes from ($+$) to ($-$); hence, the mixture of glucose and fructose is termed invert sugar.

**optical rotation** See *optical activity*.

**Opuntia** See *pear, prickly*.

**orange** Fruit of *Citrus sinensis*. Of nutritive value mainly because of its vitamin C content. The juice has the same composition.

Analysis per 100 g: carbohydrate 8.5 g, protein 0.6 g, kcal 30 (150 kJ), Ca 40 mg, Fe 0.3 mg, carotene 50 μg, vitamin C 40–60 mg.

Blood oranges are coloured by the presence of anthocyanins (cyanidin-3-glucoside and delphinidin-3-glucoside) in the juice vesicles.

**orange, bitter** *Citrus aurantium*; known as Seville orange in Spain, bigaradier in France, melangol in Italy and khush khash in Israel.

Used mainly as root stock, because of its resistance to the gummosis disease of citrus. Fruit is too acid to be edible, used in manufacture of marmalade; the peel oil is used in the liqueur curaçao; the peel and flower oils (neroli oil) and the oils from the green twigs (petit-grain oils) are used in perfumery.

**orange butter** Chopped whole orange cooked, sweetened and homogenised.

**orange colours** Orange G – disodium salt of 1-phenylazo-2-naphthol-6,8-disulphonic acid. Stable to reducing agents.

Orange RN – sodium salt of 1-sulphylazo-2-naphthol-6-phenolic acid.

**orange-flower water** Neroli oil is made from the flowers of the bitter orange by steam distillation. The condensed water layer from the distillation is orange-flower water.

**orange oil**  The peel oil, 90% limonene, main odoriferous constituent n-decylic aldehyde (decanal), also linalool and nonylic alcohol.

Oil of bitter orange is similar but contains a glucoside that confers the bitterness. See also *terpenes*.

**orange Pekoe**  See *tea*.

**orcanella**  See *alkannet*.

**orchil**  Red colour obtained from lichens of the *Roccella* species; legally permitted in food in most countries. Colouring principle is orcin (dihydroxy toluene) and orcein, slightly soluble in water to give wine-red solution, yellower with acid, blue with alkalies.

**oreganum**  Or Mexican sage. See *marjoram*.

**organic**  When used appertaining to chemicals, means those that contain carbon in the molecule (with the exception of carbonates and cyanides).

Substances of animal and vegetable origin are organic, minerals are inorganic.

**organic acids**  Acids occurring naturally in foods that contain, as do all organic compounds (apart from carbonic acid and carbonates) carbon, e.g. lactic, fumaric, citric, malic acids. As distinct from the inorganic acids they can be metabolised in the body to provide 3 kcal (13 kJ)/g.

**organoleptic**  Affecting a bodily organ or sense; used particularly of the combination of taste (perceived in the mouth) and aroma (perceived in the nose). There are four tastes – acid, bitter, salt and sweet, with the additional aspect of astringency.

**ormer**  See *abalone*.

**ornithine**  Amino acid that is part of the urea cycle, which see; not of nutritional importance, since it is not found in protein foodstuffs.

**ornithine–arginine cycle**  See *urea cycle*.

**orotic acid**  Uracil-4-carboxylic acid; an intermediate in the biosynthesis of pyrimidines; a growth factor for certain micro-organisms and called vitamin $B_{13}$.

**ortanique**  Citrus fruit; cross between orange and tangerine.

**orthophenyl phenol**  See *diphenyl*.

**oryzanin**  Obsolete name for thiamin (vitamin $B_1$).

**oryzenin**  The major protein of rice; classed as one of the glutelins.

**osazones**  Derivatives formed by reaction of aldehydes and ketones with phenylhydrazone. Used to distinguish between sugars, since the corresponding osazones of the different sugars have different crystal shape (glucose and fructose form the same osazone).

**Oslo breakfast**  Introduced into Oslo, Norway, 1929, for school children before classes started: requires no preparation.

Rye-biscuit, bread made of high extraction flour, butter or vitaminised margarine, whey cheese and cod liver oil paste, ⅓ litre of milk, raw carrot, apple, half orange.

**osmazome** Old (obsolete) name given to an aqueous extract of meat which is soluble in alcohol – regarded as the pure essence of meat.

**osmophiles** Micro-organisms that can flourish under conditions of high osmotic pressure, e.g. jams, honey, brine pickles; especially osmophilic yeasts also called xerophilic yeasts.

**osmosis** Passage through a semi-permeable membrane. See *membrane, semi-permeable*; *osmotic pressure*.

**osmosis, reverse** Passage of water from a more concentrated to a less concentrated solution through a semipermeable membrane by the application of pressure. Used for desalination of sea-water, concentration of fruit juices and processing of cheese whey. Membranes commonly cellulose acetate or polyamide of very small pore size, $10^{-4}$–$10^{-3}$ µm.

**osmotic pressure** The attractive power exerted by a solution for water molecules.

Usually demonstrated by placing a solution of a salt in a vessel separated by a semi-permeable membrane (e.g. pig's bladder) from pure water. Water passes across the membrane to dilute the salt solution until the hydrostatic pressure of the solution counterbalances the attractive power of the solution for the water, i.e. its osmotic pressure.

See *membrane, semi-permeable*.

**ossein** Organic structure of the bone left behind when the mineral salts are removed by solution in dilute acid. Chemically similar to collagen and hydrolysed by boiling water to gelatin; hence the manufacture of glue from bones – known as ossein gelatin.

**osseomucoid** Mucoid substance forming part of the structure of bone.

**osteomalacia** Bone disorder in adults equivalent to rickets in children; due to shortage of vitamin D leading to inadequate absorption of calcium and loss of calcium from the bones.

**Ostermilk** Trade name (Glaxo Laboratories) for dried milk for infant feedings. Ostermilk No. 1 is half-cream; No. 2 is normal.

**ovalbumin** The albumin of egg-white; comprises 55% of the total solids.

**Ovaltine** Trade name (A. Wander Ltd) for a preparation of malt extract, milk, eggs, cocoa and soya, for consumption as a beverage when added to milk. Fortified with vitamin $B_1$, vitamin D and nicotinic acid.

**oven spring** The sudden increases in the volume of a dough during the first 10–12 minutes of baking – due to increased rate of fermentation and to expansion of gases.

**overrun** Term used in ice-cream manufacture – the percentage increase in the volume of the mix caused by the beating-in of air. Optimum overrun, 70–100%.

To prevent excessive aeration United States regulations state that ice-cream must weigh 4.5lb per gallon.

**ovoflavin** Name given to substance isolated from eggs, shown to be identical with riboflavin.

**ovomucin** A carbohydrate–protein complex in egg-white, 1–3% of the total solids. Responsible for the firmness of egg-white.

**ovomucoid** A protein of egg-white, 12% of the total solids. Acts as a specific inhibitor of the digestive enzyme trypsin, but is destroyed by the stomach enzyme pepsin.

**oxalated blood** See *blood, oxalated*.

**oxalic acid** Lowest member of dicarboxylic acid series, COOHCOOH. Poisonous, but not in small doses; present in spinach, chocolate and rhubarb. The toxicity of rhubarb leaves is due to their high content of oxalic acid.

Oxalic acid is normally excreted in human urine, 15–20mg per day, increased in diabetes and liver disease.

**oxidase, phenol** See *phenol oxidases*.

**oxidases** Enzymes that oxidise compounds by removing hydrogen and adding it to oxygen to form water. They thus differ from dehydrogenases, since the latter cannot pass the hydrogen directly on to oxygen, but only to an intermediate.

See also *intermediate hydrogen carrier*.

**oxidation** Gain in oxygen, or loss of hydrogen or (covering all cases such as oxidation of ferrous chloride to ferric chloride when neither oxygen nor hydrogen is involved) loss of electrons.

See *intermediate hydrogen carrier*; *oxidases*.

**oximetry** The continuous measurement of the amount of oxygen in the circulating blood.

**Oxo** Trade name (Oxo Ltd) for a dried preparation of hydrolysed meat, meat extract, salt and cereal in cube form, used as a drink or a gravy.

Analysis per 100g: protein 9.5g, fat 3.4g, carbohydrate 12.0g, Ca 180mg, Fe 25mg, kcal 115 (0.5MJ).

**oxybiontic** Term applied to micro-organisms that can utilise molecular oxygen.

**oxycalorimeter** Instrument for measuring the oxygen used and carbon dioxide produced when a food is burned (as distinct from the bomb calorimeter, which measures the heat produced).

**oxyhaemoglobin** Form in which oxygen is transported from the lungs to the tissues; a loose combination of oxygen with the haemoglobin, which is readily decomposed.

**oxymyoglobin**   Myoglobin is the coloured protein in muscle which serves as a store of oxygen; it takes up oxygen to form oxymyoglobin, which is bright red, while myoglobin itself is purplish-red. The surface of fresh meat which is exposed to oxygen is bright red from the oxymyoglobin, while the interior of the meat is darker in colour where the myoglobin is not oxygenated.

**oxyntic cells**   Or parietal cells; glands in the stomach that produce hydrochloric acid of the gastric juice.

**oyster**   Marine bivalve mollusc, *Ostreidae* and *Crassostrea* species. Analysis per 100 g; protein 10 g, traces of fat and carbohydrate (some glycogen when alive) iron 6 mg, zinc 50 mg, vitamin $B_{12}$ 15 µg, only traces of other vitamins (contrary to popular superstition), 50 kcal (200 kJ).

**ozone**   Chemically, composed of three atoms of oxygen, $O_3$. Powerful germicide, used to sterilise water, in antiseptic ice for preserving fish, few ppm in the atmosphere to preserve eggs, etc.

# P

**P.4000**   A class of synthetic sweetening agents, chemically nitro-amino alkoxybenzenes. One member of the group, propoxy-amino nitrobenzene is 4100 times as sweet as saccharine, but these compounds are not considered harmless and are not permitted in foods.

   Dutch name is Aros.

**PA 3679**   Designation of a putrefactive anaerobic microbe widely used in investigations of heat sterilisation.

**PABA**   Abbreviation for para-amino benzoic acid, which see.

**pacificarins**   Compounds present in foods (of microbial origin or synthesised by the plant) that resist micro-organisms. Another name is phytoncides (or these may be similar substances).

**paddy**   Rice in the husk after threshing; also known as rough rice. See *rice*.

**palatinose**   6-*O*-glucosyl fructose (isomaltulose).

**Palestine bee**   See *bee wine*.

**palmitic acid**   One of the long-chain saturated fatty acids, $CH_3(CH_2)_{14}COOH$. Occurs as triglyceride in many animal and vegetable fats, including spermaceti and beeswax.

**palm kernel oil**   Oil extracted from the kernel of the nut of *Elaeis guineensis*. The oil from the pulp is termed palm oil, which see. Used for margarine and cooking fat.

**palm oil**   Oil extracted from the pericarp or outer pulp beneath the outer skin of the nut from the oil palm, *Elaeis guineensis*.

Coloured red because of high content of alpha-carotene (24 mg per 100 g) and beta-carotene (30 mg) together with about 60 mg tocopherols. Only 5–12% polyunsaturated fatty acids – linoleic acid.

One of the major oils of commerce, and widely used in cooking fats and margarines.

**palm, wild date** *Phoenix sylvestris*, relative of the true date palm, *P. dactylifera*, grown in India as a source of sugar, obtained from the sap.

**panada** Mixture of fat, flour and liquid (such as stock or milk) mixed to a thick paste; used to bind mixtures such as chopped meat and also as the basis of soufflés and chou pastry.

**panary fermentation** Yeast fermentation of dough in bread-making.

**pancreas** A gland in the abdomen with two functions; it secretes (a) the hormone insulin, (b) the pancreatic juice.

Known by the butcher as sweetbread, or gut sweetbread, in distinction from chest sweetbread, which is thymus.

**pancreatic juice** Digestive juice produced by the pancreas and secreted into the duodenum; slightly alkaline, contains the enzymes trypsinogen, chymotrypsinogen, carboxypeptidase, aminopeptidase, lipase, amylase, maltase, sucrase, lactase and nucleases.

**pancreatin** Preparation made from the pancreas of animals and therefore containing the enzymes of pancreatic juice. Used as an aid to digestion.

**pancreozymin** Hormone produced by the intestinal mucosa which stimulates the pancreas to secrete enzymes. See also *secretin*.

**panettone** Italian, half bread–half cake.

**pangamic acid** *N*-di-isopropyl derivative of glucuronic acid. Powerful methylating agent concerned with respiratory enzymes in cells. Also termed vitamin $B_{15}$, but no evidence that it is a dietary essential.

**panthenol** Alcohol form of pantothenic acid with similar activity.

**pantothenic acid** A vitamin with no numerical designation; chemically, beta-alanine plus pantoic acid. Is part of the structure of coenzyme A, needed for the transfer of acetyl groups and therefore essential for the metabolism of fats and carbohydrates. An unstable oil usually used as calcium or sodium salt.

Dietary shortage never arises; universally distributed in all living cells, best sources being liver, kidney, yeast, bees' royal jelly and fresh vegetables.

Deficiency symptoms in rats include greying of the hair, dermatitis, adrenal damage; in chicks, dermatitis; in dogs, gastrointestinal symptoms; but no definite pathological lesions in man.

On the basis of the needs of animals, human requirements would be 6–8 mg per day.

Also known as filtrate factor.

**pantoyltaurine** Similar to pantothenic acid but with the carboxyl group replaced by a sulphonic acid group; acts as an antagonist to the vitamin.

When given to man, leads to dizziness, postural hypotension, tachycardia, drowsiness and anorexia. Also called thiopanic acid.

**papain** Proteolytic enzyme from the juice of the papaya (*Carica papaya*) used in tenderising meat; sometimes called vegetable pepsin. Rate of reaction slow at room temperature, increase at 55–75 °C, maximum activity at 80 °C and rapidly inactivated at temperatures higher than this; hence, the papain continues to tenderise the meat during the early stages of cooking.

**papaya** See *pawpaw*.

**Papin's digester** Early version of the pressure cooker. Named after Papin, French physicist 1647–1712; originally invented for the purpose of softening bones for the preparation of gelatin.

**paprika** See *pepper*.

**para-amino benzoic acid** Essential growth factor for micro-organisms and therefore classed as a vitamin. No deficiency symptoms in higher animals except greying of the hair (achromotrichia) in rats.

Is part of the molecule of folic acid and it is assumed that one of the functions of para-amino benzoic acid is the formation of folic acid.

Sulphanilamide is chemically very similar and kills bacteria by blocking access to the vitamin.

Occurs in yeast, wheat germ; smaller amounts in meat, liver, vegetables. Also called the anti-grey hair factor.

**parabens** Methyl, ethyl and propyl esters of *p*-hydroxybenzoic acid used together with their sodium salts as antimicrobials in food. Effective over a wide range of pH; more effective against moulds and yeast than bacteria.

**paracasein** Obsolete name used in the USA for milk casein after it was precipitated.

**paraffin, medicinal** See *medicinal paraffin*.

**Paraflow** Trade name (APV Co. Ltd) for a plate heat exchanger used for pasteurising liquids.

**parakeratosis** Disease of swine characterised by cessation of growth, erythema, seborrhoea and hyperkeratosis of the skin; due to zinc deficiency, and essential fatty acids may be involved.

**paralactic acid**  See *sarcolactic acid*.

**paralytic shellfish poisoning**  Caused by shellfish which have accumulated toxins from certain species of the dinoflagellate plankton, *Gonyaulax*.

**parathormone**  See *parathyroid glands*.

**parathyroid glands**  Four glands situated in the neck near to the thyroid gland but not connected with its function. They secrete the parathyroid hormone (parathormone) which controls the levels of the calcium in the blood and the excretion of phosphate in the urine. An overactive parathyroid causes withdrawal of calcium from the bones, so raising the blood level and causing excretion in the urine. When there is a fall in serum calcium, the parathyroid responds by reducing blood phosphate by excreting it in the urine.

**parboil**  Partially cook. Of special interest in nutrition is the parboiling of brown rice, that is steaming of the rice in the husk before milling. The water-soluble B vitamins diffuse from the husk into the grain. When the rice is then polished, the white rice contains far more of these vitamins than polished raw rice.

**parchita**  See *passion fruit*.

**parenteral nutrition**  Slow infusion of solution of nutrients into the veins through a catheter.

**parietal cells**  See *oxyntic cells*.

**parillin**  Highly toxic glycoside from sarsaparilla root; consists of glucose, rhamnose and parigenin. Also known as smilacin.

**parsley**  The leaves of the herb *Petroselinum crispum* or *P. hertense*, widely used as a garnish and flavouring. Rich in carotene and vitamin C but the amount consumed is too little to make a contribution to the diet. Turnip-rooted parsley is the root of *Petroselinum crispinum* var. *tuberosum*, also known as Hamburg parsley.

**parsnip**  Root of *Pastinaca sativa*, eaten as a vegetable.

Analysis per 100 g, boiled: 13 g carbohydrate, 2.5 g dietary fibre, 1.3 g protein, 55 kcal (240 kJ) 5–20 mg vitamin C.

**parts per million**  (ppm) Method of describing small concentrations and means exactly what the terms says. Mg per kg is also ppm.

Usually used with regard to traces of metallic impurities and food additives, e.g. jam must not contain more than 40 ppm of sulphur dioxide.

**passion fruit**  Also known as parchita, granadilla and water lemon; fruit of the tropical American vine, *Passiflora* species. Purple or greenish-yellow when ripe, watery pulp containing small seeds; used in fruit drinks.

Analysis per 100 g: carbohydrate 16 g, protein 1.2 g, carotene 60 μg, vitamin C 20 mg.

**pasta**  See *alimentary pastes*.

**pasteurisation**  Vegetative forms of many bacteria can be killed by mild heat treatment, pasteurisation, whereas total destruction of all bacteria and spores, sterilisation, requires higher temperatures for longer periods, often spoiling the product in the process. Pasteurisation will prolong the storage life of foods but usually only for a limited period.

Pasteurisation of milk destroys all the pathogens, and although the milk will sour within a day or two, it is not a source of disease.

Legally, pasteurisation of milk means maintaining at 145–150°F (63–66°C) for 30 minutes, followed by immediate cooling, or so-called 'high-temperature short-time process', 161°F (72°C) for 15 seconds.

See also *flash-pasteurisation*; *methylene blue dye-reduction test*; *phosphatase test*.

**pasteuriser**  Equipment used to pasteurise liquids such as milk, fruit juices, etc. They function, in effect, as heat-exchangers. The material to be pasteurised is passed continuously over heated plates, or through pipes, where it is heated to the required temperature, maintained at that temperature for the required time, then immediately cooled.

**patent flour**  See *extraction rate*.

**pathogens**  Disease-causing bacteria, as distinct from those that are harmless.

**patri**  See *clay*.

**patulin**  Mycotoxin found in fruit juices from fruits infected with one of a variety of moulds (*Penicillium expansum*, *Aspergillus calvatus*, *A. terreus* and *Byssochlamys nivea*). Removed by fermentation and also pasteurisation.

**patum peperium**  See *Gentleman's relish*.

**Pavlov pouch**  Surgical technique, introduced by Pavlov, in which a portion of the stomach is brought to the body wall. It is then possible to take a sample of the stomach contents directly from this pouch, as the secretion of the pouch is identical with that into the main part of the stomach.

**pawpaw** (papaya)  Large green or yellow melon-like fruit of the *Carica papaya*, a tree similar to the palm. It is the commonest tropical fruit second to the banana and is a rich source of vitamin A and C.

Analysis per 100 g: water 89 g, carbohydrate 9 g, kcal 40 (0.16 MJ), carotene 800 μg, vitamin C 80 mg.

The proteolytic enzyme, papain, is obtained as the dried latex of the skin of the fruit by scratching it while still on the tree, and collecting the flow. In the tropics meat is often tenderised by wrapping in pawpaw leaves.

**payusnaya**   Coarse, pressed caviare including skins of ovaries (Russia and Eastern Europe).

**PCM**   Protein-calorie malnutrition. See *protein-energy malnutrition*.

**pea, garden**   Also called green pea; seed of the legume *Pisum sativum*.

Analysis, fresh, raw, per 100 g: 4 g sugars, 7 g starch, 5 g dietary fibre, 6 g protein, 80 kcal (180 kJ), 2 mg Fe, 300 µg carotene, 0.3 mg thiamin, 0.15 mg riboflavin, 2.5 mg niacin, 15–35 mg vitamin C.

Widely available in frozen, dried and canned forms.

See also *petit pois* and *legumes, food*.

**pea, processed**   Garden peas (*Pisum sativum*) that have matured on the plant and subsequently been canned.

**peanut**   Also known as ground nut, earth nut and monkey nut. Seed of the legume *Arachis hypogaea*; Spanish and Virginia types have 2 kernels per pod, Valencia has 3–4.

The nuts serve as an important source of protein in many tropical diets. The oil, known as arachis oil, is used for cooking, as salad oil, for canning sardines and for margarine manufacture. The residue after oil extraction is a valuable source of protein for animal feed.

Analysis per 100 g: 26 g protein, 40 g fat, 550 kcal (2.3 MJ), 2 mg Fe, 1 mg vitamin $B_1$, 0.1 mg vitamin $B_2$, 16 mg nicotinic acid.

See also *Bambarra groundnut*.

**peanut butter**   Ground, roasted peanuts; commonly prepared from a mixture of Spanish and Virginia peanuts, since the first alone is too oily and the second is too dry. Separation of the oil is prevented by partial hydrogenation of the oil and the addition of emulsifiers.

**pear**   Fruit of many species of *Pyrus*; cultivated varieties all descended from *P. communis*.

Analysis per 100 g: 0.4 g protein, 0.3 g fat, 50 kcal (0.2 MJ), very small amounts of carotenoids, B vitamins and vitamin C.

**pear, prickly**   Fruit of the cactus *Opuntia*, also called Indian fig, barberry fig, and tuna – an important part of the diet in certain areas of Mexico.

Analysis per 100 g: water 81 g, protein 1 g, carbohydrate 26 g, vitamin C 15 mg, kcal 70 (280 kJ).

**peas**   See *legumes, food*.

**pectase**   Enzyme in the pith of citrus fruits which removes the methoxyl groups from pectin to form water-insoluble pectic acid. The intermediate compounds with varying numbers of methoxy groups are pectinic acids.

Also known as pectin esterase, pectin methyl esterase and pectin methoxylase.

**pectin** Plant tissues contain protopectins (which are chemically hemicelluloses) cementing the cell walls together. As fruit ripens, there is maximum protopectin present; thereafter it breaks down to pectin, pectinic acid and finally pectic acid under the influence of enzymes, and the fruit loses its firmness and becomes soft as the adhesive between the cells breaks down.

Pectin is the setting agent in jam. Soft fruits, as strawberry, raspberry and cherry, are low in pectin; plum, apple and bitter orange are rich. Apple pulp and orange pith are the commercial source of pectin. Used to add to jams, confectionery, chocolate; added to ice-cream as an emulsifier and stabiliser instead of agar; in making jellies; and as anti-staling agent in cakes.

See *firming agents*; *jam*.

**pectinase** Enzyme present in the pith (albedo) of citrus fruits, which hydrolyses pectins or pectic acids into smaller polygalacturonic acids, and finally galacturonic acid and its methyl ester.

Also known as pectolase and polygalacturonase.

**pectinesterase** Alternative name for pectase, which see.

**pectin methoxylase** See *pectase*.

**pectins, low-methoxyl** Partially de-esterified pectins which can form gels with little or no sugar and therefore used in low-calorie jellies.

**pectolase** Alternative name for pectinase, which see.

**pectosase** See *protopectinase*.

**pectosinase** Alternative name for protopectinase, which see.

**Pekar test** A comparative test of flour colour. The flour is pressed on a board with a smooth applicator and colour comparisons are made immersed in water.

**Pekoe** See *tea*.

**pelagic fish** Refers to those that swim near the surface, compared with demersal fish, which live on the sea bottom. Pelagic fish are mostly of the oily type (herring, mackerel, pilchard), containing up to 20% oil.

**pellagra** Disease due to deficiency of nicotinic acid. Symptoms include characteristic symmetrical dermatitis on exposed surfaces such as face and back of hands, mental disturbances and digestive disorders. (Students' mnemonic – dermatitis, dementia and diarrhoea – arising from diet of meat, maize and molasses.)

**PEM** Protein-energy malnutrition

**pemmican** Mixture of dried, powdered meat and fat.

Analysis per 100 g: 3 g water, 40 g protein, 45 g fat, 560 kcal (2.4 MJ).

Used as concentrated food source, e.g. on expeditions.

**penicillin**  The first of the antibiotics, isolated from the culture fluid of the mould *Penicillium notatum*, 1929. Active against a wide range of bacteria and of great value clinically. Not used as food preservative in case repeated small doses cause penicillin resistance.

*Penicillium*  See *moulds*.

**pentosans**  Complex carbohydrates widely distributed in plants, e.g. fruit, wood, corncobs, oat hulls. Not digested in the body but broken down by acid to yield the 5-carbon sugars or pentoses.

**pentose**  Simple sugar with 5 carbon atoms. The most important is ribose.

**pentosuria**  Unexplained excretion of pentose sugars in the urine without any ill-effects. An inherited metabolic disorder almost wholly restricted to Ashkenazi (N. European) Jews.

**P-enzyme**  Potato phosphorylase, specific for 1,4-alpha links.

**pepper**  Three types.

(1) Sweet pepper, paprika, bell pepper, bullnose pepper, Spanish name pimiento (not the same as pimento or allspice); fruits of the annual plant *Capsicum annum*. Red, yellow or brown fruits, often eaten raw in salads when green and unripe; very variable size and shape; some varieties can be spicy but mostly non-pungent.

Analysis per 100 g: 2 g protein, 0.5 g fat, 6 g carbohydrate, 40 kcal (0.16 MJ), 1 mg Fe (green peppers 40 µg carotene, red peppers 300 µg), 0.06 mg vitamin $B_1$, 0.08 mg vitamin $B_2$, 1 mg nicotinic acid, 150 mg vitamin C (range 50–300).

(2) Red pepper, chilli (or chili), small red fruit of *Capsicum frutescens*, bushy, perennial plant. Usually sun-dried and therefore wrinkled, very pungent, ingredient of curry powder, pickles and tabasco sauce. Cayenne pepper is made from the powdered dried fruits.

Analysis per 100 g (dried): 15 g protein, 11 g fat, 33 g carbohydrate, 25 g fibre, 290 kcal (1.2 MJ), 9 mg Fe, 300 µg carotene, 0.6 mg vitamin $B_1$, 0.5 mg vitamin $B_2$, 12 mg nicotinic acid, 10 mg vitamin C.

(3) Black and white pepper, fruit of climbing vine, *Piper nigrum*, grows in wet tropical conditions; fruits are peppercorns. Black pepper is made from sun-dried unripe peppercorns when red outer skin turns black. White pepper is made by soaking ripe berries and rubbing off outer skin. Pungency due to alkaloids piperine, piperdine and chavicine.

Analysis per 100 g: 12 g protein, 7 g fat, 60 g carbohydrate, 5 g fibre, 350 kcal (1.5 MJ), 0.04 mg vitamin $B_1$, 0.2 mg vitamin $B_2$, 1 mg nicotinic acid.

**pepperoni** See *sausage*.

**Pepsi-Cola** Trade name (Pepsicola Co. Ltd) of a soft drink composed of sugar, vanilla, essential oils, spices and extract of cola nut coloured with caramel. Originally made in 1896 in the USA by Caleb Bradham, druggist.

**pepsin** Proteolytic enzyme in the gastric juice which hydrolyses certain of the linkages of proteins to produce peptones. Functions only at acid pH, 1.5–2.5. Secreted as the inactive precursor pepsinogen, which is activated by acid.

**peptidases** Old name for exopeptidases, which see.

**peptides** Compounds formed when amino acids are linked together through the $-CO-NH-$ linkage. Two amino acids so linked form a dipeptide, three a tripeptide, etc. Long chains are polypeptides.

Proteins are composed of multiple bundles of long chains of polypeptides joined by cross-linkages.

**peptones** Intermediate stage in the hydrolysis of proteins; distinguished from proteoses in not being precipitated by ammonium sulphate.

The term is often used for any partial hydrolysate of proteins as, for example, 'bacteriological peptone' used as a medium for the growth of micro-organisms.

**pericarp** In reference to cereal grain, this consists of 2–4 fibrous layers next to the outer husk and outside the testa; of low digestibility and removed from grain during milling. It is the major constituent of bran.

**perigo factor** Name given to a postulated inhibitory factor produced when bacterial growth medium is autoclaved with nitrite: it is about 10 times more inhibitory to certain bacteria than nitrite alone.

**perillartine** Non-nutritive sweetening agent derived from perillaldehyde, extracted from shiso oil (commercially available in Japan); 2000 times as sweet as sucrose.

**perimysium** See *muscle*.

**peristalsis** Method of movement along the intestine, peristaltic waves, caused by contraction of a ring of muscle, preceded by a wave of relaxation.

**pernicious anaemia** Form of anaemia due to a deficiency of vitamin $B_{12}$ needed for maturation of the red blood cells. Almost always due to a defect in the absorption of vitamin $B_{12}$ (termed the extrinsic factor), which requires the agency of a factor produced in the gastric mucosa – the intrinsic factor – for absorption. Rarely due to a dietary shortage of vitamin $B_{12}$, which see.

**peroxidase** Plant enzyme that splits hydrogen peroxide into water and oxygen, only when there is a substance present to accept the oxygen (unlike catalase, which splits peroxide into water and gaseous oxygen).

Contains haematin in the molecule, and blood itself has a peroxidase-like activity that is used in the benzidine test for blood.

**peroxide**   See *hydrogen peroxide.*

**peroxide number**   Or peroxide value; measure of the oxidative rancidity of fats by determination of the peroxides present. Measured by the amount of iodine liberated from potassium iodide: peroxide value is the number millilitres of 0.002 N sodium thiosulphate per gram of sample.

**Perrier water**   Mildly alkaline, well-aerated natural water, containing sodium bicarbonate. Obtained mainly from Les Bouillens, Vergéze, France.

**perry**   Fermented pear juice, analogous to cider from apples.

**Persian berry**   Yellow colour obtained from the berries of the buckthorn (*Rhamnus*) family; legally permitted in food in most countries. Contains the glucosides of two colouring matters, rhamnetin and rhamnazin.

**persimmon**   Or date plum. Fruit of *Diospyros kaki*, Japanese persimmon, which has the appearance of the tomato (called kaki in France); eaten raw, made into jams and jellies, and as persimmon pie made from the American persimmon (*D. virginiana*), in which the fruit is not cooked, since heating produces an acid taste.

**Peruvita**   Protein-rich baby food developed in Peru. Sweet version 30% protein, made from quinua and cotton-seed flour, with skim-milk powder, sugar, spices, vitamins A, $B_1$ and $B_2$ and calcium carbonate.

Savoury version, 35% protein, contains salt in place of sugar.

**pervaporation**   Evaporation from a colloidal suspension by heating in a collodion bag. If there are crystalloids present, they pass through the membrane and are deposited on the outside of the bag.

**PET**   Polyethylene terephthalate; plastic used in packaging, e.g. bottles for drinks.

**petechiae**   (petechial haemorrhages)   Small, pin-point bleedings in the skin; one of the symptoms of scurvy.

**petit-grain oils**   Prepared from twigs and leaves of the bitter orange by steam distillation; similar to neroli oil but less fragrant.

Petit-grain Portugal prepared from leaves of sweet orange, Mandarin petit-grain from tangerine tree leaves, and lemon petit-grain.

**petit pois**  Small peas; according to the code of practice for canned fruits and vegetables, up to and including $11/32$ inch in diameter; medium, up to $13/32$ inch; large or standard, greater than $13/32$ inch.

**PGA**  Pteroyl glutamic acid. See *folic acid*.

**pH**  Abbreviation of potential hydrogen, used to denote the degree of acidity of a substance.

Defined as the negative logarithm of the hydrogen-ion concentration in gram-atoms per litre. The scale runs from 0 (1 gram of H ion per litre), extremely strongly acid, to 14 (one hundred-million-millionth of a gram of H ions) extremely strongly alkaline.

Pure water is pH 7, which is neutral; below 7 is acid, above is alkaline.

**phaeophytin**  Formed from chlorophyll by the removal of the magnesium; occurs in acid medium. It is brownish-green in colour and accounts for the colour change when green vegetables are cooked.

**phage**  See *bacteriophage*.

**phagomania**  Morbid obsession with food; also sitomania.

**phagophobia**  Fear of food; also sitophobia.

**phase inversion**  Milk is an emulsion of fat in water; butter is an emulsion of water in fat. The change from cream to butter is termed phase inversion.

**phaseolin**  Globulin protein in kidney bean.

**phaseolunatin**  Cyanogenetic glucoside found in certain legumes (such as lima bean, chick pea, common vetch), which hydrolyses to produce glucose, acetone and hydrocyanic acid; not proved harmful when present in the diet.

**phasin**  Term originally used for the haemagglutinin from *Phaseolus vulgaris* but is now a term occasionally used for non-toxic plant agglutinins.

**PHB ester**  *p*-Hydroxybenzoic acid – ethyl and propyl esters and their sodium salts. Used as preservative in some countries.

**phenetylurea**  See *dulcin*.

**phenol oxidases**  Enzymes that oxidise phenolic compounds to quinones. For example, monophenol oxidase in mushrooms; polyphenol oxidases in potato and apple are responsible for the development of the brown colour when the cut surface is exposed to air; tyrosinase in plants and animals which is responsible for brown and black pigmentation.

**phenylalanine**  An essential amino acid. The non-essential tyrosine can partially replace phenylalanine in the diet.

It is rarely, if ever, the limiting amino acid in any food.

Inability to metabolise phenylalanine is an inherited disease and causes mental disorder, phenylketonuria, which see.

**phenylketonuria**  Inherited metabolic defect wherein the essential amino acid, phenylalanine, is incompletely metabolised and the end-product, phenylpyruvic acid, is excreted in the urine. The product affects the brain and causes imbecility. The effect can be moderated by strict limitation of the phenylalanine intake.

**phitosite**  High-calorie food.

**phloridzin**  See *phlorrhizin*.

**phlorrhizin**  Also spelled phloridzin and phlorhizin. A glycoside of plant origin; abolishes the renal threshold for glucose, which therefore appears in the urine (glycosuria). This is known as renal diabetes or phlorhizin diabetes. Used to examine the formation of glucose from other ingredients of the diet.

**phosphatase test**  For adequate pasteurisation of milk. Depends on the fact that the enzyme phosphatase, normally present in milk, is destroyed at a temperature slightly greater than that required to destroy the tubercle bacillus and other pathogens. This enzyme liberates inorganic phosphate from phenyl phosphate and its activity can be measured by either the phenol or the phosphate.

In the tintometer (see *Lovibond comparator*) more than 2.3 Lovibond blue units (phosphate estimation), under the conditions of the test, indicates inefficient pasteurisation. Can detect 0.2% raw milk in pasteurised milk.

**phosphate**  Salt of phosphoric acid, which see. See also *phosphate bond, energy-rich*; *phosphorus*; *polyphosphates*.

**phosphate additives**  See *polyphosphates*.

**phosphate bond, energy-rich**  Phosphates of organic compounds fall into two groups, depending on the amount of energy released when the phosphate portion is hydrolysed. (a) Low-energy potential, the ordinary phosphates which liberate 1.22 –1.5 kcal (e.g. phospho-sugars, phospho-glycerols, phospho-glyceric acids, phosphocholine); (b) high-energy potential or energy-rich phosphates, which liberate about 8–10 kcal (e.g. anhydrides, where phosphate is linked to phosphate, acidic enols such as phosphoenolpyruvic acid, acetyl phosphate and nitrogen linked to phosphate).

Phosphate-bond energy is the only form of energy that can be used by any living cell (muscular activity, osmotic work, the shock produced by the electric eel).

Adenosine triphosphate (ATP) is the key compound because it acts as a store of the energy-rich phosphate bonds.

**phosphatides**  Also phospholipins or phospholipids. Fatty substances including phosphoric acid and a nitrogenous base in the molecule. Include lecithins, cephalins, sphingomyelins, and cerebrosides. Part of the structure of the brain and nervous tissue and involved in fat transport.

Also combined with proteins as lipoproteins.

Are partly soluble in water as well as in fats and used in food technology as emulsifiers. From the dietary point of view they may be regarded as simple fats.

**phosphokinases** Enzymes that transfer the phosphate radical, together with its energy, to or from adenosine di- or triphosphate. Various other molecules can be involved but one of the pair of reactants is adenosine di- or triphosphate.

**phospholipins** See *phosphatides*.

**phosphoproteins** Conjugated proteins containing phosphate other than as nucleic acid (nucleoproteins) or lecithin (lipoproteins), e.g. casein from milk, ovovitellin from egg yolk.

**phosphoric acid** May be one of three types – orthophosphoric acid ($H_3PO_4$), metaphosphoric acid ($HPO_3$) or pyrophosphoric acid ($H_4P_2O_7$).

Used in acid-fruit flavoured beverages such as lemonade.

See also *phosphorus*.

**phosphorolysis** Hydrolysis in which the elements of phosphoric acid are added at the broken linkage, e.g. the enzyme phosphorylase hydrolyses glycogen not to glucose but to glucose phosphate.

**phosphorus** This element occurs in all biological tissues as phosphate, i.e. salts of phosphoric acid. In the body most of it (80%) is present in the skeleton and teeth as calcium phosphate $(Ca_3PO_4)_2$, about 10% in the muscles and 1% in the nervous sytem. It is of vital importance in metabolism, as many compounds (such as vitamins $B_1$ and $B_2$, glucose, adenosine, etc.) function as phosphates.

The parathyroid glands control the level of phosphate in the blood.

Human dietary needs (about 1.3g per day) are always met; a deficiency never occurs in man. Phosphate deficiency, however, is one of the commonest deficiencies in livestock and gives rise to osteomalacia (also known as sweeny or creeping sickness).

Phosphate is also essential for plant growth; hence the use of bone meal as fertiliser. Bone meal (calcium phosphate), is often used as a supplement in human foods but as a source of calcium rather than of phosphate.

In calculating the amount of phosphate in foodstuffs textbooks vary in expressing the value as phosphorus (P) or phosphate ($P_2O_5$); 31 parts of P are equivalent to 142 parts of $P_2O_5$.

See also *calcium–phosphate ratio*; *phosphate bond, energy-rich*; *phosphoric acid*; *phytic acid*; *polyphosphates*.

**photosynthesis** The manufacture by plants of complex foods from water and carbon dioxide under the influence of sunlight. During the first stage, hydrogen is stripped from the water molecules and subsequently oxygen is released. The hydrogen atoms serve as a source of electrons which, under the influence of light, convert the chlorophyll into a high-energy state. During the second stage this energy is released through a series of reactions to form ATP, which, in the third stage, results in the conversion of carbon dioxide into sugar (the Calvin cycle of carbon fixation).

See also *C3 plants*; *C4 plants*.

**phrynoderma** A follicular hyperkeratosis of the skin (blocked pores or toad-skin) often encountered in malnourished people. Originally thought to be due to vitamin A deficiency but possibly due to other deficiencies, and occurs mildly in well-nourished people.

**phthiocol** See *vitamin K*.

**phycotoxins** Name sometimes given to those marine biotoxins that accumulate in fish and shellfish from their diet (paralytic and ciguatera poisoning) as distinct from toxins naturally present (tetramine poisoning).

**phyllo** Paper-thin pastry of Greek origin made only from flour and water and used for savoury and sweet pies.

**phylloquinone** See *vitamin K*.

**phylloxera** An aphid which threatened to destroy the vineyards of Europe in the middle of the nineteenth century. Saved by grafting susceptible varieties on to resistant American rootstock.

**physalin** Zeaxanthin dipalmitate; a carotenoid pigment found in the fruits of the Chinese lantern, *Physalis*.

**physin** Growth factor needed by rats and occurring in liver; probably vitamin $B_{12}$.

**phytanic acid** Tetramethyl hexanoic acid, formed in the body from free but not combined phytol; traces in fats. See *Refsum's disease*.

**phytase** Phosphatase enzyme that hydrolyses phytin to inositol and phosphoric acid. Present in yeast, liver, blood, malt and seeds. If a high level of yeast is used in baking with high-extraction flours, some of the phytin is broken down. See also *phytic acid*.

**phytic acid** Inositol hexaphosphoric acid, present in cereals, particularly in the bran, dried legumes and some nuts as both water-soluble salts (sodium and potassium) and insoluble salts of calcium and magnesium. Magnesium calcium phytate is phytin – approximately 12% calcium, 1.5% magnesium and 22% phosphorus.

Possibly involved in texture changes when potatoes and pulses are cooked (through binding of calcium). Can bind calcium, iron and zinc into insoluble complexes and it is not clear how far phytate reduces the availability of these minerals in the diet, especially since there are phytase enzymes in yeasts and legumes (and possibly in the human gut) which may liberate these minerals.

**phytin** See *phytic acid*.

**phytoalexins** Substances, often harmful, which increase in plant tissues when stressed, as in physical damage, exposure to ultraviolet light.

**phytol** Methyl pentadecanol; traces in some plant tissues but mostly combined in chlorophyll and vitamins E and K. See *Refsum's disease*.

**phytoplankton** Minute plants floating in the sea which serve as the basic food for all marine life, since they photosynthesise.

**phytosterol** General name given to sterols occurring in plants, the chief of which is sitosterol (structurally closely related to cholesterol).

**phytylmenaquinone** See *vitamin K*.

**pica** Perverted appetite (eating of earth, sand, clay, paper, etc.).

**piccalilli** Mixture of chopped, brine-preserved vegetables in mustard sauce (mustard and vinegar, thickened with tapioca starch, plus other spices, coloured yellow).

**pickles, dill** Pickles that are fermented in a mixture of brine, cured dill weed, mixed spices and vinegar.

**pickling** Also called brining. Vegetables immersed in 5–10% brine undergo lactic acid fermentation, while the salt prevents the growth of undesirables. The sugars in the vegetables are broken down to lactic acid; at 25°C the process takes a few weeks, finishing at 1% acidity. See *curing of meat; halophilic bacteria*.

**pidan** See *Chinese eggs*.

**pikelets** See *dough cakes*.

**pilchard** Fatty fish, *Sardina* (*clupea*) *pilchardus*; young is the sardine.

Analysis per 100 g: 22 g protein, 11 g fat, 200 kcal (0.8 MJ), 230 mg Ca, 3 mg Fe.

**pimento** See *allspice*.

**pimiento** See *pepper*.

**pineapple** Fruit of the tropical plant *Ananas sativus*.

Analysis per 100 g: protein 0.3 g, fat 0.1 g, kcal 30 (0.13 MJ), Ca 12 mg, Fe 0.3 mg, vitamin $B_1$ 0.05 mg, vitamin $B_2$ 0.02 mg, nicotinic acid 0.1 mg, vitamin C 25 mg.

**pineapple dill** See *flavours, synthetic*.

**pint, reputed** 13⅓ fluid oz. See *quart, reputed*.

**pipe**  Cask for wine; volume varies with the type of wine, e.g. port, 115 gallons, 517 litres; Teneriffe, 100; Marsala, 93, 418 litres.

**pipecolic acid**  Chemically, piperidine-2-carboxylic acid. Occurs in fresh green beans, potatoes and mushrooms, in fresh fruit and the dried seeds of legumes. Its pharmacological effects are unknown.

**pipis**  Edible mollusc, *Plebidonas deltoides*, widely distributed around Australian coastline.

**pith**  See *albedo*.

**pits**  Stones from cherries, plums, peaches, apricots. The oil is extracted from these pits and used in cosmetics, pharmaceuticals, canning sardines and as table oil. The press cake left behind contains the bitter principle, amygdalin.

**plankton**  Minute organisms, both plant (phytoplankton) and animal (zooplankton), drifting in the sea, which serve as the basic foodstuffs of marine life.

**plansifter**  A nest of sieves mounted together so that material being sieved is divided into a number of fractions of different size. Widely used in flour milling.

**plantain**  Adam's fig; variety of banana with higher starch and lower sugar content than dessert bananas, picked when flesh is too hard to be eaten raw and used for cooking. Some varieties become sweet if left to ripen, others never develop a high sugar content.

Analysis per 100 g: 1 g protein, 0.2 g fat, 32 g carbohydrates, 130 kcal (0.05 MJ), 0.05 mg Fe, 30 µg carotene, 0.05 mg vitamin $B_1$, 0.05 mg vitamin $B_2$, 0.7 mg nicotinic acid, 20 mg vitamin C.

**plasma, blood**  Blood consists of red cells, white cells and platelets, suspended in a clear protein solution, the plasma. Plasma proteins include fibrinogen, albumins and globulins. Of the 9% total plasma solids, 7% are proteins.

**plasma lipids**  See *lipids*, *plasma*.

**plasmapheresis**  Experimental method of reducing the serum proteins to a low level by removing part of the blood and returning only the red cells to the blood stream.

**plasma proteins**  In solution in the blood plasma – three main types, fibrinogen (0.2–0.4 g per 100 ml), albumin (4.4–5.3) and globulin (1.9–2.8).

**plate count**  To estimate the number of bacteria in a sample, it is poured on to an agar plate, when each bacterial cell or group of cells multiplies to produce a colony which is visible to the naked eye. A count of the number of colonies gives the number of bacteria in that portion of the sample that was taken.

Pasteurised milk contains about 100000 bacteria per millilitre;

good-quality raw milk contains less than 500000 per millilitre.

**plato**  See *balling*.

**Pliofilm**  Trade name for varieties of rubber hydrochloride, the first transparent wrapping paper (1934) that could be heat-sealed.

**PLJ – Pure Lemon Juice**  Trade name (Beecham Foods Ltd). Lemon juice containing 53 mg vitamin C per 100 g.

**pluck**  Butchers' term for heart, liver and lungs of an animal.

**plum**  Numerous species of *Prunus*. Common European plums are *P. domestica*; blackthorn or sloe is *P. spinosa*; bullace is *P. insititia*; damson is *P. damascena*; gages are *P. italica*. Small amounts of protein, carbohydrate and fat.

Analysis per 100 g: 60 kcal (0.24 MJ), 100 µg carotene, 0.5 mg nicotinic acid, 5 mg vitamin C.

**pneumatic conveying**  Transfer of material in powder form by means of air currents. Applied to flour, sugar, cement, etc.

**pneumatic dryers**  The material is dried almost instantaneously in a turbulent stream of hot air, which also acts as a conveyor system. Applicable to powdered, granular and flaky materials.

**pneumatic ring dryer**  A pneumatic dryer (which see) in which the product travels several times through a ring duct, impelled by hot air, and the drying time, temperature and rate of flow of the material can be controlled.

Used for starch, mashed potatoes, cereals, flour, powdered soups.

**poach**  To cook for a short time in a shallow layer of liquid kept at a temperature just below the boiling point.

**POEMS**  Polyoxyethylene monostearate; see *polyoxyethylene*.

**poikilotherms**  Cold-blooded animals, those whose temperature varies with their environment.

**poisoning, food**  See *food poisoning*.

**polarimeter**  Instrument used to determine the degree of rotation of polarised light. Consists of two Nicol prisms (calcite), the first of which polarises the light and the second is used after the light has passed through the test solution to determine the rotation.

All optically active substances, such as sugars and amino acids, rotate polarised light and the degree of rotation is used as a quantitative measure of the substance.

See also *optical activity*.

**polariscope**  Alternative name for polarimeter, which see.

**polarised light**  Ordinary light vibrates in many planes; after passing through a crystal of quartz or 'polaroid', it vibrates in only one plane, i.e., it is polarised. Many naturally occurring compounds in solution possess the ability to rotate the plane of polarised light, i.e. they are optically active. See *optical activity*.

**polarogram** See *polarograph*.

**polarograph** Instrument used to measure traces of metallic ions by change in electric current.

The test solution is the electrolyte between two mercury electrodes; a continuously increasing negative potential is applied to the cathode and the change in current with voltage is recorded – the polarogram. The rise in current at a particular voltage is a measure of the concentration of the metal ion present.

**polenta** Traditional Italian porridge made from maize meal, often with cheese added. May be further cooked by baking or frying.

Also the Italian word for coarsely ground maize meal, as hominy grits is the American term.

**polished rice** See *rice*.

**pollards** See *wheatfeed*.

**polycythaemia** Increase in the number of red blood cells; results from strenuous physical exercise, residence at high altitudes, administration of drugs or cobalt, and certain diseases.

**polydextrose, modified** Randomly bonded glucose polymer molecular size 5000 or less prepared by heating glucose and sorbitol with citric acid; because of the random bonding and occasional diester linkage, it is more resistant to enzymic digestion than normal polymers and 60% is excreted in faeces undigested – so providing only about 1 kcal/g; hence, termed non-sweetening sucrose replacement, or bulking agent.

**polyglucose** See *polydextrose*.

**polymorphism** The ability to crystallise in two or more different forms. For example, depending on the conditions under which it is solidified, the fat tristearin can form three kinds of crystals, each of which has a different melting point, namely, 54, 65 and 71 °C.

**polymyxin** Antibiotic isolated 1947 from *Bacillus polymyxin* (*Bacillus aerosporin*). There are several polymyxins, of which polymyxin A is aerosporin. They are polypeptides, active against coliform bacteria; apart from clinical use, they are of value in controlling infection in brewing.

**polyols** Sugar alcohols such as glycerol, sorbitol, inositol, etc.

**polyose** Polysaccharide.

**polyoxyethylene** Monoglycerides are soluble in fat, but by reacting with ethylene oxide the resulting polyoxyethylene derivatives become water-soluble to whatever degree is required. These compounds are polyoxyethylene esters, ethers, sorbitol esters, etc. They are valuable as emulsifying agents in bakery.

One of the best-known is polyoxyethylene stearate, used as a crumb-softener.

**polypeptides**  See *peptides*.

**polyphagia**  Excessive or continuous eating.

**polyphosphates**  Complex phosphates added to foods, in particular to meat products; they prevent sausage discoloration, aid mixing of the fat, speed penetration of the brine in curing, cause protein fibres of meat to retain more water and swell (so improving texture).

Include pyrophosphate ($Na_4P_2O_7$), tripolyphosphate ($Na_5P_3O_{10}$), and longer phosphate chains of 100 phosphate units, polyphosphate glasses prepared by rapid quenching of $Na_2O-P_2O_5$ melts (e.g. Calgon, 12 unit chain length), etc.

**polysaccharides**  Complex carbohydrates formed by the condensation of large numbers of monosaccharide units, e.g. starch, glycogen, cellulose, dextrins, inulin. On hydrolysis the simple sugar is liberated.

**polysaccharose**  Polysaccharide.

**polyunsaturated fatty acids**  Long-chain fatty acids containing two or more double bonds separated by methylene bridges:

$$-CH_2-CH=CH-CH_2-CH=CH-CH_2-$$

including alpha and gamma linolenic (3 double bonds: higher plants and algae), eicosatetraenoic (arachidonic – 4 db), docosapentaenoic (clupanodonic – 5 db: fish oils), docosahexaenoic (6 db; fish oils).

**pomace**  Residue of crushed apple pulp after expressing juice; also applied to any pressed fruit pulp and to fish from which oil has been expressed.

**pombé**  African beer prepared from millet seed. The seed is sprouted to break down the starch to fermentable sugar, a process similar to malting in beer manufacture, and then allowed to ferment spontaneously.

**pomegranate**  *Punica granatum*. Juice contained in a pulpy sac surrounding each of a mass of seeds – outer skin contains tannin and therefore bitter.

Sweet juice used to prepare grenadine syrup for alcoholic and fruit drinks.

Analysis per 100 g: water 80 g, protein 1 g, carbohydrate 18 g, kcal 80 (0.32 MJ), Fe 0.7 mg, vitamin A nil, Vitamin $B_1$ 0.02 mg, vitamin $B_2$ 0.03 mg, nicotinic acid 0.2 mg, vitamin C 8 mg.

**pomelo**  Also spelled 'pomeloe' and 'pummelo'; alternative name shaddock, *Citrus grandis*, from which the grapefruit is descended.

**pomes**  Botanical name for fruit formed by the enlargement of the receptacle which becomes fleshy and surrounds the carpels, e.g.

apple, pear.

**Ponceau colours**   A series of strawberry red colours.

Ponceau MX – disodium salt of 1-(2,4- or mixed xylylazo)-2-naphthol-3,6-disulphonic acid; also called Ponceau R and 2R and RS.

Ponceau 4R – trisodium salt of 1-(4-sulpho-1-naphthylazo)-2-naphthol-6,8-disulphonic acid; also called Cochineal red A.

Ponceau SX – disodium salt of 2-(5-sulpho-2,4-xylylazo)-1-naphthol-4-sulphonic acid; called Red No. 4 in the USA.

Ponceau 3R – disodium salt of 1-pseudocumylazo-2-naphthol-3,6-disulphonic acid; called Red No. 1 in the USA; Maraschino cherry red colour.

Ponceau 6R – tetra sodium salt of 2-(6′-sulpho-1′-*m*-xylylazo)-1-naphthol-5-sulphonic acid.

**ponderal index**   An index of adipose tissue; height divided by the cube root of the body weight; high for thin people, low for fat people.

**ponderocrescive**   Foods tending to increase weight: easily gaining weight; opposite to pondoperditive – stimulating weight loss.

**pone bread**   Colloquial name for corn bread in the southern states of the USA. (Corn pone are small corn cakes, a speciality of Alabama, USA.)

**Pontefract cakes**   A round, flat sweetmeat made from liquorice originally in Pontefract in Yorkshire, England (also called Pomfret).

**poonac**   The residue of coconut after the extraction of the oil.

**popcorn**   Variety of maize, *Zea mays*, that expands on heating.

**pork carcass**   Analysis, fat, per 100 g: protein 9 g, fat 50 g, kcal 500 (2.0 MJ), Fe 1 mg, vitamin $B_1$ 0.3 mg.

Medium per 100 g: protein 10 g, fat 40 g, kcal 400 (1.7 MJ), Fe 1.2 mg, vitamin $B_1$ 0.4 mg, vitamin $B_2$ 0.10 mg, nicotinic acid 2.4 mg.

Lean per 100g: protein 12 g, fat 30 g, kcal 300 (1.3 MJ), Fe 1.4 mg, vitamin $B_1$ 0.4 mg, vitamin $B_2$ 0.1 mg, nicotinic acid 2.7 mg.

**Porphyra**   Red alga cultivated in Japan to make 'Komba'. In Great Britain it is collected from the sea to make laverbread, which see.

**porphyria**   Clinical disorder of metabolic pathway of haem synthesis in which porphyrins are excreted in the urine and faeces, and, in some disorders, deposited in the skin.

**porphyrins**   Compounds consisting of a ring system of four pyrrole nuclei joined by the =CH− bridges. Chlorophyll is a magnesium porphyrin; haem is an iron porphyrin.

**porphyropsin**   Photosensitive pigment in the retinas of the eyes of fresh-water fish, containing dehydro retinol – analogous to rhodopsin in the eyes of marine fish, mammals, birds and amphibians.

**porter** See *beer*.

**port wine** Fortified wine, 16% alcohol, 12% sugars, 160 kcal (660 kJ) per 100 ml. Designated 'ruby' (the youngest and sweetest), 'tawny' (aged in the wood) and 'vintage' (aged in the bottle).

**Poskitt index** Index of fatness in children; per cent expected weight for age, i.e. weight/50th centile weight at that age when the child's height was on the 50th centile of reference standard.

**posset** Drink made of hot milk curdled with ale or wine, sometimes thickened with breadcrumbs and spiced. Formerly used as remedy for colds.

**Postum, Instant** Trade name (General Foods Corp., USA) for a preparation of bran, wheat and molasses consumed as a beverage.

**potassium** Element widespread in nature and present in the human body in amounts of about 250 g. Mostly present inside the cells. One of the most important of the plant nutrients.

**potassium nitrate** See *nitrate*; *nitrites*; *saltpetre*.

**potassium sorbate** See *sorbic acid*.

**potato flour** Dried potato tuber.

Analysis per 100 g: starch 73 g, protein 8.5 g, fat 0.4 g, kcal 350 (1.5 MJ), Ca 30 mg, Fe 3 mg, vitamin $B_1$ 0.21 mg, vitamin $B_2$ 0.1 mg, nicotinic acid 5 mg, vitamin C 20 mg.

**potato, Irish** The tuber of *Solanum tuberosum*.

Analysis per 100 g: 76 g water, 20 g starch, 2 g dietary fibre, 2 g protein, 90 kcal (340 kJ), 600 mg potassium, 0.5 mg Fe, 0.1 mg thiamin, 1.2 mg niacin, 8–20 mg vitamin C, depending on length of time in storage.

**potato starch** Also called farina. Prepared from potato tuber and widely used as a stabilising agent when gelatinised. Large grains gelatinise very easily when heated.

**potato, sweet** Tubers of herbaceous climbing plant *Ipomoea batatas*.

The flesh may be white, yellow or pink (if carotene is present); the leaves are edible.

Analysis per 100 g: starch 22 g, protein 1 g, fat 0.3 g, kcal 100 (0.4 MJ), Fe 0.8 mg, carotene 150 µg, vitamin $B_1$ 0.08 mg, vitamin $B_2$ 0.04 mg, nicotinic acid 0.5 mg, vitamin C 20 mg.

**pot-au-feu** Traditional French dish made by stewing meat with vegetables. Soup is made from the liquor.

**potential energy** See *energy*.

**pottle** English wine measure of half a gallon.

**poultry, New York dressed**  Refers to poultry that have been slaughtered and plucked but not eviscerated.

**pound cake**  Rich cake containing a pound, or equal quantities, of each of the major ingredients.

**PP factor**  See *nicotinic acid*.

**ppm**  Parts per million.

**PP vitamin**  See *nicotinic acid*.

**praline**  (1) A paste of roasted nuts and partly caramelised sugar used on cakes or as a chocolate filling.

(2) A sugar-coated almond.

**prawn, Dublin Bay**  See *lobster*.

**prawns**  Shellfish of various tribes of suborder *Macrura*.

Large fish of species of *Palaemonidae*, *Penaeidae* and *Pandalidae* are prawns; smaller fish are shrimps.

In addition, deepwater prawn is *Pandalus borealis*; common pink shrimp is *Pandalus montagui*; brown shrimp is species of *Crangon*.

Dublin Bay prawn is lobster, which see.

Analysis per 100 g: 20 g protein, 2 g fat, 100 kcal (0.4 MJ), 150 mg calcium, 1 mg Fe.

**PRE**  Protein retention efficiency. See *protein quality*.

**precursor, enzyme**  Some enzymes are secreted as an inactive precursor that has to undergo a reaction before it shows normal activity. Thus, trypsin is secreted as inactive trypsinogen, which must react with enterokinase before it becomes active; similarly pepsinogen and chymotrypsinogen.

**premier jus**  Best-quality suet prepared from oxen and sheep kidneys. The fat is chilled, shredded and heated at moderate temperature.

When pressed, premier jus, like rendered tallow, separates into a liquid fraction (oleo oil or liquid oleo) and a solid fraction (oleostearin or solid tallow).

**preservation**  Protection of food from deterioration by micro-organisms, enzymes and oxidation – by cooling, destroying the micro-organisms and enzymes by heat treatment, or irradiation, reducing their activity through dehydration or the addition of chemical preservatives, and by smoking, salting and pickling.

**preservatives**  Substances capable of retarding or arresting the deterioration of food; examples are sulphur dioxide, benzoic acid, specified antibiotics, salt, acids and essential oils.

**pressure cooking**  See *autoclave*.

**pressure, oncotic**  See *oncotic pressure*.

**pressure, osmotic**  See *osmotic pressure*.

**pretzels**  Hard brittle German biscuits made from flour, water, shortening, yeast and salt. The dough is fermented and chopped into lengths and shaped; they are boiled in 0.3% sodium hydroxide, salted, baked and dried.

Originally called bretzels and still made in the shape of the letter B.

**probiotics**  Organisms and substances that contribute to intestinal microbial balance (coined by R. B. Parker, 1974). Commonly used to describe certain animal feed supplements to promote growth and protect against disease but would also apply to some preparations of yoghurt for human consumption.

**Procea**  Trade name (Procea Ltd) of a white loaf with slightly increased protein content.

Analysis per 100 g: protein 10.7 g, fat 2.4 g, carbohydrate 50 g, Ca 140 mg, Fe 1.8 mg, kcal 255 (1.1 MJ).

**proenzymes**  Inactive precursors to enzymes, also called zymogens. See **precursor, enzyme**.

**profiteroles**  Small rounds of chou pastry used as a garnish for clear soups or consommés; or filled with cream, baked and sweetened with syrup and chocolate sauce.

**Proflo**  Trade name (Trader Oil Mill Co., USA) for partially defatted, cooked, cottonseed flour.

**progesterone**  See *oestrogens*.

**progoitrin**  Substances found in plant foods which are converted into goitrins, e.g. glucoside of hydroxybutenyl isothiocyanate.

**pro-insulin**  Precursor to insulin in pancreas consisting of insulin molecule combined with a peptide called C-peptide and some amino acids.

**prolamins**  Proteins insoluble in water, neutral solvents and absolute alcohol, but soluble in 70–80% alcohol; e.g. wheat gliadin, corn zein, barley hordein, malt bynin.

Low in lysine, rich in proline and glutamic acid.

**proline**  A non-essential amino acid. Chemically, pyrrolidine carboxylic acid.

**Prolo**  Protein-rich baby food (49% protein) made in Great Britain from soya flour with methionine, minerals and vitamins A, $B_1$, $B_2$ and nicotinic acid.

**Promega**  Trade name (Parke Davis) for mixture of eicosapentaenoic and docosohexaenoic acids (EPA and DHA – long chain marine fatty acids).

**Pronutro**  Protein-rich baby food (22% protein) developed in South Africa; made from maize, skim-milk powder, groundnut flour, soya flour and fish protein concentrate with yeast, wheat germ vitamins A, $B_1$, $B_2$ and nicotinic acid, iodised salt and sugar.

**proof spirit**  A method of describing the alcohol content of spirits. Proof spirit contains 57.07% alcohol by volume and 49.24% by weight in Great Britain. In the USA it contains 50% alcohol by volume.

Thus, absolute alcohol is 175.25 degrees proof UK and 200 degrees proof USA.

Spirits are described as under or over proof. A mixture 30 degrees over proof contains in 100 volumes as much alcohol as 130 volumes of proof spirit; 30 degrees under proof means that 100 volumes contain as much alcohol as 70 volumes of proof spirit.

In Germany percentage alcohol by weight is used, in Italy and France it is percentage by volume.

Proof spirit is a solution of alcohol of such strength that it will ignite when mixed with gunpowder; specifically, at 10°C it weighs $^{12}/_{13}$ parts of an equal volume of distilled water.

**propionates** Salts of propionic acid, $CH_3CH_2COOH$. The free acid and its sodium and calcium salts are used as mould inhibitors, e.g. on cheese surfaces; also to inhibit rope in bread.

Propionic acid is formed in the rumen of cattle together with acetic and butyric acids, and all three are converted into milk constituents.

In the body it is metabolised to pyruvic acid, which is normally formed in the body, and thus considered harmless.

**propyl gallate** See *antioxidants*.

**Prosparol** Trade name (Duncan and Flockhart, Edinburgh) for an emulsion containing 50% vegetable fat – 405 kcal (1.7MJ) per 100g; used as a concentrated source of energy.

**prosthetic group** See *enzyme*.

**protamines** The simplest natural proteins, containing only a limited number of amino acids, chiefly the basic ones, especially arginine. Soluble in water; not coagulated by heat; so basic that they form salts with strong mineral acids, e.g. salmine from salmon sperm, sturine from sturgeon sperm, clupeine from herring sperm, scombrine from mackerel sperm.

**proteans** Slightly altered proteins that have become insoluble, probably an early stage of denaturation.

**Protein, Alpha** Trade name for a protein isolated from soya bean, used for paper coating, water-miscible paints, leather finishing, adhesives. 88.7% protein, 8.5% water.

**proteinases** Old name for endopeptidases, which see.

**protein, Bence-Jones** Unusual protein excreted in the urine in multiple myelomatosis, leukaemia and eczema; coagulates at 55°C and redissolves on boiling.

**Protein, Beta** Trade name for a protein isolated from soya bean, mainly used to prepare adhesives for plywood.

**protein-bound iodine** See *thyroglobulin*.

**protein calories per cent**   See *protein–energy ratio*.

**protein conversion factor**   See *nitrogen conversion factor*.

**protein, crude**   Total nitrogen multiplied by 6.25. See *nitrogen conversion factor*.

**protein efficiency ratio**   A measure of the nutritive value of proteins carried out on young growing animals. Is defined as the gain in weight per gram of protein eaten. The maximum values, e.g. egg protein, are about 4.4.

Zero values are obtained for those proteins which, when fed alone, do not permit growth, but may still have some limited value.

**protein–energy malnutrition** (PEM)   A spectrum of disorders ranging from marasmus to kwashiorkor due to inadequate feeding of infants. At one time marasmus, extreme emaciation, was more specifically attributed to severe overall malnutrition and kwashiorkor, which is accompanied by gross oedema (bloating), was attributed to diets supplying adequate energy but insufficient protein. The name kwashiorkor is derived from the Ga language of Ghana to describe the illness of the first child when it is weaned (on to an inadequate diet) on the arrival of the second child; affects many children in the 1–3 year age group in developing countries.

**protein–energy ratio**   Protein content of a food or diet expressed as ratio between energy from protein and total energy. Previously termed protein calories per cent, being expressed as a percentage of total calories supplied by protein.

**protein equivalent**   A measure of the digestible nitrogen of an animal feedingstuff in terms of protein. It is measured by direct feeding or calculated from the digestible pure protein plus half the digestible non-protein nitrogen.

**protein, first class**   First and second class proteins are obsolete terms indicating those of high or low nutritive value, generally, but not invariably, animal and plant protein, respectively.

**protein milk**   Partially skimmed lactic acid milk plus milk curd (prepared from whole milk by rennet precipitation); richer in protein and poorer in fat than ordinary milk – supposed to be better tolerated in digestive disorders. Also known as albumin milk and eiweiss milch.

**protein quality**   Measure of the usefulness of a protein food for various purposes, including growth, maintenance, repair of tissue, formation of new tissues and, in animals, production of eggs, wool and milk. Various methods of measurements are used to serve as an index of quality. See *biological value*; *net protein utilisation*; *protein efficiency ratio*.

Net protein retention (NPR) is weight gain minus the weight

loss of a non-protein group of animals, divided by protein consumed.

Protein retention efficiency (PRE) is the NPR converted into a percentage scale by multiplying by 16 – it then becomes numerically the same as net protein utilisation.

Relative protein value (RPV) is a comparison of protein quality with a standard determined by a slope-assay method of nitrogen balance carried out at different levels of dietary protein.

Chemical score is the amount of the limiting amino acid compared with the amount of the same amino acid in egg protein (protein score is similar but uses an amino acid mixture as the target). Amino acid score is another term for protein score.

Essential amino acid index is the sum of all the essential amino acids compared with those in egg protein or the amino acid target mixture.

**protein rating** Term used in Canadian Food Regulations to assess overall protein quality of a food. Protein efficiency ratio multiplied by protein content of food (per cent) multiplied by the amount of food that is reasonably consumed.

Foods with rating above 40 may be designated excellent dietary sources; foods with rating below 20 are considered to be insignificant sources; 20–40 may be described as good sources.

**protein, reference** See *reference protein*.

**proteins** Essential constituents of all living cells; distinguished from fats and carbohydrates in containing nitrogen; basically composed of carbon, hydrogen, oxygen, nitrogen, sulphur and sometimes phosphorus.

All proteins are composed of large combinations of 20 amino acids (some bacterial proteins contain additional unusual amino acids). Meat, fish, eggs, cheese, hair, leather, fur and many hormones have a high protein content.

**proteins, conjugated** The molecule contains protein and a non-protein prosthetic group; e.g. nucleoproteins, glycoproteins phosphoproteins, chromoproteins, lipoproteins, which see.

**protein score** A chemical method of defining the nutritional value of proteins; the ratio of the amount of the limiting essential amino acid in the protein, to the target value. See also *chemical score*.

**protein shift** Name applied in flour milling to the phenomenon in which the protein content of the smaller particles of flour (up to 15 micrometres) is higher, namely 15–20%, than that of the flour as a whole, 8–14%, while particles of intermediate size, 15–35 micrometres, have a lower protein content than the flour as a whole.

**Protenum** Trade name (Mead, Johnson Ltd, USA) of a concentrated food preparation containing 42% protein, 46% carbohydrate and 2% fat.

**proteolysis** The hydrolysis of proteins to amino acids by alkali, acid or enzymes.

**proteoses** Partial degradation products of proteins; soluble in water. The stages of breakdown are protein–proteoses–peptones–polypeptides–amino acids. The proteoses are distinguished from peptones in that they are precipitated from solution by ammonium sulphate, whereas peptones are not.

Primary proteoses precipitated with half-saturated ammonium sulphate; secondary proteoses require full saturation.

**prothrombin** Protein of the plasma involved in coagulation of the blood, which see.

**protogen** See *lipoic acid*.

**Protone** Protein-rich baby food (24% protein), made in Great Britain and Congo from maize, skim-milk powder, yeast with added vitamins and minerals.

**protopectin** See *pectin*.

**protopectinase** The enzyme in the pith of citrus fruits which converts protopectin into pectin with the resultant separation of the plant cells from one another. Also known as pectosinase and pectosase.

**proving** In bread making this refers to stages when the dough is left to rise.

**provitamin** A substance that is converted into a vitamin, such as 7-dehydrocholesterol, which is converted into vitamin D. In the old nomenclature carotene was termed provitamin A.

**proximate analysis** Nearly complete analysis comprising protein, fat and ash, and, by subtracting these from the total, calculating 'carbohydrate by difference'. The last value may be corrected for crude fibre.

**prunes, dried** See *fruit, dried*.

**prunin** See *naringin*.

**Pruteen** Trade name (ICI Ltd) for microbial protein produced by growing bacteria, *Methylophilus methylotrophus*, on methanol (derived from methane or natural gas); 70% protein on dry weight.

**pseudoglobulin** Water-soluble globulin which is not precipitated from salt solutions by dialysis against distilled water. Pseudoglobulin fractions occur in blood serum, in animal tissues, and in milk. See also *euglobulin*.

**pseudokeratins** See *keratin*.

**P/S ratio** Ratio between polyunsaturated and saturated fatty acids. Low ratios believed to be a risk factor in atherosclerosis and coronary heart disease. Ratio in western diets about 0.6; suggested that risk reduced if the ratio is changed towards 1.0.

**psychrometric charts**   Humidity charts; show properties of mixtures of air with water vapour.

**psychrophilic bacteria**   Prefer temperatures 15–20°C (59–68°F) and will still grow at and below 0°C (32°F) – that is, in cold stores. Bacteria of the genera *Achromobacter*, *Flavobacterium*, *Pseudomonas* and *Micrococcus*; *Torulopsis* yeasts; and moulds of the genera *Penicillium*, *Cladosporium*, *Mucor* and *Thamnidium* can all develop at low temperatures.

Temperatures must be reduced to about −10°C (13°F) before growth stops, but the organisms are not killed and will regrow when the temperature rises.

**psyllium**   Also known as plantago or flea seed – *Plantago psyllium*. Small, dark reddish-brown seeds which form a mucilaginous mass with water, taken medicinally to assist the passage of intestinal contents.

**pteroyl glutamic acid**   See *folic acid*.

**ptomaines**   Loosely used name for amino compounds formed by decarboxylation of amino acids during putrefaction of animal proteins – putrescine from arginine, cadaverine from lysine, muscarine in mushrooms, neurine formed by dehydration of choline.

**ptyalin**   Old name for salivary amylase.

**pudding, black**   Also known as blood pudding. Traditional European dish made with sheep or pig blood and suet, originally together with oatmeal, liver and herbs stuffed into membrane casings shaped like a horseshoe.

**pudding, hasty**   Old dish made from oatmeal boiled with water for only 2–3 minutes; the finished dish is very low in water content.

**PUFA**   Polyunsaturated fatty acids.

**puffer fish poisoning**   See *tetrodontin poisoning*.

**puff pastry**   During preparation continuous layers of fat are formed between layers of dough; upon baking steam accumulates between the dough layers and causes them to expand, forming large spaces between thin layers of pastry.

**pulque**   Sourish beer produced by the rapid natural fermentation of aquamiel, the sweet mucilaginous sap of the agave (American aloe or century plant). Contains 6% alcohol by volume; common in Central and South America.

**pulses**   Name given to the dried seeds (matured on the plant) of legumes such as peas, beans and lentils. In the fresh, wet form they contain about 90% water, but the dried form contains about 10% water and can be stored. See *legumes, food*.

**pumpernickel** Heavy, black bread made from rye originating from Germany. Name derived from Napoleon's remark that it was 'pain pour Nicole' (his horse).

**pumpkin** See *gourds*.

**purines** Compounds containing the structure

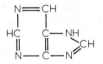

They occur in nucleic acids, which see. Caffeine and theobromine are purines. When taken in the diet, purines are excreted as uric acid. Sweetbread (pancreas) is rich in purines, followed by sardines and anchovies, then meat and fish, with little in vegetables, none in fruits and cereals.

**purothionine** Lipoprotein in wheat with fungicidal properties. May be the factor known to bakers and brewers as 'yeast poison': similar compound found in barley is called hordothionine. Used to classify yeasts.

**putrescine** Tetramethylene-diamine; formed by decarboxylation of arginine.

**pyrexia** Rise in body temperature.

**pyridine nucleotides** See *nicotinamide adenine dinucleotide*.

**pyridoxal** See *vitamin B₆*.

**pyridoxine** See *vitamin B₆*.

**pyrimidines** Compounds containing the structure

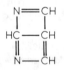

They occur in nucleic acids, which see.

**pyrithiamine** Pyridine analogue of thiamin; antagonistic to the vitamin.

**pyrocarbonate** See *diethyl pyrocarbonate*.

**pyrogens** Substances produced by living bacteria (not yeasts or moulds) which cause a rise in body temperature on injection. Thus any material that has been infected may, despite subsequent sterilisation, contain pyrogens and be unsuitable for injection. Pyrogens are not destroyed by heat and water supplies can be pyrogenic.

**pyruvate oxidation factor** See *lipoic acid*.

**pyruvic acid**  $CH_3COCOOH$. Occupies a central position in the metabolism of carbohydrate. The anaerobic breakdown of glucose produces pyruvic acid, which is then oxidised via the tricarboxylic acid cycle to carbon dioxide and water.

It accumulates in the blood in vitamin $B_1$ deficiency; it is reduced to lactic acid.

# Q

$Q_{O_2}$  Symbol used in measuring cell respiration in the Warburg manometer; the number of microlitres of oxygen consumed (or carbon dioxide or other gas produced) per mg dry weight of tissue per hour.

**Q-enzyme**  Factor isolated from potatoes that catalyses the formation of branching linkages of the 1,6-alpha type in starches; the reaction appears to be irreversible, i.e. the Q-enzyme cannot hydrolyse these 1,6-alpha linkages.

**quarg**  Low fat, acid-ripened soft cheese, 20% solids, 0–8% fat, higher fat content can be achieved by mixing with cream; originated in Germany, similar to French fromage frais.

**quart, reputed**  Customary measure in relation to bottled wine and spirits is a 'bottle' known as a reputed quart, approximately two-thirds of an imperial quart, or 26⅔ fluid ounces.

Reputed pint is 13⅓ fluid ounces.

**quebracho**  Or aspidosperma; obtained from the bark of *Aspidosperma quebrachoblanco*; used as source of tannins and alkaloids.

**queen substance**  The material secreted by the queen bee which inhibits the ovaries of the worker bees and stops them constructing queen cells. Thought to be chemically 10-hydroxy delta-2-decenoic acid.

**quenelle**  A ball of chopped spiced meat or fish.

**quercetin**  A flavone found in onion skins, tea, hops, horse chestnuts; the disaccharide derivative containing rhamnose and glucose is rutin.

**quercitol**  See *acorn sugar*.

**quercitron**  See *flavin*.

**querns**  Pair of stones used for pulverising grain (about 4000 BC to 2000 BC). The lower stone was slightly hollowed and the upper stone was rolled by hand on the lower one.

**Quetelet's index**  Index of adiposity; weight (kg) divided by square of height (metres); 25 considered 'normal'.

**quick breads**  Term for baked goods such as biscuits, muffins, popovers, griddles, cakes, waffles and dumplings, in which no yeast is used, but the raising carried out quickly with baking powder or other chemical agents.

**quick freezing**  As the term implies, a rapid freezing of food by exposure to a blast of air at a very low temperature. Unlike slow freezing, small crystals of ice are formed which do not rupture the cells of the food and so the structure is relatively undamaged.

A quick-frozen food is commonly defined as one that has been cooled from a temperature of 0°C to −5°C or lower, in a period of not more than 2 hours and then cooled to −18°C.

**quillaja**  Or soapbark; the dried bark of *Quillaja saponaria*, which contains sapotoxin, tannin and quillaja. Used to produce foam in soft drinks and shampoos and fire extinguishers.

**quince**  Pear-shaped sour fruit of *Cydonia* species, with flesh similar to that of the apple; rich in pectin and used chiefly in jams and jellies; used to be known as the apple and the vine.

Analysis per 100 g: water 83 g, protein 0.4 g, fat trace, carbohydrate 6 g, kcal 25 (0.1 MJ), vitamin C 15 mg.

**quinoa**  Glutinous seeds of a plant (*Chenopodium album*) grown in Chile and Peru; made into bread.

Analysis per 100 g: protein 12 g, fat 5 g, carbohydrate 63 g, fibre 5 g, Ca 120 mg, Fe 7 mg, vitamin $B_1$ 0.5 mg, vitamin $B_2$ 0.3 mg, nicotinic acid 1.5 mg.

**quintal**  220.46 lb (100 kg).

**Quorn**  Trade name (RHM) for myco-protein from mould *Fusarium graminearum*. Analysis per 100 g; protein 12 g, fat 3 g, fibre 5 g, 80 kcal.

# R

**rabbit**  Furry rodent, *Lepus cuniculus*.

Analysis per 100 g raw, edible meat: 75 g water, 22 g protein, 4 g fat, nil carbohydrate, 125 kcal (520 kJ), 1 mg Fe, 0.1 mg thiamin, 0.2 mg riboflavin, 8 mg niacin.

**racemic**  See *optical activity*.

**racemic compounds**  A mixture of two isomers which cancel their optical activity, which see.

**rad**  Unit of measurement of the energy absorbed from ionising radiation defined as the absorption of 100 ergs per gram of substance. Superseded by the gray, which see.

**radappertisation**  See *irradiation*.

**radiation**  See *irradiation*.

**radiation sterilisation**  See *irradiation*.

**radicidation**  See *irradiation*.

**radioallergosorbent tests** (RAST)  Tests for food allergy.

**radio frequency heating**  See *irradiation*.

**radiopasteurisation**  See *irradiation*.

**radishes**  Root of *Raphanus* genus.

    Analysis per 100 g: carbohydrate 3 g, protein 1 g, kcal 15 (60 kJ), dietary fibre 1 g, Ca 40 mg, Fe 2 mg, vitamin C 10–35 mg.

**radurisation**  See *irradiation*.

**Radyne**  Trade name (Radyne Ltd) for high-frequency heater (which see).

**raffinade**  Best-quality refined sugar.

**raffinose**  Trisaccharide found in cotton seed, sugar-beet molasses and Australian manna; also known as melitose or melitriose; hydrolyses to fructose and melibiose, which in turn hydrolyses to glucose and galactose. 23% sweetness of sucrose. Not digested.

**ragi**  See *millet*.

**raising powder**  See *baking powder*.

**raisin oil**  Obtained from seeds of Muscat grapes, which are removed before drying the grapes for raisins. The oil is used primarily to coat the raisins to prevent them sticking together, and render them soft and pliable and less subject to insect infestation.

**raisins**  Dried seedless grapes of several kinds. Valencia raisins from Spanish grapes; fruit dipped in potash lye and dried on cane trays in the sun. Thompson seedless raisins produced mainly in California from the sultanina grape (the skins are coarser than the sultana). Raisins are also produced in Australia, South Africa and the USA.

    For analysis see *fruit, dried*; see also *currants*; *muscatels*; *sultanas*.

**Ralston**  American breakfast cereal; whole wheat plus added wheat germ.

**ramekin**  (1) Porcelain or earthenware mould in which mixture is baked and then brought to the table. Paper soufflé cases nowadays called ramekin cases.

    (2) Formerly the name given to toasted cheese: now tarts filled with cream cheese are called ramekins.

**randomisation**  As used of fats, is the same as interesterification, which see.

**rape**  *Brassica napus*, closely related to garden swede. Also known as cole or coleseed. Seed used as source of edible oil, although its content of erucic acid has raised problems. Residual oilcake used for animal feed, although it contains goitrogens.

    Variety low in erucic acid is termed '0' or single low; varieties also low in glucosinolates are termed '00' or double low, both these being undesirable constituents of ordinary rapeseed.

**raspberry** Fruit of *Rubus idaeus*.

Analysis per 100 g: protein 1 g, carbohydrate 6 g, dietary fibre 7 g, kcal 25 (100 kJ), Ca 40 mg, Fe 1 mg, carotene 80 µg, vitamin C 14–35 mg.

**rastrello** Sharp-edged spoon used to cut out the pulp from halved oranges or other citrus fruit.

**ratafia** Flavouring essence made from bitter almonds; also a small light macaroon biscuit used in trifles; also a liqueur made from plum, peach and apricot kernels and bitter almonds.

**ravioli** Square envelope of pasta stuffed with minced meat.

**raw sugar** Brown unrefined sugar, 96–98% pure, as imported for refining. Contaminated with mould spores, bacteria, cane fibre, and dirt.

**RDA** Recommended daily (or dietary) allowance or amount (of energy and nutrients).

**RDI** Recommended daily intake or recommended dietary intake (of energy and nutrients).

**rebaudioside** Very sweet substance extracted from leaves of *Stevia rebaudiana* (same source as stevioside); 400 times as sweet as sucrose. There are five chemical forms, rebaudioside A, B, C, D and E.

**reciprocal ponderal index** Height divided by cube root of weight; index of adiposity.

**Recknagel's phenomenon** Slight rise in specific gravity of milk which may continue for up to 12 hours after milking; total effect may be equivalent to 0.15% solids-not-fat in the milk. The cause has not been explained.

**recommended intakes (of nutrients)** Daily amounts of each nutrient and of energy recommended as being adequate to maintain health. Based on measured requirements plus a calculated surplus to take care of individual variation (except for energy which is based on observed average intakes). See tables at end of book.

**rectal feeding** See *nutrient enemata*.

**rectifying column** A distillation column so arranged that the vapour condenses and redistils many times before it is finally condensed to form the distillate and so is purified to a greater degree than in simple distillation.

**red blood cell** See *blood, red cells*.

**red colours** Red 10 B – disodium salt of 8-amino-2-phenylazo-1-naphthol-3,6-disulphonic acid.

Red 2G – disodium salt of 8-acetamido-2-phenylazo-1-naphthol-3,6-disulphonic acid.

Red 6B – disodium salt of 8-acetamido-2-*p*-acetamido-phenylazo-1-naphthol-3,6-disulphonic acid.

Red FB – disodium salt of 2-(4-(1-hydroxy-4-sulpho-2-naphthylazo)-3-sulphophenyl)-6-methylbenzothiazole.

Fast Red E – disodium salt of 1-(4-sulpho-1-naphthylazo)-2-hydroxynaphthalene-6-sulphonic acid.

See also *amaranth*; *carmoisine*; *erythrosin*; *Ponceau colours*.

**red herrings**   Herrings that have been well salted and smoked for about 10 days. Bloaters are salted less and smoked for a shorter time; kippers lightly salted and smoked overnight. Also called Yarmouth bloaters.

**red pepper**   See *pepper*.

**red tide**   Sudden, unexplained increase in numbers of toxic dinoflagellates which cause fish and shellfish feeding on them to become seasonally toxic.

**reducing sugars**   Sugars that contain the aldehydic or ketonic reducing group, e.g. glucose, fructose, lactose, pentoses. They are tested for by their ability to reduce reagents such as Fehling's, Benedict's.

**reductinic acid**   See *reductones*.

**reduction**   Loss of oxygen, or gain in hydrogen, or (in more general terms to cover reactions such as the reduction of ferric chloride to ferrous chloride) gain of electrons.

**reduction rolls**   See *milling*.

**reductones**   Enediols which may be formed from sugars carrying a free carboxyl group by heating in alkaline solution. The simplest is hydroxyglycolaldehyde. Reductones may be formed in carbohydrate foods during heat processing, and as they have similar properties to vitamin C they interfere with its estimation.

Similar interfering substances are the reductinic acids formed by acid treatment of pentoses.

**reference man**   An arbitrary physiological standard; defined as a man of 25 years, healthy, weight 65 kg, living in a temperate zone of a mean annual temperature of 10 °C, assumed to require an average daily intake of 3200 kcal (13.5 MJ).

**reference protein**   A theoretical concept of the perfect protein which is used with 100% efficiency at whatever level it is fed in the diet. Used as a means of expressing recommended intakes.

The nearest approach to this theoretical protein are egg and human milk proteins, which are used with 90–100% efficiency when fed at low levels in the diet (4%) but not when fed at high levels (10–15%).

**reference woman**   An arbitrary physiological standard; defined as a woman of 25 years, weight 55 kg, engaged in general household duties or light industry, using 2300 kcal (9.7 MJ) per day, and as reference man, living in a temperate zone at a mean annual temperature of 10 °C.

**refractive index**  Measure of the bending or refraction of a beam of light on entering a denser medium; the ratio between the sine of the angle of incidence of the ray of light and the sine of the angle of refraction. It is constant for pure substances under standard conditions.

Used as a measure of sugar or total solids in solution, purity of oils, etc.

**refractometer**  Optical instrument used to measure the refractive index, which see.

The Abbé refractometer consists of two prisms between which is spread the substance under examination (jam, fruit juice, sugar syrup, etc.) and light is reflected through the solution.

The immersion refractometer dips into the solution.

**refrigerants**  Cooling agents in refrigerators, initially ammonia or carbon dioxide, subsequently replaced by CFCs – chlorofluoro-carbons – one carbon atom and one or more chlorine and/or fluorine. Trade names Freons (Du Pont, USA) and Arctons (ICI, UK).

**refrigeration**  See *preservation*; *psychrophilic bacteria*.

**Refsum's disease**  Inherited inability to metabolise phytanic acid giving rise to neuropathy. Phytanic acid is formed from free phytol in foods but not when it is combined as in chlorophyll and vitamins E and K.

Previously treated by excluding all fruits and green vegetables from the diet but later found that, apart from roasted peanuts, which are very rich in phytanic acid, leafy vegetables, beans, peas, tomatoes and fruits are free from, or have very low levels of, free phytol and low levels of phytanic acid.

**Rehfuss tube**  Instrument for removing samples of food from the stomach after a test meal. It is a small-diameter tube with a slotted metal tip. Another type is the Ryle tube, which see.

**Reichert–Meissl value**  Measure of the volatile fatty acids in fats. Defined as ml of N/10 NaOH required to neutralise the distillate from 5 g of fat; =Reichert–Meissl number.

**relative humidity**  See *humidity*.

**release agents**  Substances applied to tinned or enamelled surfaces or plastics films to prevent the food adhering; e.g. fatty acid amides, microcrystalline waxes, petrolatums, starch, methyl cellulose.

**relish**  Culinary term for any spicy or piquant preparation used to enhance flavour of plain food. UK – thin pickle or sauce with vinegar base; USA – includes finely chopped fruit or vegetables with dressing of salt, sugar, vinegar, sometimes eaten as a first course (apple, garden, salad relish). See also *Gentleman's relish*.

**renal threshold**   Blood level of a particular substance at which it is excreted through the kidney. For example, renal threshold of glucose is about 180 mg per 100 ml, and diabetics excrete glucose because this level is exceeded.

Various drugs can reduce the renal threshold.

**rendering**   The process of liberating the fat from the fat cells that constitute the adipose tissue. Dry rendering, heating the fat dry, or wet rendering, when water is present.

**rennet**   Extract of calf stomach; contains the enzyme rennin which clots milk. Used in cheese-making and for junkets.

**rennet, vegetable**   Name given to proteolytic enzymes derived from plants, such as bromelain (from the pineapple) and ficin (from the fig).

**rennin**   Enzyme in the abomasum of calves and the stomach of human infants which clots milk by precipitation of the casein. No evidence that it plays any part in digestion in the adult.

To avoid confusion with the kidney enzyme, renin, it is suggested that the name rennin should be replaced by chymosin.

**rentschlerising**   Sterilising by treatment with ultraviolet light named after Dr H.C. Rentschler, who developed the lamp.

**R-enzyme**   Enzyme present in beans and potatoes that splits the 1,6 linkage between the chains in starches; similar to the amylo-1,6-glucosidase found in muscle. Also known as the 'de-branching' factor.

**resazurin test**   See *methylene blue dye-reduction test*.

**resins, ion-exchange**   See *ion-exchange resins*.

**resistant starch**   See *starch, enzyme resistant*.

**respiration**   Although commonly used to mean breathing, more specifically related to the consumption of oxygen and the production of carbon dioxide. Thus, respiratory enzymes are those involved in cell oxidations.

**respiratory quotient**   Ratio between the volume of carbon dioxide produced when a substance is oxidised, and the volume of oxygen used.

In respiration in man the oxidation of carbohydrate results in RQ of 1.0; of fat, 0.71; and of protein, 0.8.

**respirometer**   See *spirometer*.

**restoration**   With reference to food, usually means the addition of nutrients to replace those lost in processing, as in milling of cereals.

**retardin**   Substance from the pancreas claimed to regulate fat metabolism.

**reticulin**   One of the structural elements (together with elastin and collagen) of skeletal muscle. Chemically it is identical with collagen but histologically it stains black with silver, while collagen stains yellow or brown; it is thought to be a precursor or a degraded form of collagen.

**reticulocyte** Young form of the red blood cell (normocyte or erythrocyte) in which the remains of the nucleus is visible as a reticulum. Very few are seen in the normal blood; they are retained in the marrow until mature; but on remission of anaemia, when there is a high rate of production, reticulocytes appear in the blood stream (reticulocytosis).

**reticulo-endothelial system** A 'system' of cells distributed throughout the body, with phagocytic properties. Present in spleen, bone marrow, liver, and lymph nodes, and are also mobile in the tissues and blood stream. They act as scavengers of tissue débris and bacteria.

The reticulo-endothelial system also removes red blood cells when they have completed their life of 120 days. The iron is recovered for further use, and the rest of the haemoglobin is converted to bile pigments, stercobilin in the faeces and urobilin in the urine.

**reticulum** See *rumen*.

**retinal** Aldehyde of retinol; formerly termed vitamin A aldehyde.

**retinene** Obsolete name for retinal.

**retinoic acid** Acid derived from retinol, formerly vitamin A acid.

**retinol** Formerly termed vitamin A alcohol; see *vitamin A*.

**retort** In connection with food technology, an autoclave.

**retrogradation** See *staling*.

**reverse osmosis** See *osmosis, reverse*.

**RF heating** See *irradiation*.

**rhamnose** A methyl pentose sugar; 33% sweetness of sucrose.

**rheology** Study of deformation and flow of materials; in food technology involves plasticity of fats, doughs, milk curd, etc. Provides scientific basis for subjective measurements such as mouth feel, spreadability, pourability.

**rhiotin** Unidentified urinary excretion product of biotin, together with miotin and triotin.

**rhizopterin** See *folic acid*.

**rhodamine B** Hydrochloride of diethyl-*m*-amino phenol phthalein – until recently used as a red colour in meat paste and mint rock, but not now permitted in the UK and most other countries.

**rhodopsin** See *visual purple*; *vitamin A*.

**rhubarb** Leaf-stalks of perennial plant, *Rheum rhaponticum*; contains only traces of protein and carbohydrate, 6 kcal (20 kJ) per 100 g, 10 mg vitamin C raw, 7 mg cooked. High content of oxalate; leaves are toxic for this reason.

**Ribena**  Trade name (Beecham Foods Ltd) for a preparation of black currant juice and sugar syrup plus added vitamin C. Very rich source of vitamin C, 206 mg per 100 g; 61% sugar, 230 kcal (1 MJ).

**riboflavin**  Vitamin $B_2$.

**ribonucleic acid**  See *nucleic acids*.

**ribose**  Pentose sugar of outstanding physiological importance; it is part of vitamin $B_2$, of coenzyme I and II, of adenylic acid, and in the nucleoproteins either as ribose or desoxyribose.

**ribosomes**  Particles found in animal cells, plants, yeasts, and as a major constituent of bacterial cytoplasm – believed to be the site of protein sythesis; composed of ribonucleic acid.

**Ribotide**  Trade name (Takeda Chemical Industries, Japan) for a mixture of disodium inosinate and disodium guanylate used as a flavour enhancer for savoury dishes.

**rice**  Grain of *Oryza sativa*; major food in many countries. Rice when threshed is known as paddy, and is covered with a fibrous husk comprising nearly 40% of the grain. When the husk has been removed, brown rice is left. When the outer bran layers up to the endosperm and germ are removed, the ordinary white rice of commerce or polished rice is obtained (usually polished with glucose and talc).

Analysis of brown rice, including the germ, per 100 g: carbohydrate 87 g, protein 7.5 g, fat 1.8 g, Ca 10 g, Fe 1 mg, kcal 360 (1.5 MJ), vitamin $B_1$ 0.3 mg, vitamin $B_2$ 0.05 mg, nicotinic acid 4.6 mg.

In conversion to polished rice there is considerable loss of vitamin $B_1$ (and nicotinic acid); hence the widespread occurrence of beriberi among rice-eating peoples.

Analysis of white rice per 100 g: carbohydrate 87 g, protein 6.7 g, fat 0.7 g, Ca 10 mg, Fe 1 mg, kcal 360 (1.5 MJ), vitamin $B_1$ 0.08 mg, vitamin $B_2$ 0.03 mg, nicotinic acid 1.6 mg.

**rice, American**  Bulgur, which see.

**rice diet**  See *Kempner diet*.

**rice, glutinous**  For most purposes separate rice grains are wanted that do not stick together in a glutinous mass. Glutinous rice is rich in soluble starch, dextrin and maltose and on boiling the grains adhere in a sticky mass; this rice is used for sweetmeats and cakes.

**rice grass, Indian**  See *Indian rice grass*.

**rice, hungry**  A variety of millet, *Digitaria exilis*, important in West Africa.

**Rice Krispies**  Trade name (Kellogg Co.) for a breakfast cereal prepared by 'explosion puffing' of rice.

Analysis per 100 g: 6 g protein, 84 g available carbohydrate,

0.7 g fat, 245 kcal (1.4 MJ), 2 g dietary fibre, 1.3 g Na, 7 mg thiamin, 1.5 mg riboflavin, 16 mg niacin, 1.8 mg vitamin $B_6$, 2.8 μg vitamin D.

**rice paper** Smooth white paper made from the pith of a tree peculiar to Taiwan. It is edible, and macaroons and similar biscuits are baked on it and the paper can be eaten with the biscuits.

**rice, parboiled** Rice that has been partially cooked before milling, so that some of the water-soluble B vitamins migrate into the grain and less is lost when the rice is subsequently milled to white rice.

**rice, red** West African species, *Oryza glaberrima*, with red bran layer.

**rice, synthetic** See *tapioca-macaroni*.

**rice, unpolished** Rice which has been undermilled in that the husk, germ and bran layers have been partially removed. Term used in the USA.

**rice, wild** Also known as zizanie, Tuscarora rice, Indian rice and American wild rice (American rice is bulgur); *Zizania aquatica*. Native to E. North America, grows 12 feet high; long, thin, greenish grain; little is grown and difficult to harvest, so is strictly a gourmet food.

Higher in protein content than ordinary rice at 14%, fat 7.0%, carbohydrate 74%.

**rice wine** See *saké*.

**ricing** Culinary term meaning cutting into small pieces about the size of rice grains.

**rickets** Malformation of the bone in growing children due to shortage of vitamin D leading to poor absorption of calcium. In adults the equivalent is osteomalacia. See *vitamin D*.

**rickets, refractory** Rickets that does not respond to normal doses of vitamin D but requires massive doses; it is suggested that refractory rickets is a congenital abnormality.

**riffle flumes** Washing equipment consisting of stepped channels along which the product being washed is carried in a flow of water; stones and grit are retained on the steps.

**rigor mortis** Stiffening of muscle that occurs after death. As the flow of blood ceases, anaerobic metabolism leads to the formation of lactic acid and the soft, pliable muscle becomes stiff and rigid. If meat is hung in a cool place for a few days (i.e. 'conditioned'), the meat softens again. Fish similarly undergo rigor mortis but is usually of shorter duration than in mammals.

**Ringer's solution** Solution of the chlorides of sodium, potassium and calcium in which isolated tissues will continue to survive (960 ml of 0.154 M NaCl, 20 ml 0.154 M KCl and 20 ml 0.11 M $CaCl_2$.)

**RNA** Ribonucleic acid; see *nucleic acids*.

**roast** Originally meant to cook meat over an open fire on a spit; now refers to cooking in an enclosed oven, and so is 'dry-heating'. With meat the juices are squeezed out and evaporate on the surface, producing the Maillard complex characteristic of roasted meat.

**Robison ester** Name given to a mixture of glucose-6-phosphate and fructose-1-phosphate, which are intermediary stages in glucose metabolism, which see.

**rocambole** *Allium scordoprasum*, a mild variety of garlic, also called sand leek.

**Rochelle salt** Potassium sodium tartrate; used to combine with the copper in Fehling's test for reducing sugars.

**roe** Hard roe is the eggs of the female fish; soft roe is from the male fish, also known as milt.

**Rohalase** Trade name (Röhm Technologies Enzymatiques) for bacterial and fungal amylases used in brewing.

**rokelax** Scandinavian term for smoked salmon.

**roller dryer** The material to be dried is spread over the surface of internally heated rollers and drying is complete in a few seconds. The rollers rotate against a knife that scrapes off the dried film as soon as it forms.

There is little damage by this method; for example, roller-dried milk is not scorched, but there is some loss of vitamin $B_1$ and C, more than in spray drying.

**roller mill** Pairs of horizontal cylindrical rollers, separated by only a small gap and revolving at different speeds. The material is thus ground and crushed in the one operation. Used in flour milling.

**roll-on closure (RO)** Aluminium or lacquered tinplate cap for sealing on to narrow-necked bottles with a threaded neck. The unthreaded cap is moulded on to the neck of the bottle and forms an air-tight seal.

**rooibos tea** Fermented leaves of a bushy plant, *Aspalathus linearis*, indigenous to S. Africa. Contains a unique polyphenol, aspalathin, which becomes red during preparation and produces a reddish herbal tea; free from caffeine and theaflavin.

**root beer** Non-alcoholic carbonated beverage flavoured with oil of sassafras and oil of wintergreen.

**rope** Bacteria of the type *B. mesentericus* and *B. subtilis* occur on wheat and thence in flour. These organisms form spores that can survive baking and then are present in the bread. Under the right conditions of warmth and moisture the spores will germinate and the mass of bacteria convert the bread into sticky, yellowish patches which can be pulled out into rope-like threads

– hence the term ropy bread. The bacterial growth is inhibited by acid substances.

Can also occur in milk and carbonated beverages.

**Rose–Gottlieb test**  For fat in milk; accurate gravimetric method, by extracting the fat with solvent.

**rose hips**  The fruit of the rose; a rich source of vitamin C from which rose hip syrup is prepared.

**rose hip syrup**  Extract of rose hip with added sugar, used as source of vitamin C – 150 mg per 100 mg.

**rosemary**  A bushy shrub, *Rosmarinus officinalis*, cultivated commercially for its essential oil, used in medicine and perfumery. The dried leaves are used to flavour soups, sauces and meat.

**rotary louvre dryer**  Hot air passes through a moving bed of the solid inside a rotating drum.

**Roth–Benedict spirometer**  See *spirometer*.

**roughage**  See *dietary fibre*.

**roux**  Preparation of flour and butter for thickening gravies and sauces.

**Rovimix**  Trade name (Hoffman La Roche) for stabilised forms of vitamins, including A, D and E as beadlets coated with a gelatin–starch mixture.

**royal jelly**  The food on which bee larvae are fed and which causes them to develop into queen bees. Richest known source of pantothenic acid (100 μg per g dry weight): also contains vitamin $B_6$ and 2% of its dry weight is 10-hydroxy-delta-2-decenoic acid.

Claimed, without foundation, to have rejuvenating virtues for human beings.

**RPV**  Relative protein value. See *protein quality*.

**RQ**  Respiratory quotient, which see.

**rubble reel**  Machine for cleaning materials such as wheat. The material is fed into a long inclined reel made of perforated metal that rotates inside a frame. The perforations become larger nearer the bottom, so that there is a graded sieving of the material as it passes down the reel.

**Rubner factors**  Factors used to calculate the energy content of foods in kilocalories after allowing for losses of urinary nitrogen but not allowing for incomplete absorption, therefore greater than Atwater factors; protein 4.1, fat 9.3, carbohydrates 4.1. See also *energy*.

**rum**  A spirit distilled from fermented molasses. There are three main categories, Cuban, Jamaican and Dutch East Indies.

**rumen**  Ruminating animals, such as the cow, sheep and goat, possess four stomachs, in distinction from monogastric animals, such as man, pig, dog and rat. The four are: the rumen, or first stomach, where bacterial fermentation produces lower fatty acids, and whence the food is returned to the mouth for further mastication (chewing the cud); the reticulum, where further bacterial fermentation produces lower fatty acids; the omasum; and the abomasum or true stomach.

The bacterial fermentation allows ruminants to obtain nourishment from grass and hay which cannot be digested by monogastric animals.

**ruminant**  See *rumen*.

**rumpbone**  Cut of meat (USA) = aitchbone (UK) = loin or haunch.

**rush nut**  See *tiger nut*.

**rutabaga**  American name for swede.

**rutin**  A disaccharide (rhamnose and glucose) derivative of quercetin; found in grains, tomato stalk, elderberry blossom. See *vitamin P*.

**rye**  Grain of cereal *Secale cereale*, the predominant cereal in some parts of Europe; very hardy and withstands adverse conditions better than wheat.

Rye flour is dark and the dough lacks elasticity; rye bread is usually made with sour dough or leaven rather than yeast. See also *crispbreads*; *pumpernickel*.

Analysis per 100 g: protein 8 g, fat 1.5 g, kcal 350 (1.5 MJ), Ca 25 mg, Fe 3.5 mg, vitamin $B_1$ 0.27 mg, vitamin $B_2$ 0.1 mg, nicotinic acid 1.2 mg.

**Ryle tube**  Instrument for removing samples of the contents from the stomach at intervals after a test meal. It is a narrow rubber tube with a blind end containing a lead weight, with holes above this level. Another type is the Rehfuss tube, which see.

**Ryvita**  Trade name (Ryvita Co. Ltd) for a crisp bread (which see).

Analysis per 100 g: protein 7 g, fat 2 g, carbohydrate 77 g, Ca 40 mg, Fe 4 mg, kcal 345 (1.45 MJ). Phytic acid phosphorus 54% of total P (295 mg/100 mg).

# S

**saccharases**  A group of enzymes that attack sugars to liberate glucose or fructose depending on the type of saccharase. See *invertase*.

**saccharic acid**  Dibasic acid derived from glucose.

**saccharimeter**  Polarimeter used to determine the purity of sugar; graduated on the International Sugar Scale – degrees sugar.

26% solution of pure sucrose reads 100° sugar in a 200 mm tube.

See also *optical activity*.

**saccharin**  Chemical, benzoic sulphimide, 550 times as sweet as cane sugar. Soluble saccharin is the sodium salt. Has no food value; useful as a sweetening agent for diabetics and slimmers. Discovered in the USA in 1879.

**saccharometer**  Floating device used to determine the specific gravity of sugar solutions (distinct from saccharimeter).

**saccharose**  Sucrose.

**safe allowances**  Alternative term for recommended intakes.

**saffron**  Dried stigma of *Crocus sativus* (related to garden crocus). Contains glycoside picrocrocin, and colouring principles crocin and crocetin. Used as natural dyestuff (permitted food colour) and spice. Very soluble in water.

**sage**  Dried leaf of the Dalmatian sage, *Salvia officinalis*, of the mint family; fragrant and spicy and is the most important herb used in the kitchen for flavouring meat and fish dishes and in poultry stuffing. Other sages (Greek, Spanish, English) differ in flavour from the Dalmatian variety. Also sage oil from the same source by steam distillation. Contains the essential oil thujone together with α-pinene, cineol, borneol and D-camphor.

**sago**  Starchy grains prepared from the pith of the sago palm (*Metrozylon sago*); almost pure starch free from protein.

Analysis per 100 g: protein 0.5 g, fat negligible, carbohydrate 88 g, trace of B vitamins.

**St Anthony's Fire**  See *ergot*.

**St John's Bread**  See *carob seed*.

**saithe**  *Polachius virens*. Also known as coley and coal fish. Apart from being eaten cooked, it is smoked, salted and dyed red, when it is similar to smoked salmon.

**saké**  Japanese wine made from rice. Cooked whole rice grains are fermented with a yeast-like fungus culture for 10–14 days and stored in wooden barrels. Contains about 17% alcohol, by volume.

**salad cream**  Oil-in-water emulsion made from vegetable oil, vinegar, salt, spices, emulsified with egg yolk and thickened.

Legally, in the UK, must contain not less than 25% by weight of vegetable oil and not less than 1.35% egg-yolk solids. Mayonnaise usually contains more oil, less carbohydrate and water.

By USA regulations salad dressing contains 30% vegetable oil and 4% egg yolk; mayonnaise contains 65% oil plus egg yolk.

**salad dressing**  See *French dressing*.

**salamagundi**  Old English dish consisting of diced fresh and salt meats mixed with hard-boiled eggs, pickled vegetables and spices, dressed on a bed of salad.

**salinometer**  Or salimeter, or salometer. Hydrometer to measure concentration of salt solutions.

**Salisbury cure**  Exclusive protein diet, supposed to cure or alleviate a number of diseases.

**Salisbury steak**  Similar to hamburger – minced lean beef mixed with bread, eggs, milk and seasoning, shaped into cakes and fried.

**saliva**  Secretion of the salivary glands in the mouth. There are three pairs of glands – parotid, submandibular and submaxillary. Dilute solution of the protein mucin and the enzyme amylase, with small quantities of urea, potassium thocyanate, sodium chloride and bicarbonate.

One to 1.5 litre per day secreted of solution of 0.5% solids. The mucin lubricates the food, and the amylase hydrolyses starch to maltose.

**salivary glands**  See *saliva*.

**Sally Lunn**  A sweet, spongy, yeast cake, named after a girl of that name who sold her tea cakes in the streets of Bath 1788.

**salmon**  *Salmo salar*; cherry salmon – *Onchorhynchus masou*; chum or keta salmon – *O. keta*; medium red or Coho salmon – *O. kisutch*; pink – *O. gorbuscha*; red or sockeye – *O. nerka*; Spring or King or Chinook – *O. tschwytscha*. See *fish, fatty*.

**Salmonella**  Genus of bacteria of family Enterobacteriaceae. Common cause of food poisoning, which see. Found in eggs from infected hens, sausages, etc.; can survive in brine and in the refrigerator; destroyed by adequate heating.

**salt**  Usually refers to sodium chloride, i.e. common salt or table salt (although any compound of acid and alkali is a salt). See *salt-free diets*; *sodium*.

**salt content**  See *salt-free diets*.

**salt-free diets**  More correctly these are diets low in (never completely free from) sodium, but as most of the sodium of the diet is consumed as sodium chloride or salt, they are referred to as low-salt diets. It is the sodium and not the chloride that is of importance.

Sodium controls the retention of fluid in the body, and reduced retention, aided by low-sodium diets, is required in cardiac insufficiency accompanied by oedema, in certain kidney diseases, toxaemias of pregnancy and hypertension.

The average sodium intake is about 3.5 g (9 g NaCl) per day, and restricted diets are usually about 2.3 g and can be as low as 0.6 g.

To improve the palatability of such diets 'salt' mixtures are available containing potassium and ammonium chlorides together with citrates, formates, phosphates, glutamates, as well as herbs and spices.

Foods low in salt (0–20 mg/100 g): sugar, flour, fruit, green vegetables, macaroni, nuts. Medium salt (50–100 mg/100 g): chicken, fish, eggs, meat, milk. High salt (500–2000 mg/100 g): corned beef, bread, ham, bacon, kippers, sausages, cheese.

**saltlicks** An adequate intake of sodium chloride is necessary to all animals. Grass is relatively poor in sodium, and its high potassium content induces excretion of sodium in the urine. This loss causes a craving for sodium which is satisfied by natural or artificial saltlicks.

**saltpetre** (Bengal saltpetre) Potassium nitrate.

**salts, bile** See *bile*.

**salts, Indian** Greek and Roman name for sugar.

**sambol** Name given to a curry of fairly solid consistency in India and other parts of the East.

**Sami** Socially acceptable monitoring instrument. A small, heart-rate counting apparatus used to estimate energy expenditure of human subjects.

**samna** See *ghee*.

**samp** Coarsely cut portions of maize with bran and germ partly removed.

**Sanatogen** Trade name (Fisons) for a preparation of casein and sodium glycerophosphate for consumption as a beverage when added to milk.

**Sanecta** Trade name (Holland Sweetener Co.) for aspartame.

**Sanka** Trade name (Maxwell House) for a decaffeinated instant coffee.

**sapodilla** Fruit of the sapodilla tree (*Achras sapota*); size of a small apple, rough-grained, yellow to greyish pulp.

Analysis per 100 g: water 75 g, protein 0.4 g, fat 1 g, carbohydrate 22 g, kcal 100 (0.4 MJ), Fe 0.8 mg, vitamin $B_2$ 0.03 mg, nicotinic acid 0.2 mg, vitamin C 15 mg.

Chicle, the basis of chewing gum, is made from the latex of the same tree.

**saponification** Splitting of fat into its constituent glycerol and fatty acids by boiling with alkali. The fatty acids will be present as the sodium salts, also called the sodium soaps.

Method of concentrating vitamin A from oils, because the vitamin does not saponify and can then be separated from the rest of the fat in the so-called non-saponifiable fraction. The latter also contains mineral oils and higher alcohols such as cholesterol.

**saponification value**  Used with reference to fats as an indication of the nature (molecular weight) of the fatty acids present.

Defined as the number of milligrams of potassium hydroxide required to saponify 1 g of fat. Values greater than 200 are short-chain fatty acids; below 190 are of high molecular weight.

**saponins**  Group of substances that occur in plants and can produce a soapy lather with water. Extracted commercially from soapwort or soapbark and used as foam producer in beverages and fire extinguishers, as detergent and for emulsifying oils. Bitter in flavour.

There is a second group, the steroid saponins, which are cardiac active and are used as a starting material for the synthesis of sex hormones.

**Saracen corn**  See *buckwheat*.

**saran**  Generic name for thermoplastic materials made from polymers of vinylidine chloride and vinyl chloride. They are clear transparent films used for wrapping food, resistant to oils and chemicals; can be heat-shrunk on to the product.

**sarcolactic acid**  Old name for the form of lactic acid which turns the plane of polarised light to the right, i.e. (+) lactic acid; found in muscle, as distinct from the inactive lactic acid (mixture of (+) and (−) found in sour milk. Also known as paralactic acid.

**sarcolemma**  See *muscle*.

**sarcoplasm**  See *muscle*.

**sarcosine**  $N$-methylglycine; found in starfish and sea urchins; intermediate in the synthesis of antienzyme agents in toothpaste.

**sardell**  Anchovy.

**sardine**  Young pilchard, *Sardina* (*Clupea*) *pilchardus*.

Analysis of canned product per 100 g: 20 g protein, 23 g fat, 300 kcal (1.3 MJ), 400 mg Ca, 4 mg Fe, 30 µg vitamin A, 8 µg vitamin D, 0.2 mg vitamin $B_2$, 5 mg nicotinic acid.

**Saridele**  Protein-rich baby food (26–30% protein) developed in Indonesia; extract of soya bean with sugar, calcium carbonate, vitamins $B_1$, $B_{12}$ and C.

**sarsaparilla**  Flavour prepared from oil of sassafras and oil of wintergreen or oil of sweet birch; used in a carbonated beverage.

**sassafras oil**  Used to flavour root beer and similar beverages. Main component is safrole, believed to be a weak hepatic carcinogen and banned in some countries.

**saturation humidity**  See *humidity*.

**sauerkraut**  Prepared by lactic fermentation of shredded cabbage. In the presence of 2–3% salt, acid-forming bacteria thrive and convert sugars in the cabbage into acetic and lactic acids, which then act as preservatives.

**sauerteig** See *bread, black.*

**sausage** Chopped meat, mostly beef or pork, seasoned with salt and spices, mixed with cereal (usually wheat rusk prepared from crumbed unleavened biscuits) and packed into casings made from the connective tissue of animal intestines or cellulose.

There are six main types – fresh, smoked, cooked, smoked and cooked, semi-dry and dry. Frankfurters, Bologna, Polish and Berliner sausages are made from cured meat and are smoked and cooked. Thuringer, soft salami, mortadella and soft cervelat are semi-dry sausages. Pepperoni, chorizos, dry salami, dry cervelat are slowly dried to a hard texture.

**sausage casings** Natural casings are made from hog intestines for fresh frying sausages, and from sheep intestines for chipolatas and frankfurters. Skinless sausages are prepared in cellulose casing, which is then peeled off.

**sausage factor** See *meat factor.*

**sauté** Toss in hot fat without browning (sauté potatoes usually cooked first and browned).

**savarin** See *baba.*

**saveloy** Highly seasoned smoked sausage; the addition of salt-petre gives rise to the bright red colour. Originally a sausage made from pig's brains.

**savory** Plant with strongly flavoured leaves used as seasoning in sauces, soups, salad dishes. Summer savory is an annual, *Satureja hortensis*; winter savory is a perennial, *Satureja montana*. The plants are cut down at flowering time and dried for later use.

**Saxin** Trade name (Burroughs Wellcome Ltd) for saccharin.

**scald** Defect occurring in stored apples, consisting of formation of brown patches on the skin, with browning and softening of the tissues underneath. Due to accumulation of gases given off during ripening.

**scallops** Marine bivalve molluscs of *Pectinidae* species; Queen scallop *Chlamys opercularis*, France – coquille St Jacques.

Analysis per 100 g: protein 25 g, fat 1 g, carbohydrate 0, iron 3 mg, 100 kcal (400 kJ).

**scampi** Norway lobster or Dublin Bay prawn. See *lobster.*

**Scenedesmus** See *algae.*

**Schardinger's enzyme** The same as xanthine oxidase, which oxidises a whole range of aldehydes to acids, and also xanthine and hypoxanthine to uric acid.

**Schilling Test** Test for vitamin $B_{12}$ nutritional status by measuring the urinary excretion of a dose of labelled $B_{12}$ given orally accompanied by large parenteral dose of non-labelled $B_{12}$.

**scombroid poisoning**   Apparently caused by bacterial spoilage of fish including many of the scrombidae (tuna, bonito, mackerel) but also non-scombroid fish and other foods. Symptoms (including skin rash, nausea, tingling) resemble histamine poisoning and previously thought to be due to bacterial formation of histamine, now doubted.

**scone**   A variety of tea cake originally made from oatmeal and sour milk, in Scone, Scotland.

**SCP**   Single cell protein.

**scrapple**   Meat dish prepared from pork carcass trimmings, maize meal, flour, salt and spices – cooked to a thick consistency.

**scrod**   Young cod.

**scuppernong**   Name of the most widely cultivated of the muscadine grapes, used chiefly in wine rather than as a dessert grape.

**scurvy**   See *vitamin C*.

**scurvy, Alpine**   Pellagra.

**scurvy grass**   A herb, *Cochlearia officinalis*, recommended as far back as the late sixteenth century as a remedy for scurvy.

**scutellum**   Area surrounding the embryo of the cereal grain; scutellum plus embryo is the germ. Rich in vitamins.

**SDA**   See *specific dynamic action*.

**SDS**   Sucrose distearate. See *sucrose esters*.

**SE**   Starch equivalent.

**sea slub**   See *bêche-de-mer*.

**seaweed**   Algae of interest as food. Irish moss, laver bread and kelp are eaten to some extent in different communities and serve as a mineral supplement in animal feed.

**secretin**   Hormone, secreted by the intestinal mucosa, which travels via the blood stream to the pancreas and stimulates this organ to secrete. Is a small, basic polypeptide, destroyed by pepsin and trypsin, and therefore ineffective when given by mouth.

**sedoheptulose**   A 7-carbon sugar. Also called sedoheptose. See *hexosemonophosphate shunt*.

**Seitz filter**   Asbestos disc with pores so fine that they will not permit passage of bacteria; thus solutions filtered through a Seitz filter emerge sterile.

**selenium**   Dietary essential, since it is part of the enzyme glutathione peroxidase, but toxic in excess. Can replace vitamin E in some but not all its functions.

First shown to be of nutritional importance in 1941 in preventing liver necrosis in rats on certain diets – an effect shown by vitamin E, cystine and an extract of yeast, which was therefore termed Factor 3, subsequently identified as an organic form of selenium. (The cystine contained selenium as a contaminant.)

**self-raising flour** See *flour, self-raising*.

**semolina** The inner, granular, starchy endosperm of hard or durum wheat (not yet ground into flour); used to make pasta and semolina milk pudding.

**sequestrants** Substances that combine with a metal ion or acid radical and render it inactive, e.g. citrates, tartrates, phosphates, and various calcium salts. See also *ethylenediamine tetra-acetic acid*.

**Sequestrene** Trade name (Geigy Industrial Chemicals, USA) for ethylenediamine tetra-acetic acid, disodium and disodium calcium salts.

**serendipity berry** *Dioscoreophyllum cumminsii*, Nigerian berry. West African fruit with an extremely sweet taste. Active principle called monellin.

**serine** A non-essential amino acid; amino hyroxypropionic acid.

**serosal** In reference to the intestine, means the outer side of the intestinal wall, as distinct from the inner or mucosal side.

**serotonin** See *5-hydroxytryptamine*.

**serum** Clear liquid left after the protein has been clotted; reference both to blood and to milk. The serum from milk, occasionally referred to as lacto-serum, is whey.

**serum, blood** Blood plasma without the fibrinogen. When blood clots, the fibrinogen is converted to fibrin, which is deposited in strands that trap the red cells and form the clot. The clear liquid that is exuded is the serum.

**serum butter** See *butter, whey*.

**sesame** *Sesamum indicum*. Tropical and sub-tropical plant, also known as sim-sim in East Africa and benniseed in West Africa. Seeds are small and, in most varieties, white; used whole in sweetmeats, in stews and to decorate cakes and bread, and for extraction of the oil.

Analysis per 100 g: 20 g protein, 50 g fat, 16 g carbohydrate, 5 g fibre, 600 kcal (2.5 MJ), 1 mg vitamin $B_1$, 0.25 mg vitamin $B_2$, 5 mg nicotinic acid.

**Seven Foods Plan** See *basic 7 foods plan*.

**Seville orange** Spanish term for the bitter orange, which see, under *orange, bitter*.

**sex hormones** See *hormones, sex*; *oestrogens*.

**sfumatrice** Machine for obtaining the oil from the peel of citrus fruit. Based on the principle that the natural turgor of the oil sacs forces out the oil when the peel is folded.

**shaddock** Alternative name for pomelo, *Citrus grandis*, from which grapefruit is descended (named after Captain Shaddock, who introduced it into West Indies).

**shandy**   A mixture of lemonade and beer, originally shandy-gaff. Ginger beer may be used – ginger beer shandy. Contains 1% alcohol.

**Sharples centrifuge**   Continuous high-speed centrifuge (15000–30000 rev/min) consisting of vertical cylinder. Used to separate liquids of different densities or to clarify by sedimenting solids.

**sharps**   See *wheatfeed*.

**shashlik**   Similar to shishkebab, omitting steeping the meat in wine. According to some recipes the same as shishkebab.

**shea butter**   See *vegetable butters*.

**shearling**   Sheep 15–18 months old.

**shellfish, edible**   Include prawns, shrimps, lobsters, crayfish and crabs.

Zoologically they are of the order Decapoda, sub-order Macrura (prawns, shrimps, lobsters and crayfish) and sub-order Brachyura (crabs).

See under separate entries.

**sherbet**   Arabic name for water-ice (sugar, water and flavouring), also known by French name, sorbet, and the Italian name, granits. Used to be served between courses during a meal to refresh the palate.

**shishkebab**   Lamb (although beef sometimes used) cut into cubes steeped in onion, garlic and wine for a few hours, impaled on a skewer; pieces of meat alternating with tomatoes, mushrooms, or pieces of eggplant, dusted with flour and then broiled.

**shortening**   Soft fats that produce a crisp, flaky effect in baked products. Lard possesses the correct properties to a greater extent than any other single fat.

Unlike oils, shortenings are plastic and disperse as a film through the batter and prevent the formation of a hard, tough mass.

Shortenings are compounded from mixtures of fats or prepared by hydrogenation and are still called lard compounds or lard substitutes.

**Shoyu**   Soy sauce.

**shrimp**   The pink shrimp commonly sold at fishmongers is *Pandalus montagui*. See *prawns*.

Analysis per 100 g, without shell: protein 22 g, fat 2 g, carbohydrate 0, kcal 100 (0.42 MJ), Ca 320 mg, Fe 1.8 mg, vitamin $B_1$ 0.03 mg, vitamin $B_2$ 0.03 mg, nicotinic acid 3 mg.

**sialic acid**   Group of compounds derived from neuraminic acid which are constituents of certain mucoproteins in the tissues; they include acetyl and glycolyl neuraminic acids. Also termed lactaminic and gynaminic acids.

**sialogogue**   Substance that stimulates the flow of saliva.

**siderophilin** Or transferrin, an iron carbonate–protein complex, the form in which iron is transported in the blood plasma.

**siderosis** Accumulation of the iron–protein complex, haemo-siderin, in liver, spleen and bone marrow in cases of excessive red cell destruction and on diets exceptionally rich in iron. It is common among Bantu, apparently owing to intakes of about 100 mg of iron daily from iron cooking pots and kaffir beer.

**sikor** See *clay*.

**sild** Young herring, *Clupea harengus*.

**silica gel** Drying agent.

**silicones** Organic compounds of silicon; in the food field they are used as antifoaming agents, as semi-permanent glazes on baking tins and other metal containers, on non-sticking wrapping paper.

**silver** Not of interest in foods apart from its use in covering 'nonpareils' – the silver beads used to decorate confectionery. Present in traces in all plant and animal tissues but has no function nor is enough ever absorbed to cause toxicity. See also *oligodynamic*.

**Simon's metabolites** Name given to two compounds found (by Simon and co-workers) in the urine of rabbits as metabolites of vitamin E. Called Simon's metabolites in place of the long chemical names but now known by the trivial names of tocopheronic acid and tocopheronolactone.

**Simplesse** Trade name (Nutrasweet) for low calorie fat substitute made from milk or egg white. Consists of particles $0.1$–$2.0\,\mu m$ which create the feeling of creaminess in the mouth but cannot be used for cooking. Provides 1.3 kcal/g compared with 9 for fats.

**sim-sim** See *sesame*.

**single cell protein** Collective term used for biomass of bacteria, algae and yeast, and also (incorrectly) moulds, of potential use as animal or human food.

**sinharanut** See *chestnut, water*.

**sippet** A small piece of bread, fried or toasted, served as a garnish to a mince or hash.

**Sippy diet** For peptic ulcer patients; hourly feeds of small quantities, 150 ml of milk, cream or other milky food. See also *Lenhartz diet*; *Meulengracht diet*.

**Sister Laura's Food** Trade name (Sister Laura Food Co.) for an infant food comprising wheat flour, sugar and salt. No vitamins are claimed.

**sitapophasis** Refusal to eat as expression of mental disorder.

**sitology** Science of food (from the Greek *sitos*, food).

**sitomania** Mania for eating.

**sitophobia**  Fear of food, also phagophobia.

**sitosterol**  The main sterol found in vegetable oils, similar in structure to cholesterol with an extra ethyl group.

**skin factor**  Obsolete name for biotin.

**skinfold thickness**  Index of subcutaneous fat. Measured at four sites, biceps (midpoint of front upper arm), triceps (midpoint of back upper arm), subscapular (directly below point of shoulder blade at angle of 45 degrees), supra-iliac (directly above iliac crest in mid-axillary line).

Rapid surveys often involve only biceps.

**skyr**  See *milks, fermented*.

**sliwowitz**  Plum brandy, originating in Yugoslavia. Some of the stones are included with the fruit and produce a characteristic bitter flavour from the hydrocyanic acid (0.008% HCN is present in the finished brandy).

**sloe**  Wild sour plum of the blackthorn (*Prunus spinosa*); almost only use is for the preparation of sloe gin.

**SLR factor**  *Streptococcus lactis* factor. See *folic acid*.

**SM**  Protein-rich baby food (15% protein) made in Ethiopia from teff, peas, chick peas, lentils and skim-milk powder.

**SMA**  Trade name (John Wyeth Ltd) for a milk preparation for infant feeding modified to resemble the composition of human milk.

**smell**  See *organoleptic*.

**smoke point**  Term used with reference to frying oils; the temperature at which the decomposition products become visible (bluish smoke). The temperature varies with different fats and ranges between 160 and 260°C.

See also *fire point*; *flash point*.

**smoking**  Meat and fish are often smoked after pickling to assist preservation and improve the flavour. Hard woods, oak, elm, and ash, produce a smoke containing aldehydes, phenols and acids with a preservative action; surface dehydration also helps preservation.

**smörgåsbord**  Scandinavian; table laden with delicacies such as fish, meat and cheese, as traditional gesture of hospitality.

**smörrebrod**  Danish open sandwiches; literally means smeared bread.

**SMS**  Sucrose monostearate. See *sucrose esters*.

**smut**  Group of fungi that attack wheat; includes loose or common smut (*Ustilago tritici*) and stinking smut or bunt (*Tilletia tritici*).

**sn**  Stereochemical numbering – used in nomenclature of lipids to indicate that the system of numbering the glycerol carbon atoms is being used in place of the DL system.

**SNF**  See *solids-not-fat*.

**snibbing**  Topping and tailing of gooseberries.

**SO₂**  See *sulphur dioxide*.

**soapstock**  In the refining of crude edible oils the free fatty acids are removed by agitation with alkali. The fatty acids settle to the bottom as alkali soaps and are known as soapstock or 'foots'.

**soda bread**  Made from flour and whey, or butter milk, using sodium bicarbonate and acid in place of yeast. Common in Ireland.

**sodium**  A dietary essential which is almost invariably satisfied by the normal diet. The body contains about 100 g of sodium and the average diet contains 3–6 g, equivalent to 10 g of sodium chloride. The intake varies enormously in different individuals and the excretion varies accordingly.

Vegetables are relatively poor in sodium and rich in potassium. Animal foods are rich in sodium.

See also *salt-free diets*; *sodium–potassium ratio*; *water balance*.

**sodium bicarbonate**  See *baking powder*.

**sodium chloride**  Common salt – the commonest form in which sodium is consumed. See *salt-free diets*; *sodium*.

**sodium glutamate**  See *glutamic acid*.

**sodium-potassium ratio**  The ratio of sodium (in the extracellular fluid) to the body potassium (in the cell water) is about 2:3. The ratio in unprocessed food, no salt added, is much lower, and when salt is added during processing it is much higher. Unproven suggestions have been made for the benefits of controlling the sodium–potassium ratio in the diet.

**soft drinks**  Term applied to non-alcoholic, usually fruit and fruit-flavoured drinks. Various concentrations and preparations are termed squash, crush and cordial, which usually require dilution before drinking; others are ready-to-drink.

In the USA cider refers to unfermented apple juice (a soft drink), while the fermented product is termed hard cider.

**sol**  A colloidal solution, i.e. a suspension of particles intermediate in size between ordinary molecules (as in a solution) and coarse particles (as in a suspension). A jelly-like sol is a gel.

**Solanaceae**  Family of plants including potato (*Solanum tuberosum*), aubergine (*S. melongena*), Cape gooseberry (*Physalis peruviana*), tomato (*Lycopersicon esculentum*).

**solanine**  Heat-stable toxic glycoside of the alkaloid solanidine, found in small amounts of potatoes, and larger and sometimes toxic amounts in sprouts and in skin when potatoes become green through exposure to light. 20 mg solanine per 100 g fresh weight of potato tissue is accepted as the upper limit. Causes gastrointestinal disturbances and certain neurological disorders; *in vitro* it inhibits cholinesterase.

**solids-not-fat**  Refers to the solids of milk excluding the fat, i.e. protein, lactose and salts. SNF serves as an index of milk quality and is determined by measuring the specific gravity in the lactometer.

Normal specific gravity is 1.032 at 60°F (15.5°C).

Percentage total solids = 0.25 × SG + 1.2 × percentage fat + 0.14.

**somatomedins**  Group of growth-promoting peptide hormones in fetal tissues; related to insulin and previously termed 'insulin-like growth factor' (IGF).

**sorbet**  See *sherbet*.

**sorbic acid**  Hexadienoic acid, $CH_3CH=CHCH=CHCOOH$. Used together with its sodium, potassium and calcium salts as fungistat in wine, cheese, soft drinks, low-sugar jams, flour confectionery, etc.

**Sorbistat**  Sorbistat K. Trade names (Pfizer) for sorbic acid, which see, and its potassium salt.

**sorbitol**  Six-carbon sugar alcohol formed by the reduction of fructose; old names glycitol and glucitol. Although it is metabolised in the body with the liberation of 4 kcal per gram, it is absorbed from the intestine only slowly and is tolerated by diabetics. Found in plum, apricot, cherry and apple; used in place of sucrose to make jam suitable for diabetics; 60% as sweet as sucrose.

**sorcerer's milk**  See *witches' milk*.

**Sorenson titration**  Method of titrating amino acids and ammonium salts by adding formaldehyde, which combines with the amino groups, and titrating the carboxyl groups (or acidic radical of the ammonium salt).

**sorghum**  *Sorghum vulgare*. A cereal that thrives in semi-arid regions; important human food in tropical Africa, central and N. India and China. Sorghum produced in the USA and Australia is used for animal feed. Also known as kaffir corn (in South Africa), guinea corn (in West Africa), jowar (in India), Indian millet and millo maize. The white grain variety is eaten as meal, red grained has a bitter taste and is used for beer; sugar syrup is obtained from the crushed stems of the sweet sorghum.

Analysis per 100 g: 10 g protein, 3 g fat, 70 g carbohydrate, 2 g fibre, 4.5 mg Fe, 0.5 mg vitamin $B_1$, 0.12 mg vitamin $B_2$, 3.5 mg nicotinic acid.

**sorghum syrup**  The concentrated juice from a sweet variety of sorghum.

**Souchong**  See *tea*.

**soursop**  See *custard apple*.

**souse**  To steep or cook a food such as herring in vinegar or white wine.

**sous-vide**  French-originated term for cooking in special pouches under vacuum; shelf-life of weeks; claimed also to retain flavour and nutrients.

Derived from French culinary method, cooking en papillote, i.e. in a sealed container (parchment paper case).

**Soxhlet**  An apparatus for the extraction of solids, mostly used for the extraction of fat. The solid is contained in a 'thimble' and is percolated by fresh solvent continuously. The fat-laden solvent siphons over into a flask from which it is boiled off to be repercolated, while the fat is left in the flask.

**soya**  A bean (*Glycine max*) of importance as a source of both oil and protein. The protein is of high biological value, higher than that of many other vegetable proteins, and is of great value for animal and human food.

When raw it contains a trypsin inhibitor destroyed by heat.

Native of China, where it has been cultivated for 5000 years; grows 2–3 ft high with 2–3 beans per pod. The original variety was 20% protein with no fat, but modern varieties contain 40% protein and 20% fat.

**soybean curd**  Precipitate from soybean milk.

Analysis per 100 g: water 85 g, protein 7 g, fat 4 g, carbohydrate 3 g, fibre 0.1 g, kcal 80 (0.32 MJ), Fe 1.8 mg, vitamin $B_1$ 0.05 mg, vitamin $B_2$ 0.04 mg, nicotinic acid 0.5 mg.

**soybean flour**  Dehulled, ground soya bean. The unheated material is a rich source of amylase and proteinase and is useful as a baking aid. The heated material has no enzymic activity but is a valuable food.

Analysis per 100 g, full fat: protein 40 g, fat 20 g, kcal 360 (1.5 MJ), Ca 200 mg, Fe 6 mg, carotene 40 µg, vitamin $B_1$ 0.8 mg, vitamin $B_2$ 0.3 mg, nicotinic acid 2 mg.

Defatted: protein 46 g, fat 5 g, kcal 260 (1 MJ), Ca 250 mg, Fe 7 mg, carotene 30 µg, vitamin $B_1$ 0.7 mg, vitamin $B_2$ 0.3 mg, nicotinic acid 2 mg.

There is about 25% carbohydrate in the bean, of which 12% is polysaccharide (dextrins, galactans and pentosans) and 12.5% sugars (6% sucrose, 5% stachyose and 1.5% raffinose).

**soybean milk**  Extract of the bean.

Analysis per 100 g: water 93 g, protein 3 g, fat 1.5 g, carbohydrate 1 g, fibre 0.4 g, kcal 30 (0.13 MJ), Fe 0.6 mg, vitamin $B_1$ 0.1 mg, vitamin $B_2$ 0.04 mg, nicotinic acid 0.2 mg.

**Soyolk**  Trade name (Soya Foods Ltd) for full fat soya flour.

**soy sauce**  The fermented soya bean commonly eaten in China and Japan. Traditionally the bean, often mixed with wheat, is fermented with *Aspergillus oryzae* over a period of 1–3 years. The modern process is carried out at a high temperature or in an autoclave for a short time.

Analysis per 100 g: water 68 g, protein 6 g, fat 1 g, carbohydrate 5 g, kcal 50 (0.2 MJ), Ca 100 mg, Fe 5.5 mg, vitamin $B_1$ 0.02 mg, vitamin $B_2$ 0.06 mg, nicotinic acid 0.3 mg.

**spaghetti**  See *alimentary pastes*.

**Spanish toxic oil syndrome**  Widespread disease in Spain, 1981–83, with 450 deaths due to consumption of an oil including aniline-denatured crude rape seed oil sold as pure olive oil. The disease appears to be unique and the precise cause is unknown.

**Spans**  Trade name (Atlas Co.) for non-ionic surface agents derived from fatty acids and hexahydric alcohols. Oil soluble, in contrast to Tweens (which see), which are water-soluble or well-dispersible in water. Used in bread as crumb-softeners (antistaling) to improve doughs, cakes and biscuits and as emulsifiers.

**specific dynamic action**  The term applied to the increase in metabolism (as indicated by heat output) following ingestion of food. In modern terminology it is referred to as thermogenesis or the thermic effect, thought to be due to stimulation of brown fat. Earlier term, Luxus Konsumption. Possible means whereby constant body weight is maintained despite variations in food intake.

**specificity**  In relation to enzymes, refers to the ability of an enzyme to catalyse only a limited range of reactions, or, in some cases, a single reaction. Specificity is the main distinction between enzymes and catalysts, as the latter are non-specific.

Examples: arginase will hydrolyse L-arginine only, not even the D-isomer; esterase will hydrolyse the whole group of compounds containing the ester linkage, but no others.

**specificity, stereochemical**  Used in reference to enzymes; those that will attack one stereochemical isomer but not the other. Thus there are distinct L- and D-amino acid oxidases which will attack only the corresponding isomer and leave the other untouched.

**spectrophotometer**  Optical instrument that measures the amount of light absorbed at any particular wavelength. Used extensively to measure substances that have specific absorption in the infrared or ultraviolet range, or are coloured, or can react to form colour derivatives. Similar in this way to the absorptiometer.

**spelt**  Coarse type of wheat, mainly used as cattle feed.

**spent wash**  Liquor remaining in the whisky still after distilling the spirit. A source of unidentified growth factors detected by chick growth. When dried is known as distillers' dried solubles.

**sphingomyelins**  Complex phosphatides found in brain and nerve tissue and as part of cell structure; composed of the base sphingosine plus fatty acids, phosphoric acid and choline.

**spices** Distinguished from herbs only in that part instead of the whole of the aromatic plant is meant, such as root, stem, seeds.

Originally used to mask putrefactive flavours. Some have preservative effect because of their essential oils, e.g. cloves, cinnamon and mustard.

Consumed in too small a quantity to provide any nutrients, except possibly for curry powder, which contains 22 mg iron per ounce.

**spinach** Leaves of *Spinacia oleracea*. A rich source of carotene and vitamin C; also contains oxalic acid, which renders calcium insoluble and non-available.

Analysis boiled per 100 g: protein 5 g, carbohydrate 1.5 g, kcal 30 (130 kJ), Ca 600 mg, Fe 4 mg, carotene 6 mg, vitamin C 10–60 mg.

**spinach beet** Swiss chard.

**spirits** Made by distillation of yeast fermentation liquors, subsequently diluted. Alcohol content, w/v, of brandy, gin, rum, whisky, 31.7% (termed 70 degrees proof), with traces of nitrogen, minerals and sugars; now more usually 40% alcohol.

**spirit, silent** Highly purified alcohol, or neutral spirit, distilled from any fermentable material.

**spirometer** (respirometer) Apparatus used to measure the amount of oxygen consumed (and in some instances the amount of carbon dioxide produced) from which to calculate the energy expended (indirect calorimetry). There are several types, including the Benedict–Roth spirometer, the Kofranyi–Michaelis spirometer and the integrating motor pneumotachograph (IMP).

**Spirulina** Blue-green alga which can make use of atmospheric nitrogen; eaten for centuries round Lake Chad in N. Africa and in Mexico. See *algae*.

**spores** In relation to bacteria, they are the resting state; thick-walled, highly resistant to damage by heat. Under suitable conditions they germinate to produce bacteria.

Not all bacteria can form spores; the so-called spore-bearers are a hazard in pasteurisation and sterilisation, as the spores can remain undamaged in the processing and the material is consequently not sterile.

**sprat** *Sprattus sprattus (Clupea sprattus)*, related to the herring; young is brisling.

Analysis per 100 g (fried weighed with head): 20 g protein, 33 g fat, 400 kcal (1.7 MJ), 600 mg Ca, 4 mg Fe.

**spray dryer** Equipment in which material to be dried is sprayed as a fine mist into a hot-air chamber and falls to the bottom as dry powder. Period of heating is very brief and so damage is avoided. Dried powder consists of hollow particles of low density. Widely applied to many foods (e.g. milk) and pharmaceuticals.

**spreading factor** See *hyaluronidase*.

**springers** See *swells*.

**sprue** Disease in which the villi of the small intestine are atrophied and food is incompletely absorbed, followed consequently by undernutrition and weight loss. In tropical sprue (see *sprue, tropical*) folic acid is thought to be involved and possibly an infective agent.

**sprue, tropical** Name given (by Dutch in Java) to tropical disease of unknown origin characterised by fatty diarrhoea and sore mouth, with signs of undernutrition due to poor absorption of nutrients.

**squalene** A hydrocarbon, $C_{30}H_{50}$, found in liver of shark and rat; suggested as a possible intermediate in the synthesis of cholesterol in the body.

**squash** See *gourds*.

**squash, fruit** See *soft drinks*.

**stabilisers** See also *emulsifying agents*. Substances that stabilise emulsions of fat and water, e.g. gums, agar, egg albumin, cellulose ethers; used to produce the texture of meringues and marshmallow, lecithin for crumb-softening in bread and confectionery, glyceryl monostearate and polyoxyethylene stearate for crumb-softening.

The legally permitted list includes also superglycerinated fats, propylene glycol alginate and stearate, methyl-, methylethyl-, and sodium carboxymethyl-celluloses, stearyl tartrate, sorbitan esters of fatty acids.

Bread may contain only superglycerinated fats and stearyl tartrate.

**stachyase** Enzyme that hydrolyses the tetrasaccharide stachyose to fructose and a mannosaccharide consisting of glucose and two molecules of galactose. Found in the digestive juices of crustaceans and molluscs.

**stachyose** Tetrose sugar composed of two units of galactose and one each of fructose and glucose. Not hydrolysed in the human digestive tract and passes to the large intestine, where it is fermented by bacteria. Present in soya beans, some other legumes, including lupins, and the tuber of *Stachys tubifera*; gives rise to the flatulence commonly associated with eating beans.

Also known as mannotetrose and lupeose.

**stackburn** Name given to the deterioration in colour and quality of canned foods which have not been sufficiently cooled after canning and then stored in stacks which cool slowly.

**staling** Starch has a crystalline structure which is lost during baking. Subsequently the starch recrystallises, i.e. it retrogrades and, in the instance of bread, the crumb loses its softness and the bread goes stale. Staling can be delayed by emulsifiers (crumb softeners) such as polyoxyethylene and monoglyceride derivatives of fatty acids.

Retrogradation of starch also takes place in dehydrated potatoes.

**staphylococcal poisoning** See *food poisoning*.

**staple food** The principal food, e.g. wheat, rice, maize, etc.

**starch** Complex polysaccharide composed of unit of glucose; consists of about one-quarter amylose and three-quarters amylopectin; the form in which carbohydrate is stored in the plant, and does not occur in animal tissue. (Glycogen is sometimes referred to as animal starch.)

All starches are broken down by acid or enzymic hydrolysis, or during digestion, first to maltose and then glucose, but the various starches such as potato, maize, cereal, arrowroot, sago, etc., have different structures.

It is the principal carbohydrate of the diet and, hence, the major source of energy for man and animals.

See also *amylase*; *amylopectin*.

**starch, A and B** Refers to larger granules of wheat starch, A, 25–35 µm, and smaller particles, B, 2–8 µm.

**starch, animal** See *glycogen*.

**starch, arum** From root of the arum lily; similar to sago.

**starch, derivatised** See *starch, modified*.

**starch, enzyme-resistant** A glucan formed when starch is heated (apparently formed after gelatinisation by spontaneous self-association of the hydrated amylose component).

Escapes digestion in the small intestine but can be fermented in the large intestine. According to the method of analysis of dietary fibre enzyme-resistant starch can be included.

**starch equivalent** A measure of the energy value of animal feedingstuffs; the number of parts of pure starch that would be equivalent to 100 parts of the ration as a source of energy.

Determined by direct feeding experiments or may be calculated from the formula: SE per 100 lb = 0.44 × digestible protein plus 2.41 × digestible fat plus digestible carbohydrate plus fibre.

Protein has SE 0.94, crude fibre 1.0, ether extract of oilseeds 2.4. 1 lb starch equivalent has a net energy value of 1071 kcal; 1 kg = 9.9 MJ.

**starches, waxy** Those containing a high percentage of amylopectin; they do not form rigid gels when gelatinised but soft pastes. See also *maize starches*, *waxy*.

**starch, inhibited**  See *starch, modified*.

**starch, modified**  Starch altered by physical or chemical treatment to give special properties of value in food processing, e.g. change in gel strength, flow properties, colour, clarity, stability of the paste.

Acid-modified starch – acid treatment reduces the viscosity of the paste (used in sugar confectionery, e.g. gum drops, jelly beans.)

Oxidised starch – peroxide, permanganate, chlorine, etc., alter viscosity, clarity and stability of the paste (major use is outside the food industry).

Derivatised starch – chemical derivatives such as ethers and esters show properties such as reduced gelatinisation in hot water and greater stability to acids and alkalies ('inhibited' starch); useful where food has to withstand heat treatment, as in canning or in acid foods. Further degrees of treatment can result in starch being unaffected by boiling water and losing its gel-forming properties.

See also *starch, pregelatinised*.

**starch, oxidised**  See *starch, modified*.

**starch, pregelatinised**  Raw starch does not form a paste with cold water and therefore requires cooking if it is to be used as a food thickening agent. Pregelatinised starch, mostly maize starch, has been cooked and dried.

Used in instant puddings, pie-fillings, soup mixes, salad dressings, sugar confectionery, as binder in meat products. Nutritional value the same as that of the original starch.

See also *starch, modified*.

**starch syrup**  See *glucose syrups*.

**starter**  Culture of bacteria used to inoculate or start growth in, e.g. milk for cheese production, or butter to develop the flavour, or any fermentation.

**steam baking**  In baking an even temperature is maintained in the oven by means of closed pipes through which steam circulates. This is sometimes erroneously believed to mean that the bread is baked in live steam.

**steapsin**  Obsolete name for pancreatic lipase.

**stearic acid**  Saturated long-chain fatty acid with 18 carbon atoms – octadecenoic acid, $C_{17}H_{35}COOH$; present in most animal and vegetable fats in the triglycerides. Used in pharmacy and cosmetics.

**steatorrhoea**  Excess of fat in the stools. May be due to lack of bile, lack of lipase in the digestive juices, or defective absorption of fat. Treatment by feeding low-fat diet.

See also *coeliac disease*.

**steer**   Bull castrated when very young; if castrated after reaching maturity, known as a stag.

**stercobilin**   One of the brown pigments of the faeces; formed from the bile pigments, which, in turn, are formed as break-down products of the haemoglobin of obsolete red blood cells.

**stereoisomerism**   Occurs when compounds have the same molecular formula, and the same structural formula, but with the atoms arranged differently in space. There are two sub-divisions, namely, optical isomerism (see *optical activity*) and geometrical isomerism (see *cis–trans isomerism*).

**sterigmatocystin**   See *mycotoxins*.

**sterile**   Free from all micro-organisms – bacteria, moulds and yeasts.

When foods are sterilised, as in canning, they are preserved indefinitely, as they are protected from recontamination in the can, and also from chemical and enzymic deterioration.

**sterilisation, cold**   Applied to preservation with sulphur dioxide or with ionising radiation. See *irradiation*.

**sterilisation, radiation**   See *irradiation*.

**sterility, commercial**   Term applied to canned foods which are not sterile but which will not spoil during storage, because of the high acid content of the food, or the presence of pickling salts, or a high concentration of sugar.

**steroids**   Compounds that contain the cyclopenteno-phenanthrene ring system

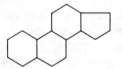

include vitamin D, male and female sex hormones, hormones of the adrenal cortex, sterols such as cholesterol, toad poisons, cardiac glycosides of the digitalis group, and some of the carcinogenic hydrocarbons.

The steroid alcohols, i.e. steroids carrying the −OH alcoholic grouping, are sterols.

**sterols**   Alcohols derived from the steroids, which see. Include cholesterol, widely distributed in animal tissue, including brain and egg yolk; coprosterol in faeces; ergosterol in yeast, which is the precursor for the synthetic vitamin $D_2$; and sitosterol and stigmasterol in plants.

**stevioside**   Naturally occurring glucoside of steviol, a steroid derivative, which is 300 times as sweet as sucrose. Isolated from leaves of a Paraguayan shrub, *Stevia rebaudiana* – yerba dulce.

**Stevix**   Trade name (Japan) for mixture of the sweet glycosides extracted from stevia leaves. See also *stevioside*; *rebaudioside*.

**stew**   To cook foods in an enclosed pan; temperature below boiling point, about 90 °C (195 °F). Such slow cooking is useful for low-quality meat (rich in connective tissue), since it slowly breaks down the connective tissue to gelatin and so softens the meat.

**stickwater**   The aqueous fraction from pressing cooked fish in the manufacture of fish meal. Contains amino acids, vitamins and minerals, and is added to animal feed or mixed back with the fish meal and dried.

Also known as fish solubles.

**stilboestrol**   Synthetic substance with potent activity as female sex hormone; widely used clinically and for food production (for chemical caponisation of cockerels and to stimulate the growth of cattle).

**stiparogenic**   Foods that tend to cause constipation.

**stiparolytic**   Foods that tend to prevent or relieve constipation.

**stobb**   Strawberry stalk.

**stockfish**   Unsalted fish that has been dried naturally in air and sunshine; mostly prepared in Norway. Contains 12–15% water, and 1 lb is made from 4½ lb of fresh fish.

Analysis per 100 g, after boiling: protein 30 g, fat 1 g, carbohydrate nil, kcal 140 (0.6 MJ), Ca 20 mg, Fe 2 mg.

**stock; meat, vegetable, bone stock**   Liquid in which the meat or bone or vegetable, or a mixture of these, has been boiled until most of the water-soluble matter has been extracted.

Meat and bone contain collagen, which is converted into gelatin by prolonged boiling; hence, the stock may set to a gel on cooling.

The main nutritive value of stock is the mineral content.

**storage, gas**   See *gas storage*.

**stork process**   The name given to the process of ultra-high temperature sterilisation of milk followed by sterilisation again inside the bottle.

**stout**   See *beer*. So-called milk stout merely has added lactose (milk sugar).

**strandin**   A substance isolated from brain tissue which dries in long strands; composed of fatty acid, sphingosine, carbohydrate and a small proportion of neuraminic acid.

**strawberry**   Fruit of *Fragaria* species, a perennial herb of American origin, introduced into Europe about 1600. 40–90 mg vitamin C per 100 g; trace of carotene.

Alpine strawberry is *Fragaria vesca semperflorens*, a variety of the European wild strawberry.

**strepogenin**  Name given to a peptide-like fraction from natural sources, claimed to be essential for micro-organisms and higher animals. The need for special peptides for the latter has not been confirmed.

**streptococcal poisoning**  See *food poisoning*.

**Streptococcus lactis factor**  A fermentation product of the mould *Rhizopus nigricans*, known as rhizopterin, which is essential to *S. lactis* R. Related to folic acid, which see.

**streptodornase**  See *streptokinase*.

**streptokinase**  Proteolytic enzyme prepared from haemolytic streptococci. Used clinically to liquefy thick pus in empyemata and to remove the fibrin clot covering wounds. Streptodornase is a similar enzyme preparation that attacks pus cells.

**struvite**  Small crystals of magnesium ammonium phosphate which occasionally form in canned fish – resemble broken glass.

**Stubbs and More factor**  Factor for estimating amount of fat-free meat from total nitrogen content.

**substrate**  In relation to enzymes, refers to the substance on which the enzyme acts. Thus, the substrate for the enzyme amylase is starch, which is hydrolysed to maltose.

Substrate can also mean the medium on which micro-organisms grow.

**subtilin**  Antibiotic isolated from a strain of *Bacillus subtilis* grown on a medium containing asparagine. Used as a food preservative (not permitted in Great Britain), as it reduces the thermal resistance of spores and is effective against thermophilic flat sours; thus, subtilin permits a reduction in the processing time.

**Sucaryl**  Trade name (Abbott Laboratories) for sodium or calcium salt of cyclohexyl sulphamate.

**succory**  Another name for chicory.

**succotash**  Stew of green maize and Lima beans (butter beans), an American-Indian dish.

**succus entericus**  Intestinal juice, which see.

**suchar**  Activated carbon, used to decolorise solutions.

**Sucralose**  Trade name (Tate & Lyle) for synthetic chlorinated sucrose (trichlorogalactosucrose) 2000 times as sweet as sucrose, stable to heat and acid.

**sucrase**  See *invertase*.

**sucrol**  See *dulcin*.

**Sucron**  Trade name (Accepted Foods Ltd) for mixture of saccharine and sucrose, four times as sweet as sucrose alone.

**sucrose**  Cane sugar or beet sugar. A disaccharide composed of a molecule of glucose linked to one of fructose (α-D-glucopyranosyl β-fructofuranoside or β-D-fructofuranosyl α-Dglucopyranoside ($C_{12} H_{22} O_{11}$)); these two monosaccharides are formed by the hydrolysis of sucrose.

Crude brown sugar is 97% carbohydrate, and contains, per 100 g, 1 g water, 0.2 g protein, 2 mg Fe, 0.02 mg vitamin $B_1$, 0.1 mg vitamin $B_2$, 0.3 mg nicotinic acid.

Refined white sugar is close to 100% pure and contains no minerals or vitamins.

**sucrose distearate**  See *sucrose esters*.

**sucrose esters**  Di- and trilaurates and mono- and distearates of sucrose. Used as emulsifiers, wetting agents and surface active agents, e.g. for washing fruits and vegetables, as anti-spattering agents, anti-foam agents and anti-staling or crumb-softening agents.

**sucrose intolerance**  See *disaccharide intolerance*.

**sucrose monostearate**  See *sucrose esters*.

**sucrose polyesters (SPE)**  Mixtures of hexa-, hepta- and octa-esters of sucrose and common fatty acids (C12 to C20 and above). Can replace conventional fats and oils in foods and food preparation but pass through the gastrointestinal tract without being absorbed.

**suet**  Fat prepared from the kidneys of oxen and sheep.

**sufu**  Fermented product made by inoculating sterilised cubes of soybean curd with the mould, *Actinomucor elegans*; stored after adding salt and alcohol.

**sugar**  Although the term is commonly used to refer to table sugar or sucrose, there are a large number of sugars, e.g. fruit sugar (fructose), grape (glucose), which are monosaccharides; malt sugar (maltose), milk sugar (lactose), which are disaccharides; and also higher multiples.

Table sugar (sucrose) is extracted from the sugar beet or sugar cane, concentrated and refined. Molasses is the residue left after the first stage of crystallisation and is bitter and black. The residue from the second stage is treacle, less bitter and less viscous than molasses. The first crude crystals are Muscovado or Barbados sugar, brown and sticky. The next stage is light brown, Demerara sugar.

**sugar alcohols**  Differ from sugars in including a hydroxyl group in place of the aldehyde or ketonic grouping (C=O). They occur in nature but glucose can be converted into sorbitol, galactose into dulcitol, etc.). They provide 2.4 kcal/g (10 kJ), differ in metabolic function and, for labelling purposes in UK, are included with carbohydrates not sugars.

**sugar beet**  *Beta vulgaris* subsp. *cicla*, the most important source of sugar (sucrose) in temperate countries; contains 15–20% sugar; biennial related to the garden beetroot but with white, conical roots.

**sugar cane**   The plant, *Saccharum officinarum*, from the juice of which sugar is prepared.

**sugar, caster**   Ordinary sugar (sucrose) crystallised in small crystals.

**sugar doctor**   To prevent the crystallisation or 'graining' of sugar in sugar confectionery, a substance called the sugar doctor or candy doctor is added. This may be a weak acid, such as cream of tartar, which 'inverts' part of the cane sugar during the boiling, or invert sugar or starch syrup.

**sugar esters**   See *sucrose esters*.

**sugar, icing**   Powdered sucrose.

**sugaring, of dried fruits**   A type of deterioration of dried fruit on storage, most frequently on prunes and figs. A sugary substance appears on the surface or under the skin, consisting of glucose and fructose, with traces of citric and malic acids, lysine, asparagine and aspartic acid.

When occurring under the skin of prunes, it is called 'red sugar'.

**sugar, London Demerara**   White sugar coloured with molasses to resemble partly refined sugar.

**sugar maple**   *Acer saccharum*; the sap is evaporated down to a syrup, maple syrup, and crystallised to sucrose, maple sugar.

**sugar palm**   *Arenga saccharifera*; grows wild in Malaysia and Indonesia. Sugar (sucrose) is obtained from the sap.

**sugar tolerance**   See *glucose tolerance*.

**sulpha drugs**   Group of synthetic drugs derived from sulphanilamide (or aminobenzenesulphonamide) used to combat bacterial infection.

Sulphanilamide itself functions as an antivitamin to bacteria, as it inhibits the uptake of para-amino benzoic acid, an essential nutrient. These drugs include sulphapyridine, sulphadiazine, sulphathiazole, etc.

**sulphate**   The mineral sulphur occurs in foods and in the body in two main forms, (1) as sulphate – salts of sulphuric acid, and (2) in the amino acids methionine and cystine. See *sulphur*.

**sulphites**   Salts of sulphurous acid used as sources of sulphur dioxide, which see.

**sulphur**   An element that is part of the amino acids cystine and methionine and is therefore present in all proteins. It is also part of the molecules of vitamin $B_1$ and biotin.

Apart from its presence as part of these compounds, there appears to be no dietary need for sulphur in any other form and no deficiency has ever been observed, although it is essential for plants.

Not only was the old-fashioned remedy of sulphur and molasses quite unnecessary but also elemental sulphur is probably not used by the body.

**sulphur amino acids** Cysteine and methionine; methionine is essential but can be partially replaced by cysteine, so the amounts of the two in a protein food are usually added together.

**sulphur dioxide** Preservative used in gaseous form or as salts or sulphite for fruit drinks, wine, comminuted meat, as processing aid to control physical properties of flour; also prevents enzymic and non-enzymic browning. Protects vitamin C but destroys thiamin.

Prepared by ancient Egyptians and Romans by burning sulphur and used to disinfect wine.

**sulphuring** Preservation by sulphur dioxide.

**sulphur in urine** Three groups of sulphur compounds are excreted: inorganic sulphates (sodium, potassium, calcium, magnesium, and ammonium), organic sulphates (sulphuric esters of phenolic compounds), neutral sulphur (thiosulphates, thiocyanates, mercapturic acids, urochrome).

**sultanas** Made by drying the golden sultana grapes (Turkey, Greece, Australia, and South Africa); the bunches are dipped in alkali, washed, sulphured and dried. Sultanas of the European type produced in the USA are termed seedless raisins.

For analysis see *fruit, dried*; see also *currants*; *muscatels*; *raisins*.

**Sunett** Trade name (Hoechst) for acesulfame K.

**sunflower** *Helianthus annuus*. Seed used as source of edible oil, rich in polyunsaturated fatty acids; residual oilcake used for animal feed. Seeds also eaten raw.

Analysis per 100 g: 27 g protein, 36 g fat, 23 g carbohydrate, 540 kcal (2.2 MJ), 100 mg Ca, 7 mg Fe, 1.9 mg vitamin $B_1$, 0.2 mg vitamin $B_2$, 5.8 mg nicotinic acid.

**sunlight flavour** Name given to unpleasant flavours developing in foods after exposure to sunlight. In milk it is said to be due to the breakdown of methionine in the presence of vitamin $B_2$; in beer due to a change in the bitter principles from the hops.

**superchill** Cool to temperature −1 to −4°C (chill temperature usually +2°C).

**superglycerinated fats** Normal fats are triglycerides, i.e. three molecules of fatty acid to each molecule of glycerol. Mono- and diglycerides are known as superglycerinated.

Glyceryl monostearate (GMS) is solid at room temperature, flexible and non-greasy; used as a protective coating for foods, as plasticiser for softening the crumb of bread, to reduce spattering in frying fats, as emulsifier and stabiliser.

Glyceryl mono-oleate (GMO) is semi-liquid at room temperature.

**suprarenal glands**  See *adrenal glands*.

**Supro**  Protein-rich baby food (24% protein) made in East Africa from maize or barley flour with torula yeast, skim-milk powder and flavouring.

**surface area**  Heat loss from the body, and therefore basal metabolism, is related to surface area. Calculated by formula of Du Bois or Meeh.

Du Bois: Area ($cm^2$) = weight (kg) to power of 0.425 × height (cm) to power of 0.725 × 71.84.

Meeh: Area=11.9 × weight to power of 2/3.

**surfactants**  Surface active agents which are hydrophilic or have hydrophilic and hydrophobic portions of their structure and so have affinity for both fats and water and act as emulsifiers. Used in baked goods, as wetting agents for powders, to clean and peel fruits and vegetables, and in comminuted meat products. See also *Spans*; *Tweens*.

**surimi**  Water extract of minced flesh of low-oil fish (mostly myofibrillar protein) with gelling properties, used to prepare a range of foods. It is relatively tasteless, odourless and white.

Introduced from Japan into the United States in 1979, as the basis for seafood analogues but with broad potentialities.

**susceptor plates**  Special metallic films (usually powdered aluminium) deposited inside the packets of foods intended for microwave cooking; they concentrate the energy on the outside of the food and brown and crisp it.

**suspensoids**  See *colloids, lyophobic*.

**Sustagen**  US trade name (Mead Johnson Laboratories) of food concentrate in powder form, also usable for tube feeding; mixture of whole and skim milk, casein, maltose, dextrins and glucose.

Analysis: protein 24%, fat 8%, carbohydrate 68%; vitamins A, $B_1$, $B_2$, nicotinic acid, C, D, E, $B_{12}$, calcium pantothenate, pyridoxine plus choline, calcium and iron.

**sweat**  Solution of salt (about 0.3%), urea 0.03%, lactate 0.07%. Varies in composition but hypotonic to blood plasma.

**swede**  Root of *Brassica rutabaga* or Swedish turnip; called rutabaga in the USA.

Analysis per 100 g: 91 g water, 4 g sugars, 3 g dietary fibre, 1 g protein, 20 kcal (90 kJ), 15–40 g vitamin C.

**sweetbread**  See *pancreas*.

**sweeteners, bulk**  Used to replace sucrose and glucose syrups. One example is hydrogenated glucose syrup, in which the free aldehyde groups of glucose units have been reduced to sorbitol by catalytic hydrogenation; effectively a mixture of glucose and sorbitol. Used in soft drinks and sugar confectionery, and in some diabetic foods as a partial substitute for sorbitol; 70–80% as sweet as sucrose.

**sweeteners, non-nutritive** Refers to sweetening agents which are not sugars and have no food value, such as saccharin and cyclamate.

**sweetening agents** Three groups: (1) The sugars, of which the commonest is sucrose. Fructose has 173% of the sweetness of sucrose; glucose, 74%; maltose, 33%; and lactose, 16%. (2) Synthetic non-nutritive sweeteners such as saccharin (550 times as sweet as sucrose), dulcin (250 times), sucaryl (30 times), P4000 (4000 times) – see under individual headings. (3) Various other chemicals such as glycerol and glycine (70% as sweet as sucrose), and certain peptides.

**Sweetex** Trade name (Boots Ltd) for saccharin.

**sweet sop** See *custard apple*.

**swells** Applied to infected canned foods when gases produced by fermentation inside the can cause the ends to swell.

A 'hard swell' has permanently extended ends. If the ends can be moved under pressure, but not forced back to the original position, they are 'soft swells'. 'Springers' can be forced back, but the opposite end bulges.

A 'flipper' is a can of normal appearance in which the end flips out when the can is struck.

Hydrogen swells are harmless, and due to acid fruits attacking the can.

**Swift stability test** See *active oxygen method*.

**Swiss chard** *Beta vulgaris* var. *cicla*, also known as leaf beet, leaf chard, sea kale beet, silver beet, white leaf beet, spinach beet. Grown for green leaves (spinach-like) and broad mid-rib (can be cooked).

Analysis per 100 g; 2.5 g protein, 4.5 g carbohydrate, 25 kcal (100 kJ), 3 mg iron, 2 mg retinol equivalent, 30 mg vitamin C. Term also used for blanched summer shoots of globe artichoke and for inner leaves of cardoon, *Cynara cardunculus*.

**syllabub** Also sillabub. Elizabethan dish made of milk or cream mixed with wine or brandy, sweetened and whipped.

**syneresis** Oozing of liquid from gel when cut and allowed to stand (e.g. jelly or baked custard).

**Synsepalum** See *miracle berry*.

**synthalin** Decamethylene-diguanidine; lowers blood sugar and used experimentally in the treatment of diabetes, but is toxic.

**syntonin** Old name given to degradation products of proteins.

**syrup** A solution of sugar which may be from a variety of sources such as maple, corn, sorghum, and stages in refining such as top syrup, refiners syrup and sugar syrup.

Analysis of the product of refining called golden syrup: 20% water, sugar 79%, protein 0.03%, fat nil, kcal 297 (1.25 MJ), Fe 1.5 mg; vitamins present only in traces.

The sugar solutions used for canning fruit are also syrups: light syrup – 15° Brix; syrup – 20 or 30° Brix; heavy syrup – 30 or 40° Brix; extra heavy syrup – 40 or 50° Brix. (Degrees Brix = percentage sugar.)

**syrup, corn**   See *glucose syrups*.

# T

**T3**   Tri-iodothyronine.

**T4**   Thyroxine (tetraiodothyronine).

**tabasco sauce**   Hot sauce made from chillis, salt and vinegar.

**tachycardia**   Rapid heart-beat; a symptom, among other causes, of certain vitamin deficiencies.

**tachyphagia**   Rapid eating.

**tachyphylaxis**   Decreased effects on repeated injections of a substance.

**tachysterol**   One of the compounds produced (along with vitamin $D_2$ or calciferol) by ultraviolet irradiation of ergosterol. It has no anti-rachitic activity until it has been reduced to dihydro-tachysterol, also called AT-10.

AT-10 is also used for the treatment of deficient thyroid function.

**taette**   See *milks, fermented*.

**tafia**   Spirit similar to rum made from sugar cane.

**takadiastase**   Or koji, an enzyme preparation produced by growing the fungus *Aspergillus oryzae* on bran, leaching the culture mass with water and precipitating with alcohol.

Contains a mixture of enzymes, largely diastatic; used for the preparation of starch hydrolysates.

**Talin**   Trade name (Tate & Lyle Ltd) for thaumatin, an extract of the berry *Thaumatococcus danielli*, about 3000 times as sweet as sucrose. See *katemfe*.

**tallow, rendered**   Beef or mutton fat prepared from parts other than the kidney, by heating with water in an autoclave. When pressed, separates to a liquid fraction, oleo oil, used in margarine, and a solid fraction, oleostearin, used for soap and candles.

**tallow, solid**   See *premier jus*.

**tamales**   Flat, Mexican, cornmeal pancakes similar to tortillas, rolled around spiced meat or fish or fruit.

**tamarind**  Leguminous tree, *Tamarindus indica*, with pods containing seeds embedded in brown pulp, eaten fresh and used in seasonings and curries.

Analysis per 100 g: 2 g protein, 74 g carbohydrate, 2 g fibre, 300 kcal (1.25 MJ), 3 mg Fe, 0.4 mg vitamin $B_1$, 0.15 mg vitamin $B_2$, 1.5 mg nicotinic acid, 10 mg vitamin C.

**tammy**  Cookery term meaning to strain through a fine woollen cloth – a tammy cloth.

**tangelo**  Cross between tangerine and grapefruit.

**tangerine**  *Citrus reticulata*, also called mandarin. Similar fruits which are varieties of tangerine are satsumas and king orange.

**tankage**  Ground, dried residue from slaughter house excluding all the useful tissues.

**tannia** (also tanier)  Corm of *Xanthosoma sagittifolium*; known as new cocoyam in West Africa and as yautia: same family as taro.

Analysis per 100 g; 2 g protein, 0.3 g fat, 31 g carbohydrate, 130 kcal (0.55 MJ), 1 mg Fe, 0.1 mg vitamin $B_1$, 0.03 mg vitamin $B_2$, 0.5 mg nicotinic acid, 10 mg vitamin C.

**tannins**  Any polyphenolic substance with molecular weight greater than 500. Classified as hydrolysable (to yield sugar residue and phenolcarboxylic acid) and condensed or compound tannins, which are polymeric flavonoids (also called catechin tannins).

Present in dark-coloured sorghum, carob bean, unripe fruits, tea; give an astringent effect in the mouth; precipitate proteins and used to clarify beer and wines. Also called tannic acid and gallotannin.

**tansy**  *Tanacetum vulgare*. Leaves and young shoots used for flavouring puddings and omelettes. Tansy cakes made with eggs and young leaves used to be eaten at Easter. Tansy tea made by infusing the herb formerly used as tonic and for intestinal worms. Root, preserved in honey or sugar, was used for gout.

**tapioca**  Starch prepared from the root of the cassava plant. The starch paste is heated to burst the granules, then dried either in globules resembling sago or in flakes. The term is also used of starch in general, as in manioc tapioca and potato flour tapioca.

**tapioca-macaroni**  A mixture of 80–90 parts tapioca flour, with 10–12 parts of peanut flour, or tapioca, peanut, semolina, 60:15:25, baked into shapes resembling rice grains or macaroni shapes; developed in India. Also referred to as synthetic rice.

**tares**  Traditional English name for the vetches, which are pulses, which see.

**taro**  Corm of *Colocasia esculenta* and *C. antiquorum*; called eddo or dasheen in West Indies, old cocoyam in West Africa.

Analysis per 100 g: 2 g protein, 26 g carbohydrate, 110 kcal

(500 kJ), 1 mg Fe, 0.1 mg vitamin $B_1$, 0.03 mg vitamin $B_2$, 1 mg nicotinic acid, 5 mg vitamin C.

**tarragon**   Dried leaves and flowering tops of the bushy perennial plant *Artemisia dracunculus*. Has an anise-like flavour and is used to flavour vinegar, and pickles, and is one of the ingredients of *fines herbes*.

Tarragon vinegar is made by steeping the fresh herb in white wine vinegar and is used in making sauce tartare and French mustard.

**tartar**   Name given by the alchemists to animal and vegetable concretions, such as wine lees, stone, gravel and deposits on teeth, as they were all attributed to the same cause.

**tartar emetic**   Potassium antimonyl tartrate, produces inflammation of the gastrointestinal mucosa and used to be used as an emetic.

**tartaric acid**   A dibasic acid, dihydroxysuccinic COOHCHOH-CHOHCOOH. Occurs in fruits, the chief source is grapes; used in preparing lemonade, added to jams when the fruit is not sufficiently acidic (citric acid also used) and in baking powder.

Tartar emetic is the potassium antimonyl salt, and Rochelle salt is potassium sodium tartrate.

See also *argol*; *cream of tartar*.

**tartrazine**   Yellow colour, trisodium salt of 5-hydroxy-1-*p*-sulphophenyl-4-*p*-sulphonphenyl-azopyrazole-3-carboxylic acid; called Yellow No. 5 in the USA.

**tartronate**   Salt of tartronic (or hydroxymalonic) acid. Suggested as coenzyme in the decarboxylation of oxalosuccinic acid in the citric acid cycle and also claimed as a dietary essential for the rat but not confirmed.

**taste**   See *organoleptic*.

**taste buds**   Situated mostly on the tongue; about 9000 elongated cells ending in minute hairlike processes, the gustatory hairs.

**taurocholic acid**   See *bile*.

**tea**   Prepared from the young leaves, leaf buds and internodes of varieties of *Camellia sinensis*, originating from China.

Green tea is dried without further treatment. Black tea is fermented (actually an oxidation) before drying; Oolong tea is lightly fermented.

Among the black teas, Flowering Pekoe is made from the top leaf buds, Orange Pekoe from first opened leaf, Pekoe from third leaves, and Souchong from next leaves.

**teaseed oil**   Oil from the seed of *Thea sasangua*, cultivated in China; used as salad oil and for frying; similar in properties to olive oil.

**teeth, mottled**   See *mottled teeth*.

**TEF** Thermal effect of food. Same as thermogenic effect, see *specific dynamic action*.

**teff** Millet-like cereal grain; major protein of the diet of Ethiopia. See *millet*.

**teg** Two-year-old sheep.

**tempeh** Soya bean fermented by a mould, *Rhizopus* (Indonesia).

**Temptein** Trade name (Miles Lab., USA) for textured vegetable protein.

**tenderiser** Usually refers to the enzyme papain, when used to tenderise meat. Weak acids such as vinegar and lemon juice and 2% sodium chloride also tenderise meat.

**tenderometer** Instrument to measure the stage of maturity of peas to determine whether they are ready for canning. Measures the force required to effect a shearing action.

**tenuate** See *anorectic drugs*.

**tepary bean** *Phaseolus acutifolius*, also known as Mexican haricot bean, frijole and pinto. Able to grow during drought.

**tequila** Distilled liquor obtained from a fermented mash made from the cultivated cactus, *Agave tequilana*; 90–100 degrees proof; common in Mexico.

Mescal is similar but made from the mescal agave, which grows wild and is much cheaper.

**teratogen** Substance able to deform the fetus in the womb and so induce birth defects.

**terpeneless oil** See *terpenes*.

**terpenes** Components of the essential oils of citrus fruits; hydrocarbons of the general formula $C_{10}H_{16}$; also sesquiterpenes, $C_{15}H_{24}$. Include limonene, alpha, beta, and gamma terpinene, alpha and beta phellandrene. Limonene is 90% of oil of orange.

Although terpenes constitute 90–95% of citrus oils, they are not responsible for the characteristic flavour, and as they readily oxidise and polymerise to produce unpleasant flavours, they are removed from citrus oils by distillation or solvent extraction, leaving the so-called terpeneless oils. Further, the terpenes are not very soluble, so that unless they are removed the oils cannot be used for flavouring beverages and clear jellies.

**terramycin** Antibiotic isolated 1950 from *Streptomyces rimosus*. Now known as oxytetracycline. See *tetracyclines*.

**testa** In reference to cereal grains, the testa is a fibrous layer between the pericarp and the inner aleurone layer.

**test meal** See *fractional test meal*.

**tetany** Oversensitivity of motor nerves to stimuli; particularly affects face, hands and feet. Caused by reduction in the level of ionised calcium in the blood stream and can accompany severe rickets.

**tetracyclines** Group of closely related antibiotics, tetracycline, oxytetracycline (aureomycin). The last two are used in some countries for preserving food and, when added to animal feed at the rate of a few mg per ton, improve growth.

Of special use for eviscerated poultry; the bird is dipped in solution of 10ppm, and, when stored at 34–37°F, shelf life is extended from 10–14 to 17–21 days. 2ppm left in the poultry, much reduced on cooking.

Also of great value in extending the storage life of fresh fish by 2–3 days, by adding 5ppm antibiotic to the ice or chilled water, or by dipping fillets into water containing 5–20ppm.

**tetraenoic acid** Fatty acid with four double bonds, e.g. arachidonic acid.

**tetramine poisoning** Caused by a toxin in the salivary glands of red whelks, *Neptunea antiqua* (effects similar to curare); distinct from the edible whelk *Buccinum undatum*.

**tetrodontin poisoning** Caused by toxin, tetrodotoxin, in fish of the Tetrodontidae family (puffer fish) and amphibia of the Salamandridae family. Occurs in Japan from Japanese puffer fish or fugu (*Fuga rubripes*), eaten for its gustatory and tactile pleasure since traces of the poison cause a tingling sensation in the extremities (larger doses cause respiratory failure).

**tewfikose** Name given to a sugar isolated from a sample of buffalo milk obtained from Egypt in 1892, later found to be an artefact; named after Tewfik Bey Pasha, Governor of Egypt.

**Texgran** Trade name (Swift Edible Oil Co., USA) for textured vegetable protein.

**Texatrein** Trade name (Cargill, Inc., USA) for textured vegetable protein made by extrusion.

**texture** Combination of physical properties perceived by senses of kinaesthesis (muscle-nerve endings), touch (including mouth feel), sight and hearing. Physical properties may include shape, size, number and conformation of constituent structural elements (British Standard 5098: 1975).

**textured vegetable protein** Spun or extruded vegetable protein made to simulate meat.

**texture profile** Organoleptic analysis of the complex of food in terms of mechanical, geometrical, fat and moisture content characteristics, including the order in which they appear from the first bite to complete mastication.

**TGS** Trichlorogalactosucrose. See *sucralose*.

**theaflavins** Reddish-orange pigments formed in tea during fermentation by condensation of *o*-quinones and reaction with gallates. Responsible for the colour of tea extracts and part of the astringent flavour.

**theanine** γ-*N*-ethylglutamine, the major free amino acid in tea, 1–2% dry weight of leaf.

**theine** Alternative name for caffeine.

**thaumatin** See *katemfe*.

**theobromine** Dimethylxanthine, an alkaloid found in cocoa in amounts ranging between 0.8 and 1.3% (together with caffeine, trimethylxanthine, 0.14–0.7%).

**theophylline** Alkaloid in tea, 1, 3-dimethyl xanthine.

**therapeutic diets** Those formulated to treat disease or metabolic disorders.

**thermic effect** See *specific dynamic action*.

**thermisation** Heat treatment, less severe than pasteurisation, e.g. heat treatment of milk for cheese-making whereby the number of organisms is diminished.

**thermoduric** Bacteria that are heat resistant but not thermophilic. Found in milk. They survive pasteurisation temperatures but do not develop at them. Usually not pathogens but indicative of insanitary conditions.

**thermogenesis** See *specific dynamic action*.

**thermogenic drugs** Substances that stimulate body heat output.

**thermopeeling** A method of peeling tough-skinned fruits in which the fruit is rapidly passed through an electric furnace at about 900°C then sprayed with water.

**thermophiles** Bacteria that prefer temperatures of 55°C (131°F) and above; can tolerate temperatures up to 75–80°C (167–176°F). Some strains reported to survive boiling 24 hours at pH 6.1.

Include the 'flat sours' that produce acids from carbohydrates but no gas (*Bacillus stearothermophilus*), anaerobes not producing $H_2S$ (*Clostridium thermosaccharolyticum*) and anaerobes producing $H_2S$ (*C. nigrificans.*)

Thermophilic bacteria are responsible for spontaneous combustion in hay stacks.

**thiamin** Vitamin $B_1$.

**thiaminase** An enzyme present in many species of fish which hydrolyses thiamin and can therefore cause vitamin $B_1$ deficiency. See *Chastek's paralysis*.

**thiochrome** Compound to which vitamin $B_1$ can be oxidised (for example, by potassium ferricyanide) and which gives a strong blue fluorescence in ultraviolet light. This is used as an assay of the vitamin.

**thioctic acid** α-Lipoic acid, which see.

**thiopanic acid** Pantoyltaurine, which see.

**thirst** See *water balance*.

**threonine** An essential amino acid; the latest of the amino acids to be discovered, 1935; amino hydroxybutyric acid.

**thrombin** Plasma protein involved in coagulation of the blood, which see.

**thrombokinase** Or thromboplastin. Liberated from damaged tissue and blood platelets; converts prothrombin to thrombin in coagulation of the blood, which see.

**thromboplastin** Or thrombokinase See *coagulation, blood*.

**Thunberg tube** A test-tube carrying a curved hollow stopper which is used to hold one of the reactants; the whole tube can be evacuated through a side-arm. It is used to study oxidation reactions where it is necessary to keep the reactants separate until the oxygen has been removed from the system.

**thuricide** Name given to a living culture of *Bacillus thuringiensis* which is harmless to man but kills off insect pests. Known as a microbial insecticide. Used to treat certain foods and fodder crops to destroy pests such as corn earworm, flour moth, tomato fruit worm, cabbage looper, etc. The bacillus is mass-produced and stored like a chemical.

**thyme** Dried leaves and flavouring tops of *Thymus vulgaris* used in sausage and as flavouring in soup, meat, fish and poultry dressing.

**thymine** See *pyrimidines*.

**thymonucleic acid** Alternative name for deoxyribonucleic acid. See *nucleic acids*.

**thyroglobulin** The protein-bound form in which thyroxine and tri-iodothyronine exist in the thyroid gland; it is broken down under the influence of the thyroid-stimulating hormone of the pituitary gland to liberate the free hormones, which pass into the blood stream. Here they travel in combination with plasma protein as the so-called protein-bound iodine (PBI). The concentration of PBI in the blood is thus an index of thyroid activity.

**thyroid gland** Endocrine gland situated in the neck, which traps iodine from the blood stream and produces the thyroid hormones, mono- and di-iodotyrosines, and tri- and tetra-iodothyronines (the last being thyroxine). Controls the basal metabolic rate of the body. See also *cretinism*; *goitre*.

**thyrotoxicosis** Also known as Jodbasedow, Basedow's disease and Graves' disease. Iodine-induced thyrotoxicosis affecting mostly elderly people who have lived for a long time in iodine-deficient areas and have had a long-standing goitre, and then been given extra iodine.

**thyroxine**  Hydroxyphenyl-tetra-iodotyrosine; hormone from the thyroid gland (which see), converted into the more active tri-iodothyronine in the tissues.

**tierce**  Obsolete measure of wine cask; one-third of a pipe, i.e. about 35 imperial gallons (160 litres).

**tiger nut**  Tuber of *Cyperus esculentus*, also earth almond, chufa nut, rush nut (USA); usually available in partly dried condition.

Analysis per 100 g dry matter: 5 g protein, 17 g sucrose, 30 g starch, 25 g fat, 19 g dietary fibre (compare dietary fibre in carrot 31 g per 100 g dry matter, and beet, 22 g).

**tin**  Appears to be a dietary essential for rats but is so widely distributed in foods that no deficiency has been reported in man.

In the absence of oxygen tin is resistant to corrosion; hence, widely used in tinned cans for food containers.

**tintometer**  Instrument for measuring depth and shade of colour visually by comparison with a range of coloured glass sides. The Lovibond tintometer is the best-known.

Used for the chemical determination of substances that can be converted to coloured compounds, e.g. many minerals and vitamins.

**tipsy cake**  Sponge cake soaked in wine and fruit juice, made into a trifle and reassembled into the original tall shape. The wine and fruit juice may cause the cake to topple sideways in drunken (tipsy) fashion.

**tisane**  French term for a medicinal tea or infusion made from herbs (camomile, lime blossoms, fennel seeds, etc.).

**TLC**  See *chromatography*.

**tocol**  See *vitamin E*.

**tocopherol**  See *vitamin E*.

**tocopheronic acid**  Water-soluble degradation product of alpha-tocopherol (vitamin E) isolated from the urine of animals fed tocopherol, together with tocopheronolactone, the lactone of tocopheronic acid, which is highly vitamin-E active.

Tocopheronic acid is 2-(3-hydroxy-3-methyl-5-carboxyl)-pentyl, 3, 5, 6-trimethyl benzoquinone.

**tocotrienol**  See *vitamin E*.

**toffee**  A sweetmeat that is essentially a dispersion of minute globules of fat in a supersaturated sugar solution; made from fat, milk, sugar and confectioners' glucose. No real distinction between toffees and caramels except that toffees are boiled at a slightly higher temperature, 260–270°C compared with 250–255°C for caramels (and originally did not include milk).

Analysis per 100 g: water 4.8 g, sugars 70 g, protein 2 g, fat 17 g, kcal 430 (1.8 MJ), Ca 95 mg, Fe 1.5 mg.

**tofu**  A Japanese product, soybean curd. Contains 5–8% protein, 3–4% fat, 2–4% carbohydrate and 84–90% water.

**tomatine** An antifungal substance isolated from wilt-resistant tomatoes.

**tomato** Fruit of *Lycopersicon esculentum*.

Analysis per 100 g: protein 1.1 g, carbohydrate 3 g, kcal 20 (80 kJ), Ca 11 mg, Fe 0.6 mg, carotene 200 μg, vitamin $B_1$ 0.06 mg, vitamin $B_2$ 0.04 mg, nicotinic acid 0.5 mg, vitamin C 23 mg.

**Topfer's reagent** Dimethylamino-azobenzene; an indicator with a pH range 2.9–4.0, changing red to yellow. Often used in titration of the acidity of gastric contents, as it changes colour only in the presence of free hydrochloric acid.

**toppings** See *wheatfeed*.

**Torry kiln** Machine developed by the Fisheries Research Station at Torry (UK) for the controlled smoking of fish.

**tortilla** Large, flat pancake made from ground maize, commonly eaten in Mexico.

**Torula** See *yeasts*.

**torularhodin** Carotenoid pigment in red yeast, *Torula rubra*, with vitamin A activity.

**torulin** Antibiotic produced during aerobic culture of *Torula utilis*.

**total parenteral nutrition** Dependence entirely on parenteral nutrition.

**tous-les-mois** Queensland arrowroot, used as a source of starch.

**toxins** Harmful substances (although many dietary essentials, including some vitamins, are toxic in large amounts). Generally refer to: (a) substances such as cyanide which inhibit metabolic processes; (b) those produced by food-poisoning bacteria; (c) heavy metals; (d) a large number of substances occurring in foods which affect nervous sytem, cause liver damage or are carcinogenic. See also *endotoxins*; *exotoxins*; *food poisoning*.

**TPN** (1) Abbreviation for triphosphopyridine nucleotide; obsolete name for nicotinamide adenine dinucleotide. (2) Total parenteral nutrition, which see.

**trace elements** Refers to mineral salts needed in small amounts of the order of micrograms or milligrams per day – iodine, copper, manganese, magnesium, zinc, chromium, etc., as distinct from those needed in the 100 mg range such as calcium, potassium, sodium. Iron is sometimes included as a trace element.

**tragacanth** A gum obtained from shrubs of the genus *Astragalus*. Used as emulsifying agent in pharmaceutical preparations and as a thickener.

**trans** See *cis–trans isomerism*.

**transaminase (aminotransferase) test** See *enzyme activation tests*.

**transamination** Transfer of the amino group, $-NH_2$, from one compound to another, usually under the influence of an enzyme, transaminase. Thus, glutamic acid under the influence of glutamic-alanine-transaminase conveys its amino group to pyruvic acid to form alanine, leaving keto-glutaric acid.

The prosthetic group of the enzyme is pyridoxal, vitamin $B_6$, which acts as an intermediate amino carrier.

**transferrin** Or siderophilin, an iron carbonate–protein complex, the form in which iron is transported in the blood plasma.

**transketolase test** See *enzyme activation tests.*

**treacle** First product of refining of molasses from beet or sugar cane is black treacle, slightly less bitter; will not crystallise.

Analysis per 100 g: 67 g sucrose, about 0.2 g N, 500 mg Ca, 9 mg Fe (traces of other minerals), 260 kcal (1.1 MJ).

**trehalose** Mushroom sugar, also called mycose, a disaccharide: α-D-glucopyranosyl-glucopyranoside; found in some fungi (*Amanita*), manna and insects; hydrolysed to glucose.

**tremorgens** Name given to a group of neurotoxins produced by various species of moulds (*Penicillium*, *Aspergillus*, *Claviceps*) which cause sustained whole body tremors leading to convulsive seizures which may be fatal (alfatrem from *A. flavus*, penitrem from *Penicillium* species). Possible cause of certain endemic afflictions in human beings in Nigeria and India.

**trepang** Bêche-de-mer.

**tricarboxylic acid cycle** See *citric acid cycle.*

**trichinosis** (trichiniasis) Disease due to *Trichinella spiralis*, a worm that is a parasite in pork muscle. Destroyed by heat and by freezing: caused by eating undercooked pork or sausage meat.

**Trifyba** Trade name (Labaz; Sanofi UK) for processed wheat bran from husk of *Testa triticum tricum* containing 80 g dietary fibre/100 g with reduced content of phytate.

**triglycerides** See *glycerides.*

**trigonelline** The betaine of nicotinic acid, the form in which nicotinic acid is excreted in the urine; formula $C_7H_7NO_2$; has no vitamin activity.

Also found in seeds of fenugreek and in coffee.

**tri-iodothyronine** The active hormone of the thyroid gland into which thyroxine is converted in the tissues. It is synthesised in the body from the amino acid tyrosine and iodine. See *thyroid gland*; *thyroglobulin.*

**triotin** Unidentified urinary excretion product of biotin, together with miotin and rhiotin.

**tripe** Lining of the stomach of ruminants, usually calf or ox. According to the part of the stomach used, there are various kinds such as blanket, honeycomb, book, monk's hood and reed tripe.

Contains large amounts of connective tissue which is converted into gelatin on boiling; sold 'dressed' i.e. cleaned and treated with lime.

Analysis per 100 g: 88 g water, 9 g protein, 3 g fat, 60 kcal (250 kJ), only traces of B vitamins.

**tripeptide**  See *polypeptides*.

**triphosphopyridine nucleotide**  See *nicotinamide adenine dinucleotide phosphate*.

**triticale**  Cross between wheat (*Triticum*) and rye (*Secale*) which combines the winter hardiness of the rye with the special properties of wheat.

**tritium**  See *hydrogen, heavy*.

**tropical oils**  Suggested term (USA) to classify vegetable oils that contain little polyunsaturated fatty acids, such as coconut and palm oils.

**truffle**  Edible fungus that grows underground and is detected by trained dogs or pigs.

The French black or Perigord truffle (*Tuber melanosporum*) is the most highly prized for its aroma and is used in pâté de foie gras and for larding chicken and game. White truffle (*T. album* and *T. niveum*) is held in lower regard.

**Trusoy**  Trade name (British Soya Products Ltd) for full-fat soya flour, heat-treated.

**trypsin**  Proteolytic enzyme of the pancreatic juice which attacks parts of the protein molecule left unattacked by pepsin. Functions at alkaline pH, 8–11. Secreted as the inactive precursor, trypsinogen; liberated by enterokinase.

**tryptophan**  Amino indole propionic acid, an essential amino acid. Destroyed by acid; therefore protein analysis requires a separate alkaline hydrolysis.

**TSP**  Trade name (Spillers Ltd) for textured soya protein in extruded form.

**tuberin**  The protein of potato, a globulin.

**tuber**  Underground storage organ of some plants, e.g. potato, Jerusalem artichoke, sweet potato, yam.

**tun**  Obsolete measure; large cask holding 216 imperial gallons (972 litres) of ale; 252 gallons (1134 litres) of wine.

**tuna**  Or tunny. Fatty fish, species of *Thunnus* and *Neothunnus*. Also name for prickly pear.

**turbidity test for milk**  See *milk, turbidity test*.

**turkey X disease**  See *aflatoxins*.

**turmeric**  Dried rhizome of *Curcuma longa* (ginger family), grown in India and S. Asia. Deep yellow and used both as condiment and (permitted) dyestuff. Used in curry powder and in prepared mustard.

Its pigment is used as a dye under the name curcumin or Indian saffron.

**turnip** Root of *Brassica campestris*.

Analysis per 100g: protein 0.8g, fat trace, carbohydrate 3.8g, kcal 20 (80kJ), Ca 60mg, Fe 0.4mg, vitamin $B_1$ 0.05mg, vitamin $B_2$ 0.04mg, nicotinic acid 0.8mg, vitamin C 15–40mg.

**turtle, mock** Gelatinous soup, similar in consistency to turtle soup, made from calf's head, ham, shin of beef, etc., seasoned and clarified.

**Tuxford's index** Formula for relating height to weight in children; heavier than average have an index greater than 1; lighter, have an index below 1.

For boys

$$\frac{W}{H} \times \frac{336 - m}{270}$$

For girls

$$\frac{W}{H} \times \frac{308 - m}{235}$$

$W$ is weight in pounds; $H$ is height in inches; $m$ is age in months.

**TVP** Textured vegetable protein.

**Twaddell** Scale for measurement of density.

1% salt – 1.4° Twaddell – 1.007 SG.
2% salt – 2.8° Twaddell – 1.014 SG.
4% salt – 5.6° Twaddell – 1.028 SG.
10% salt – 14.6° Twaddell – 1.073 SG.
20% salt – 30.2° Twaddell – 1.151 SG.

Only used for densities greater than 1;

$$\text{density} = 1 + \frac{\text{degrees}}{200}$$

**Tweens** Trade name (Atlas Co.) for nonionic surface agents derived from Span products (which see) by adding polyoxyethylene chains to the non-esterified hydroxyls, so making them water-soluble. Polysorbate 80 is a mixture of polyoxyethylene esters of oleic esters of sorbitol anhydrides used in medicinal products as an emulsifying agent.

**tyramine** 4-Hydroxyphenethylamine, also called tyrosamine, formed by decarboxylation of the amino acid tyrosine. Found in ripened cheese; stimulates the sympathetic system and can cause increased blood pressure and may be a cause of migraine.

Normally destroyed by monoamine oxidases, but certain drugs inhibit these enzymes and patients on such drugs must avoid cheese and other foods which contain similar amines, including wine, chocolate and yeast preparations.

**tyrosinase** Enzyme that oxidises tyrosine and other phenolic compounds, with the ultimate production of brown and black pigments. Absent in albinos, and from the white areas of piebald animals.

It is present in the potato and is responsible for the dark colour produced when raw potatoes or the juice are allowed to autoxidise in air.

**tyrosine** Non-essential amino acid that has some sparing action on the essential amino acid phenylalanine. Very little soluble and crystallises out of solutions of protein hydrolysates.

Tyrosine is the starting material for the formation of melanin, the pigment in the hair and skin, increased after sunburn. Chemically amino hydroxyphenyl propionic acid.

**tyrosinosis** An inborn error of metabolism in which there is failure of the enzyme p-hydroxyphenylpyruvate hydroxylase, so that the normal metabolic path of tyrosine to homogentisic acid cannot be followed and tyrosine, hydroxyphenylpyruvate, lactate and acetate are excreted in the urine. The defect appears to be harmless.


# U


**ubi-chromenol** Cyclised form of ubiquinone, which see.

**ubiquinones** A number of derivatives of benzoquinone with 6–10 isoprene side-chains; widely distributed in nature; function as part of the respiratory chain.

Also known as coenzyme $Q_6$–$Q_{10}$, and as mitoquinones.

**UFA** See *non-esterified fatty acids*.

**ugli** Citrus fruit, cross between grapefruit and tangerine.

**UHT** Ultra high temperature or ultra heat-treated. A continuous process at 132–150°C (depending on the type of food) for only 1–2 seconds; causes less damage to palatability of the food and to nutrients.

**ullage** Liquid left in cask or bottle after some has been removed or lost through defective container.

**ultracentrifuge** Centrifuge operating at very high speeds; will separate particles of different size in a colloidal suspension. Used to separate the different fractions of cells.

Ultracentrifuged milk has been treated for a few seconds at 15000–16000 rev/min, when spore-forming bacteria are sedimented.

**ultrafiltration**   A pressure-driven membrane process similar to reverse osmosis (see *osmosis, reverse*) but using a more open membrane – pore size $10^{-3}$–$0.5\,\mu m$. It allows inorganic salts and small molecules to pass through with the water and holds back only the larger molecules. Used to separate materials on basis of molecular size and shape, whereas reverse osmosis is used for water removal, i.e. concentration.

**ultra high temperature sterilisation**   See *UHT*.

**ultrasonic homogeniser**   Super-high-speed vibrator giving a cavitation force of 60 tons per square inch in the liquid. Used to cream soups, disperse dried milk, disperse essential oils in soft drinks, stabilise tomato purée, prepare peanut butter, etc.

**ultraviolet irradiation**   Lethal to bacteria (wavelength 2900–2100 Angstrom units) but of poor penetrating power and only of value for surface sterilisation or sterilising the air. Also used for tenderising and aging of meat, curing cheese, and prevention of mould growth on the surface of bakery products.

**umbles**   Edible entrails of any animal (more particularly deer) which used to be made into pie – umble pie or humble pie.

**unesterified fatty acids**   See *non-esterified fatty acids*.

**UNICEF**   The United Nations Children's Fund (UNCF), originally the United Nations International Children's Emergency Fund.

**unsaturated fatty acids**   See *fatty acids*.

**uperisation**   A method of sterilising milk by injecting steam under pressure to raise the temperature to 150 °C. The added water is evaporated off.

**uracil**   See *nucleic acids*; *pyrimidines*.

**urea**   The waste nitrogen of most mammals is excreted in the urine as urea, $CO(NH_2)_2$. Formed in the liver by the urea cycle (which see) and excreted by the kidneys.

**urea cycle**   Sequence of reactions in which the amino group of unwanted amino acids is converted to urea, the nitrogenous excretion product. Formulated by Krebs, and known as the Krebs urea cycle (not to be confused with the Krebs tricarboxylic acid cycle).

The cycle is: ornithine + ammonia + $CO_2 \rightarrow$ citrulline; citrulline + ammonia $\rightarrow$ arginine; arginine, under the influence of arginase$\rightarrow$urea and ornithine.

The synthesis of urea takes place in the liver and it is excreted by the kidneys.

**urease**   Enzyme that hydrolyses urea to ammonia and carbon dioxide; appears to be absolutely specific for urea and used for the quantitative determination of urea in body fluids, etc.

Obtained from the jack bean and water-melon seed; the first enzyme to be crystallised.

**ureotelic**  Animals that excrete their waste nitrogen as urea, e.g. the mammals.

**urethane**  Ethyl carbamate, $NH_2COOC_2H_5$. Used as intermediate in organic syntheses and as solubiliser. Found in small amounts in liqueurs made from stone fruits, wines and some distilled spirits where it is formed by reaction between ethanol and N compounds; cause for concern since it is genotoxic.

**uric acid**  End-product of nitrogen metabolism in birds and reptiles and of purine metabolism in man and the anthropoid apes. Other mammals posses the enzyme uricase, which converts the uric acid to allantoin. See also *purines*.

**uricase**  See *uric acid*.

**uricotelic**  Animals that excrete their waste nitrogen as uric acid, e.g. birds and reptiles.

**urobilinogen**  Pigment in urine derived from the bile pigments, which, in turn, are formed from haemoglobin. When urine is left to stand, the urobilinogen is oxidised in air to urobilin.

**urogastrone**  Hormone similar to gastrin found in urine; little known of its function.

**uropepsin**  Proteolytic enzyme in urine; produced by acidification of uropepsinogen, which is identical with gastric pepsinogen. Urinary output serves as a measure of the amount of peptic glandular tissue.

# V

**vac-ice process**  Alternative name for freeze-drying.

**vacreation**  Deodorisation of cream by steam distillation under reduced pressure (see also *deodorisation*); developed in New Zealand.

**vacuum contact plate process**  Method of dehydrating food in a vacuum oven in which material is heated by hot plates both above and below. As the material shrinks owing to water losses, continuous contact is maintained by closing of the plates. Has the advantage over a simple vacuum oven of supplying heat more effectively to the food. (Also known as VCD – vacuum contact dryer.)

**valine**  An essential amino acid, rarely, if ever, limiting in foods. Chemically, amino isovaleric acid.

**valzin**  See *dulcin*.

**vanadium**  Element not shown to be essential but found in several animal tissues, and believed to play a biological role.

**vanaspati**  Purified, hydrogenated, vegetable oil, used in India and similar to margarine; fortified with vitamin A and vitamin D.

**vanilla**   Extract of the vanilla bean, fruit of the orchid *Aracus aromaticus* (or *Vanilla aromaticus*) and related species. Fruits are allowed to ferment, when the beans become dark brown in colour; they are crushed and extracted with alcohol.

Chief flavouring principle is vanillin or methyl protocatechuic aldehyde, but other substances present aid the flavour, and synthetic vanillin has not the true flavour.

Discovered in Mexico in 1571 and could not be grown elsewhere, because pollination could be effected only by a small Mexican bee, until artificial pollination was introduced in 1820. Main growing regions now Madagascar and Tahiti.

Vanilla sugar – ground bean mixed with sugar.

Ethyl vanillin – a synthetic substance, does not occur in the vanilla bean; incorrectly named – ethyl replaces methyl of vanillin; 3½ times as strong in flavour, and more stable to storage than vanillin.

**vasoconstriction**   Constriction of the blood vessels; the reverse of vasodilatation.

**vasodilatation**   Dilation of the blood vessels; the reverse is vaso-constriction. Caused by a rise in body temperature and serves to lose heat from the body.

**VCD**   See *vacuum contact plate process*.

**VDQS**   Vins Délimités de Qualité Supérieure – description of wines of superior quality, named wines from specified areas to serve as a guarantee of quality.

**veal**   Meat of the young calf, not less than 3 weeks old.

Analysis per 100 g: protein 15 g, fat 11 g, 160 kcal (0.68 MJ), Fe 1.8 mg, vitamin $B_1$ 0.1 mg, vitamin $B_2$ 0.2 mg, nicotinic acid 4.9 mg.

**vegans**   Those who consume no animal foods. (Vegetarians often consume milk and/or eggs.)

**vegetable butters**   Naturally occurring fats that melt rather sharply because they contain a preponderance of a single triglyceride.

Cocoa butter – from *Theobroma cacao*, cocoa bean, used in chocolate; Borneo tallow or green butter – from Malayan and East Indian plant, *Shorea stenoptera*, resembles cocoa butter; shea butter – from African plant, *Butyrospermum parkii*, softer than cocoa butter. Mowrah fat or illipé butter – from Indian plant, *Bassia longifolia*, used for soap and candles.

**vegetable casein**   Name once used for wheat gluten.

**vegetable protein products**   General term to include textured soya products often made to simulate meat. Basic material is termed flour when the protein content is not less than 50%; concentrate, not less than 65%; isolate, not less than 90% protein.

**vegetables**   Plants or parts of plants cultivated for food. Some foods that are botanically fruits, such as tomatoes and cucumbers, and seeds, such as peas and beans, are included with the vegetables.

As a source of nutrients most of the vegetables are useful sources of vitamin C and minerals, the root vegetables supply carbohydrate, but only the seeds are an important source of protein.

**verbascose**  A non-digestible tetrasaccharide, galactose–galactose–glucose–fructose, found in legumes; passes down the intestine, where it is fermented by bacteria and causes flatulence.

**verdoflavin**  Name given to a substance isolated from grass, later shown to be riboflavin.

**verjuice**  Originally the juice of crab apples, now lemon juice used in cooking meat or fish.

**vermicelli**  See *alimentary pastes*.

**vermouth**  Wine to which has been added a mixture of aromatic and bitter herbs, such as angelica, cinchona, coriander, wormwood, angostura, etc.

Sweet or Italian vermouth, 15–17% alcohol (by volume) and 12–20% sugar (by weight). Dry or French type 3–5% sugar, 18–20% alcohol.

**Versene**  Trade name for ethylenediamine tetra-acetic acid, which see.

**Verv**  Trade name (Patterson Co., USA) for calcium stearyl-2-lactate, used to reduce baking variations in flour. It produces a more extensible dough, more easily machined, and gives a loaf with better keeping properties and more uniform structure.

**vetches**  Old term generally applied to legumes; originally applied to *Vicia* genus.

**vicilin**  Globulin protein in pea and lentil.

**vicine**  See *favism*.

**Vienna bread**  Loaf with a very crisp, thin, highly glazed crust, with cuts on the upper surface, coarser than ordinary bread and with gas holes. It is baked in an oven which retains the steam.

**Vieth's ratio**  With reference to milk is the ratio anhydrous lactose: protein: ash, which is normally $13:9:2$.

**villi, intestinal**  Small, finger-like processes covering the surface of the small intestine in large numbers. They provide an enormous surface area for the absorption of digested food from the small intestine.

**vinasses**  The residual liquors from sugar-beet molasses; contain appreciable quantities of betaine.

**vinegar**  The product of two successive fermentations of the sugars and starches derived from malted barley (malt vinegar), apples (cider vinegar), oranges, dates, etc. Yeast ferments the sugars to ethanol – this liquor is called gyle (6–9% alcohol) – then oxidised with *Acetobacter* to acetic acid.

Vinegar is not less than 4% acetic acid with flavours derived from esters and higher alcohols, and may be coloured with caramel.

Non-brewed condiment (once called non-brewed vinegar) is a solution of 4–8% acetic acid.

**violet BNP** Sodium salt of 4,4'-di(dimethylamino)-4"-di(*p*-sulphobenzylamino) triphenylmethanol anhydride.

**viosterol** Irradiated ergosterol, i.e. vitamin $D_2$.

**Virol** Trade name (Virol Ltd) for a vitamin preparation composed of malt extract, starch syrup and egg with added vitamins.

Analysis per 100 g: protein 3.4 g, fat 12 g, carbohydrate 60 g, Ca 108 mg, Fe 27 mg, kcal 350 (1.46 MJ).

**viscogen** Thickening agent for whipping cream. Two parts of lime (CaO) in six parts of water, added to five parts of sugar in ten parts of water; used at the rate of ½–1 oz per gallon of cream.

**viscometer** Instrument for measuring the viscosity of liquids.

**viscosity** Term used of liquids to define their resistance to flow (i.e. the internal friction).

**visual purple** (rhodopsin) Pigment in the retina of the eye, consisting of retinol plus protein, which is necessary for vision in dim light. See *vitamin A*.

**vitamers** Substances structurally related to vitamins, possessing some biological activity, though often less than the true vitamin.

**vitamin** Naturally occurring organic substance essential in very small amounts for the normal functioning of the living cell. Thus, a factor essential for an animal or micro-organism and not essential for man is, nevertheless, termed a vitamin.

It is now questionable whether it is desirable to group together substances as varied in function as, for example, the B vitamins, which function as coenzymes, and substances like vitamin D, which appears to function as a hormone.

The confusion in vitamin nomenclature has been partly clarified by the recommendations of the International Union of Nutritional Sciences (*Nutr. Abstr. Rev.*, **40**, 395, 1970) and the International Union of Pure and Applied Chemistry (*Eur. J. Biochem.*, **2**, 1, 1967). There is still a difference, as shown below.

|  | IUNS | IUPAC |
|---|---|---|
| 1. Generic descriptor | Folacin | Folic acid |

Specific
compounds (a) Folic acid            Pteroyl glutamic acid
          (b) Folic acid glutamate (2)   Pteroyldiglutamic acid
          (c) Tetrahydrofolic acid      Tetrahydropteroyl
                                           glutamic acid

2. Generic
   descriptor:    Menaquinone
                  (vitamin K)

Specific
compounds: (a) Phytylmenaquinone     Phylloquinone
          (b) Multiprenyl-            Menaquinone-$n$
              menaquinones
          (c) Prenylmenaquinone-6    Menaquinone-6

For other vitamins there is agreement between the two recommendations, as follows.

A generic descriptor indicates a group of substances with the specific biological activity; thus, 'vitamin A' is used in terms of vitamin A deficiency; otherwise specific chemical names are used, as retinol (old name vitamin A alcohol), dehydroretinol (vitamin $A_2$), carotene.

Riboflavin and thiamin spelled without the final 'e'. Niacin is a generic descriptor; specific terms are nicotinic acid and nicotinamide. Vitamin $B_6$ is the generic descriptor; specific chemical substances are pyridoxine, pyridoxal and pyridoxamine. (See individual vitamins.)

**vitamin** (pronunciation)   According to Fowler's *Modern English Usage* (Oxford University Press), vītamin is the better pronunciation, in conformity with other words derived from *vita*, but seems unlikely to hold its own against the more popular vĭtamin.

**vitamin A**   Includes both retinol (previously called preformed vitamin A) and carotene (previously termed vitamin A precursor). Essential for formation of glycoproteins of the mucous tissue by acting as a carrier for the monosaccharides involved; thus, maintains normal condition of moist epithelial tissues lining mouth, respiratory and urinary tract; essential for growth. The aldehyde, retinal, is needed for vision in dim light in combination with protein to form visual purple.

Deficiency leads to night blindness, xerophthalmia (drying of tear ducts) and keratomalacia (ulceration of the cornea), blindness and stunting of growth.

Occurs as retinol in fish liver oils (cod and halibut), milk and butter, and as carotene in green vegetables, carrots and palm oil.

Daily recommended intake 750 µg for adult (2500 i.u.). Vitamin A content of foods expressed as retinol equivalents: 1 µg retinol = 6 µg beta-carotene = 12 µg other active carotenoids = 3.3 i.u. retinol = 10 i.u. beta-carotene.

**vitamin A₂** Old name for dehydroretinol, the form found in livers of freshwater fish; has 40% of biological activity of retinol.

**vitamin B complex** See under individual B vitamins. These vitamins occur together in cereal germ, liver and yeast; are all coenzymes; and historically were discovered by separation from what was know originally as 'vitamin B': hence, they are grouped together as the B complex. The vitamin B₂ complex is of purely historical origin and includes all except B₁.

**vitamin B_c** See *folic acid*.

**vitamin B_p** Called the antiperosis factor for chicks, but can be replaced by manganese and choline.

**vitamin B_T** An essential dietary factor for the mealworm, *Tenebrio molitor*, and certain related species; now known to be identical with carnitine. In higher animals carnitine plays a part in fat synthesis by transferring acetyl across the mitochondrial membrane but it is not a dietary essential.

**vitamin B_w** Or factor W; probably identical with biotin.

**vitamin B_x** Non-existent; has been used in the past for both pantothenic acid and para-amino benzoic acid.

**vitamin B₁** Thiamin. Thiamin pyrophosphate is the coenzyme, cocarboxylase, needed in oxidative decarboxylation, e.g. the conversion of ketoglutarate to succinate and of pyruvic acid to acetyl. A deficiency of the vitamin leads to impaired metabolism of carbohydrate and clinically results in the disease beriberi, in which pyruvate accumulates in the blood.

The daily requirement is related to the amount of carbohydrate oxidised (the non-fat calories) – 0.6 mg per 1000 non-fat calories or 0.4 mg per 1000 total calories (daily total approximately 1 mg). Thiamin is water-soluble and there is little storage in the body.

Occurs in cereal grains (little in white flour and white rice but these are enriched with added thiamin in many countries), in yeast, meat, especially pork, pulses, egg.

Obsolete name aneurine.

It is one of the more labile of the vitamins and is destroyed by heat under alkaline conditions and by sulphur dioxide, and is lost by leaching into the cooking water. The baking of bread can lead to 15–30% loss; up to half can be lost in cooked meat and fish, depending on the conditions.

**vitamin B₂** Riboflavin. In combination with a number of different proteins it forms a group of coenzymes called flavoproteins, essential for the oxidation of carbohydrates. Flavoproteins act as intermediary hydrogen carriers and include flavin mononucleotide, flavin adenine dinucleotide, cytochrome c reductase, etc.

A deficiency of riboflavin impairs cell oxidation and results clinically in a set of symptoms known as ariboflavinosis. These include cracking of the skin at the corners of the mouth (angular stomatitis), fissuring of the lips (cheilosis) and tongue changes (glossitis); seborrhoeic accumulations appear around the nose and eyes.

Recommended intake – 0.55 mg per 1000 kcal or an average of 1.5 mg per day. It occurs in yeast, liver, milk, eggs, cheese and pulses.

Processing losses are partly due to leaching into the water and partly to exposure to light. 50% of the riboflavin of milk can be destroyed in 2 hours by exposure to bright sunlight, and even on a dull day the losses can be 20%. The products of photoxidation of the vitamin $B_2$ destroy the vitamin C.

**vitamin $B_3$**  Non-existent; term once used for pantothenic acid and sometimes, quite wrongly, used for niacin.

**vitamin $B_4$**  Name given to what was later identified as a mixture of arginine, glycine and cystine.

**vitamin $B_5$**  Name given to a substance later presumed to be identical with vitamin $B_6$ or possibly nicotinic acid: also used for pantothenic acid.

**vitamin $B_6$**  Generic descriptor for three derivatives of 2-methylpyridine, namely the hydroxy compound, pyridoxine (previously known as adermin and pyridoxol), the aldehyde, pyridoxal, and the amine, pyridoxamine; all equally active.

Deficiency causes convulsions and acrodynia (skin disorder) in rats, abnormal red cells in dairy cattle, anaemia in dogs and epileptiform seizures in human babies.

Functions as coenzyme for specific amino acid decarboxylases and deaminases, transaminases and transmethylases.

Rarely deficient in human diets; recommended intake thought to be about 2 mg per day; occurs in nuts, meat, fish, whole grain.

Obsolete names adermin, yeast eluate factor, factor I and factor Y.

See also *transamination*.

**vitamin $B_7$**  When a new factor was discovered which was claimed to be essential for chick growth and feathering, the claimant stated that as nine factors were known the new factors should be called vitamins $B_{10}$ and $B_{11}$. In fact, the B vitamins had been numbered only up to $B_6$, hence $B_7$, $B_8$ and $B_9$ have never existed.

**vitamin B₈**  See *vitamin B₇*.

**vitamin B₉**  See *vitamin B₇*. Sometimes used for folic acid.

**vitamin B₁₀**  The names $B_{10}$ and $B_{11}$ were given to two factors claimed to be essential for chick growth and feathering; they were later shown to be a mixture of vitamin $B_1$ and folic acid.

**vitamin B₁₁**  See *vitamin B₁₀*.

**vitamin B₁₂**  Generic descriptor for the cobalamins, water-soluble organic compounds consisting of a corrin nucleus of four linked pyrrole rings linked to a cobalt atom. Hydroxocobalamin (formerly $B_{12}$a) and aquocobalamin ($B_{12}$b) are the active forms; cyanocobalamin is found in small amounts in blood plasma but does not have an active role.

Essential for nucleic acid synthesis and so for formation of red blood cells. Pernicious anaemia is due to inability to absorb the $B_{12}$ because of lack of a factor in the stomach termed the intrinsic factor, rather than a dietary deficiency of the vitamin (formerly called the extrinsic factor).

Earlier called animal protein factor, cow manure factor and zoopherin.

**vitamin B₁₃**  See *orotic acid*; not an established vitamin.

**vitamin B₁₄**  Not an established vitamin; a substance found in human urine which increases the rate of cell-proliferation in bone-marrow culture.

**vitamin B₁₅**  Pangamic acid, which see; no evidence that it is a dietary essential.

**vitamin B₁₆**  This term has never been used.

**vitamin B₁₇**  See *laetrile*.

**vitamin C**  L-xylo-ascorbic acid (the isomer, D-araboascorbic acid, or isoascorbic acid or erythorbic acid, has only slight biological activity, 1/20th, but is used as an antioxidant in foods.) Controls production of intercellular cementing substances, because it is essential for the hydroxylation of proline to hydroxyproline, a step in the synthesis of collagen. Breakdown of this matrix allows seepage of blood from capillaries, subcutaneous bleeding, weakness of muscles, soft, spongy gums leading to loss of teeth – in other words, scurvy.

Easily oxidised, especially in foods kept hot, and leached into cooking water. Recommended intake 30 mg per day according to UK and FAO authorities; 45–70 mg according to USA authorities at different times.

Occurs in fruits and vegetables; used as antioxidant and bread improver.

D-xyloascorbic acid, L-araboascorbic have zero biological activity; L-rhamno- has 1/5th of activity of vitamin C; D-arabo- has 1/20th.

**vitamin D**   Formed in the skin under the action of ultraviolet light which converts 7-dehydrocholesterol into vitamin $D_3$ or cholecalciferol. Also synthesised as vitamin $D_2$ or ergocalciferol by irradiation of ergosterol.

Term vitamin $D_1$ was given originally to an impure mixture and is not used now.

Converted into 25-hydroxy derivative in liver and then into 1,25-dihydroxy derivative in kidney. This is 10 times more potent than vitamin D and stimulates absorption of dietary calcium from intestine and calcium turnover in bone.

Deficiency causes rickets in young children, osteomalacia in adults. Not widely distributed in foods – egg yolk, butter, fatty fish and enriched margarine.

Recommended intakes 10 µg (400 i.u.) for infants and children 2.5 µg (100 i.u.) for adults. Excess can be harmful.

**vitamin E**   Generic descriptor for group of fat-soluble compounds essential for reproduction in animals. Essential for man (not for reproduction, so far as is known) but rarely, if ever, deficient in the diet. Deficiency symptoms vary considerably in different animal species – sterility in mouse, rat, rabbit, sheep and turkey; muscular dystrophy in several species; capillary permeability in chick and turkey; anaemia in monkey. Many substances have vitamin E-like activity, eight in particular (old names in parentheses): 5,7,8-trimethyl tocol (alpha-tocopherol); 5,8-dimethyl tocol (beta); 7,8-dimethyl tocol (gamma); 8-methyl tocol (delta-tocopherol); 5,7,8-trimethyl tocotrienol (alpha-tocotrienol); 5,8-dimethyl tocotrienol (beta); 7,8-dimethyl tocotrienol (gamma); and 8-methyl tocotrienol (delta). All expressed as alpha-tocopherol equivalents.

These compounds are antioxidants with varying potencies, and their natural occurrence in vegetable oils protects the latter against rancidity.

**vitamin F**   See *essential fatty acids*.

**vitamin G**   Obsolete name for vitamin $B_2$.

**vitamin H**   See *biotin*.

**vitamin K**   Fat-soluble vitamin essential for the production by the liver of prothrombin and several other factors involved in the blood clotting system. Hence, called the antihaemorrhagic vitamin.

There is a discrepancy between the nomenclature of the International Union of Pure and Applied Chemistry and that of the International Union of Nutritional Sciences (given in parentheses). Generic descriptor: menaquinone, 2-methyl-1,4-naphthoquinone. Specific compounds phylloquinone (phytyl-menaquinone), the 3-phytyl derivative, formerly called vitamin

$K_1$ – used therapeutically. Compounds with prenyl side-chains are menaquinone-$n$ (multiprenylquinones) such as menaquinone-6 (prenylmenaquinone-6). Potency expressed as phylloquinone (phytylmenaquinone) equivalents.

The old designation vitamin $K_2$ (naturally occurring) was given to 2-methyl-difarnesyl-1,4-naphthoquinone. Synthetic analogues were termed $K_3$ (menaquinone); $K_4$ or menadiol, the hydroquinone form; $K_5$, 4-amino-2-methyl-1-naphthol (used as a food preservative); $K_6$, 2-methyl-1,4-naphthalene diamine (toxic); $K_7$, 4-amino-3-methyl-1-naphthol.

Widely distributed in greenstuffs and synthesised by bacteria in the intestine but not known how much is absorbed; dietary deficiency is not encountered (except in newborn infants with a sterile intestine) only failure of absorption.

**vitamin L**   Vitamin $L_1$ and $L_2$ are factors in yeast said to be essential for lactation; they have not become established.

**vitamin M**   See *folic acid*.

**vitaminoids**   Name given to compounds with 'vitamin-like' activity; that is, considered by some to be vitamins or partially to replace vitamins – include bioflavonoids (formerly vitamin P), mesoinositol, carnitine, choline, lipoic acid and the essential fatty acids (formerly vitamin F).

**vitamin P**   Name formerly given to a group of plant flavonoid substances which affect the strength of the walls of the blood capillaries – namely, rutin (in buckwheat), hesperidin, eriodictin and citrin (in the pith of citrus fruits). (Citrin is a mixture of hesperidin and eriodictin.) Now considered that the effect is pharmacological and that they are not dietary essentials; sometimes called 'bioflavonoids'.

Called vitamin P from 'permeabilitäts vitamin'. Once claimed as a cure for the common cold.

See also *capillary fragility*; *flavonoids*.

**vitamin PP**   See *nicotinic acid*.

**vitamins** (content of foods)   According to the Code of Practice, no claims for the presence of a vitamin or mineral in a food should be made unless the amount ordinarily consumed in a day contains one-sixth of the daily requirements (UK practice).

No claim should be made that the food is a rich or excellent source unless half of the daily requirement is present; no reference to the prevention of disease unless the full day's requirement is present.

For this purpose the requirements are taken to be : vitamin A 900 µg, $B_1$ 0.9 mg, $B_2$ 1.8 mg; nicotinic acid 12 mg; vitamin C 30 mg; D 12 µg; calcium 0.75 g, iron 10 mg; iodine 0.1 mg; phosphate 0.75 g.

**vitamins, fat-soluble**  See *fat-soluble vitamins*.

**vitamins, water-soluble**  See *water-soluble vitamins*.

**vitamin T**  Factor found in insect cuticle, mould mycelia and yeast fermentation liquor, claimed to accelerate maturation and promote protein synthesis. Also known as torulitine. Said to be a mixture of folic acid, vitamin $B_{12}$ and desoxyribosides and not a new factor.

**Vita-Wheat**  Trade name (Peak Frean Ltd) for a crispbread, which see.

Analysis per 100 g: protein 8.6 g, fat 10.3 g, carbohydrate 77.8 g, Ca 44 mg, Fe 3.4 mg, kcal 423 (1.8 MJ).

Phytic acid phosphorus 59% of total phosphorus (372 mg per 100 g).

**vitellin**  One of the proteins of egg yolk; approximately four-fifths of the total protein; is a phosphoprotein and accounts for one-third of the phosphorus of egg yolk.

**VLDL**  Very low-density lipoproteins. See *lipids, plasma*.

**vodka**  Made from neutral spirit, i.e. alcohol distillate (in Russia mainly from potatoes), with little or no acid present, so that there is no ester formation and, hence, no flavour.

**Vol**  Trade name for commercial ammonium carbonate, a mixture of ammonium bicarbonate and carbamate. Used as aerating agent in baking, as it breaks down when heated to give carbon dioxide, ammonia and steam, without leaving any residue.

**volemitol**  Sweet substance found in mushrooms and roots of primroses; D-glycero-D-manno-heptitol.

**votator**  Machine used for the continuous manufacture of margarine; the fat and water are emulsified, and the subsequent conditioning process carried out in the same machine.

# W

**Warburg apparatus**  Small vessel attached to a manometer in which reactions that involve gas exchange can be followed. The vessel is immersed in a constant-temperature bath and shaken continually to equilibrate the gas in solution, where the reactions are taking place, with the gas in the gas phase, where it is being measured.

Living tissues as slices, minces, homogenates, and microorganisms are examined in this way.

**Warburg and Christian's coenzyme**  Nicotinamide adenine dinucleotide phosphate.

**Warburg's respiratory enzyme**  Enzyme postulated by Warburg as part of the cell oxidation system; later shown to be cytochrome oxidase.

**Warburg's yellow enzyme**   A flavoprotein that is part of the cell oxidation chain; passes on the hydrogen from reduced coenzyme I to cytochrome.

**water activity** ($a_w$)   Ratio between vapour pressure of water in the food and that of pure water at the same temperature.

Most bacteria cannot grow at $a_w$ below 0.9, yeasts below 0.85 and moulds below 0.7. So-called dehydrated foods have $a_w$ lower than 0.6.

**water balance**   The balance between intake and excretion. Intake as drinks averages 1–1.5 litres per day; as aqueous part of food, 0.5 litre; and formed in the body by oxidation of foodstuffs, 300–500 ml; total 2–3 litres.

Losses as water from the lungs, 400–500 ml; through the skin 400–500 ml; in faeces 80–100 ml; in urine 1–1.8 litre.

Total body water 40–44 litres (80 pints) as blood plasma (2–3 litres), extracellular water (10 litres) and intracellular water 27–30 litres).

The kidney controls the volume of extracellular water by excreting water. Ingestion of sodium chloride raises the osmotic pressure of the extracellular water, causing thirst.

**watercress**   Leaves of *Nasturtium officinale*; recommended 1597 in John Gerarde's *Herball* as cure for scurvy; not cultivated commercially until early nineteenth century.

Analysis per 100 g: 2.9 g protein, 0.7 g carbohydrate, 15 kcal 60 kJ, 220 mg Ca, 1.6 mg Fe, 3 mg carotene, 0.1 mg vitamin $B_1$, 0.6 mg nicotinic acid, 60 mg vitamin C.

**water, demineralised**   Water that has been purified by passage through a bed of ion-exchange resin which removes mineral salts. Demineralised or deionised water is as pure as, and can be purer than, distilled water.

**water, extracellular**   See *water balance*.

**water-glass**   Sodium silicate; used to preserve eggs, as a layer of insoluble calcium silicate is formed around the shell, which seals the pores.

**water hardness**   Soap-precipitating power of water due to the formation of insoluble calcium and magnesium salts of the soap. Temporary hardness is removed by boiling, permanent hardness is not.

May be measured in degrees Clarke; one degree = 1 part of calcium carbonate per 100 000 parts of water.

**water, intracellular**   See *water balance*.

**water, metabolic**   See *metabolic water*.

**water, natural**   See *mineral waters*.

**water-soluble vitamins**   All the members of the B complex (thiamin, riboflavin, nicotinic acid, pantothenic acid, pyridoxine, biotin, folic acid, para-amino benzoic acid, choline, inositol and vitamin $B_{12}$) and vitamin C.

Unlike the storage of vitamins A and D in the liver, there is no specific site for storage of the water-soluble vitamins; they are merely dispersed in solution through the blood and tissues.

See also *fat-soluble vitamins*.

**wax, apple** Peel wax contains triacontane, heptaconsanol and malol.

**waxes** Esters of fatty acids with long-chain monohydric alcohols (fats are esters of fatty acids with the three-carbon trihydric alcohol, glycerol). For example, beeswax, ester of palmitic acid with myricyl alcohol; spermaceti, cetyl palmitate.

Animal waxes are often esters of the steroid alcohol, cholesterol.

**weatings** See *wheatfeed*.

**Weende analysis** Analysis of foods and feedingstuffs for nitrogen, ether extract, crude fibre and ash together with soluble carbohydrate calculated by subtracting these values from the total.

Named after the Weende Experimental Station in Germany in 1865, which outlined the methods of analysis to be used; also called proximate analysis.

**Weetabix** Trade name (Weetabix Ltd) for a breakfast cereal prepared from wheat flakes.

Analysis per 100 g: protein 11 g, fat 3.4 g, carbohydrate 70 g, dietary fibre 13 g, 340 kcal (1.4 MJ), vitamin $B_1$ 1 mg, vitamin $B_2$ 1.5 mg, nicotinic acid 12 mg.

**weight-for-age** Standard weight-for-age is the 50th centile of the weight-for-age curves of well-fed children.

**weighting oils** See *brominated oils*.

**Wetzel Grid** Children are grouped by physique into five groups, ranging from tall and thin to short and thick-set. A healthy child will grow, as measured by height and weight, along one of these channels at a standard rate, if he deviates from the channel malnutrition is suspected.

**wey** 48 bushels of oats or 40 bushels of salt or 'corn'.

**whalemeat** Analysis per 100 g (edible portion only): protein 20 g, fat 4 g, kcal 125 (0.53 MJ), Fe 2.4 mg, vitamin $B_1$ 0.03 mg, vitamin $B_2$ 0.1 mg, nicotinic acid 4.4 mg.

**whale oil** Used, after hardening by hydrogenation, for lower-quality margarines, also in soap making.

**wheat** The most important of the cereals and one of the most widely grown crops. Many thousand varieties are known but there are three main types: *Triticum vulgare*, used mainly for bread; *Triticum durum* (Durum wheat), largely used for macaroni; and *Triticum compactum* (club wheat), too soft for ordinary bread.

The berry is composed of the outer branny husk, 13% of the grain, the germ or embryo (rich in nutrients) 2%, and the central endosperm (mainly starch) 85%.

Analysis per 100 g: protein 12–13 g, fat 2 g, carbohydrate 63 g, kcal 320 (1.3 MJ), Ca 35 mg, Fe 4 mg, vitamin $B_1$ 0.45 mg, vitamin $B_2$ 0.08 mg, nicotinic acid 5.5 mg.

See also *extraction rate*; *flour*; *wheatfeed*.

**wheatfeed** Also called millers' offal and wheat offals; by-product from milling of wheat, i.e. bran of various particle sizes and varying amounts of attached endosperm.

Originally classed according to particle size and crude fibre content as pollards, middlings, sharps and toppings but now classed as weatings (not more than 5.75% crude fibre) and superfine weatings (not more than 4.5% crude fibre).

**wheat germ** See *germ, wheat*.

**wheatmeal, national** Name given to the 85% extraction flour when introduced in UK in February 1941 (as distinct from wholemeal, which is 100% extraction). Later called national flour. It was milled to contain as much of the germ and aleurone layer as possible, having most of the nutritional properties of wholemeal flour, with higher digestibility and a more attractive loaf.

A loaf described as wheatmeal must contain not less than 0.6% fibre calculated on dry weight.

**Wheat, Puffed** Trade name of a breakfast cereal prepared by heating wheat grains under pressure and then rapidly releasing the pressure, when the superheated steam in the grain suddenly expands, so puffing or 'exploding' the grain.

Analysis per 100 g: protein 13.9 g, fat 2.0 g, carbohydrate 75.3 g, Fe 3.3 mg, vitamin $B_1$ 1.2 mg, kcal 360 (1.5 MJ).

**Wheat, Shredded** Trade name (Nabisco Ltd) of a breakfast cereal prepared from wheat grains.

Analysis per 100 g: protein 9.7 g, fat 2.8 g, carbohydrate 79 g, Fe 4.5 mg, kcal 360 (1.5 MJ).

Phytic acid phosphorus 80% of total P (287 mg/100 g).

**whelks** Several types of spiral-shelled marine molluscs, *Buccineum undatum, Fusus antiquus*. Analysis per 100 g protein 20 g, fat 2 g, carbohydrate 0, iron 6 mg, zinc 7 mg, 90 kcal (360 kJ).

**whey** The residue from milk after removal of the casein and most of the fat (as in cheese-making); also known as lacto-serum.

Contains about 1% protein (lactalbumin and lactoglobulin) together with all the lactose, water-soluble vitamins and minerals, and therefore has some food value, although it is 92% water.

Whey cheese can be made by heat coagulation of the protein, and whey butter from the small amount (0.25%) fat.

Dried whey is added to processed cheese; most whey is fed in liquid form to pigs.

**whey butter**   See *butter, whey.*

**whiskey, whisky**   A grain spirit distilled from barley, rye or other cereal which has first been malted and then fermented. Most brands of whisky are a blend of pure malt whisky with spirit distilled from grain.

Oxford Dictionary permits both spellings; the trade regards whisky as the Scotch variety and whiskey as the Irish and American varieties. The name is derived from the Gaelic *uisge beatha* – water of life.

**white blood cells**   See *leucocytes.*

**white cell count**   See *leucocytes.*

**white foots**   Fine white precipitate of calcium and other salts deposited in jars of meat cured with rock salt.

**white rice**   See *rice.*

**WHO**   World Health Organisation.

**whole-wheat meal**   Flour or meal prepared by milling the whole wheat grain, i.e. 100% extraction rate.

**whortleberry**   See *bilberry.*

**Wills' factor**   A factor in autolysed yeast effective in promoting red blood cell formation, probably folic acid.

**Wilson's formula**   See *blood volume.*

**windberry**   See *bilberry.*

**wine**   Fermented grape juice containing 9–10% w/v ethyl alcohol. Beverages made by fermenting other fruit juices and sugar in the presence of vegetables or leaves or roots are also called wines (parsnip, peapod, oak leaf wine, etc.), although the legal definition may be restricted to the fermented grape.

Fortified wines such as Madeira, sherry and port have added spirit to bring the alcohol content to 15%. See *alcoholic beverages.*

**wineberry**   *Rubus phoenicolasius*; similar to raspberry, orange-coloured.

**wine, British**   Made in Great Britain from grape juice or concentrated grape juice.

**winkles (periwinkles)**   Marine molluscs, *Littorina littorea.* Analysis per 100 g: protein 15 g, fat 1 g, carbohydrate 0, iron 15 mg, zinc 6 mg, 70 kcal (280 kJ).

**winterisation**   Applied to edible oils, meaning the removal of the more saturated glycerides so that the oil remains bright and clear at low temperatures. The oil is simply chilled and the solidified palmitates and stearates filtered off.

**witches' milk**  Secretion of the mammary gland of the newborn of both sexes; due to the presence of the hormone prolactin that travels from the blood of the mother into the fetus. Also known as sorcerers' milk.

**witchetty grubs**  Edible grubs, species of longicorn beetle of *Xylentes* species; associated with aborigines of Australia.

**witloof**  See *chicory*.

**wood alcohol**  Methyl alcohol, $CH_3OH$; highly toxic. It presence in methylated spirits accounts for the toxicity of the latter.

**Worcester sauce**  Characterised by spicy flavour, sediment and thin supernatant liquid. Recipes usually secret but basically soya, tamarinds, anchovies, garlic and spices, plus sugar, salt and vinegar, matured 6 months in oak casks.

**work**  See *energy*.

**World Food Programme**  Part of Food and Agriculture Organisation of the United Nations; intended to give international aid in the form of food from countries with a surplus.

**wort**  See *beer*.

# X

**xanthan gum**  Complex polymer made by bacterial fermentation; stable to wide range of pH and temperatures; used as thickening agent to form gels, increase viscosity in foods.

**xanthine**  2,6-Dioxypurine; formed from the purines adenine and guanine. Caffeine (coffee and tea) is 1,3,7-trimethylxanthine; theophylline (tea) is 1,3-dimethylxanthine; theobromine (cocoa) is 3,7-dimethylxanthine.

**xanthine oxidase**  An enzyme present in milk and in liver; specific for the two purines xanthine and hypoxanthine (which it oxidises to uric acid), and will also oxidise a range of aldehydes to the corresponding acids. It is identical with Schardinger's enzyme of milk.

**xanthophyll**  Yellow, hydroxy carotene derivative; occurs in all green leaves together with the chlorophyll and carotene, also present in egg yolk. Has no vitamin A activity.

Also known as lutein and luteol.

**xanthophylls**  Collective term for hydroxylated carotenoids or carotenols.

**xanthoproteic test**  For proteins (actually for the benzene nucleus of tyrosine and tryptophan which occur in nearly all proteins). Yellow colour on boiling with nitric acid, turns orange on adding ammonia.

**xenobiotic**   Substances foreign to the body, including drugs and some food additives.

**xerophilic yeasts**   See *osmophiles*.

**xerophthalmia**   Occurs in advanced vitamin A deficiency. Epithelium of the cornea and conjunctiva of the eye deteriorates because of impairment of the tear glands, resulting in dryness then ulceration.

**xylitol**   Five-carbon sugar alcohol corresponding to the sugar xylulose. As sweet as sucrose, less prone to cause dental decay and used in some 'sugar-free' products such as chewing gum.

**xyloascorbic acid**   See *ascorbic acid*.

**xyloketose**   Xylulose.

**xylose**   Pentose sugar found in plant tissues as complex polysaccharide; 40% sweetness of sucrose: wood sugar.

**xylulose**   Five-carbon sugar-alcohol derived from the pentose sugar xylose.


# Y


**yabbie**   Species of freshwater crayfish found in Australia.

**yam**   Tubers of perennial climbing plants of a number of species of *Dioscorea*; *D. rotundata*, white yam, and *D. cayenensis*, yellow or Guinea yam, water, trifoliate or Chinese yam; a major food in parts of Africa and also the Far East.

Analysis per 100 g: 73 g water, 30 g starch, 2 g protein, 130 kcal (560 kJ), small amounts of B vitamins, 10 mg vitamin C.

In the United States sweet potatoes are sometimes called yam.

**yang**   See *macrobiotic diet*.

**Yarmouth bloater**   See *red herrings*.

**yautia**   See *tannia*.

**yeast adenylic acid**   Adenosine 3-phosphoric acid. Muscle adenylic acid is adenosine-5-phosphoric acid.

**yeast eluate factor**   Obsolete name for vitamin $B_6$.

**yeast extract**   A preparation of the water-soluble fraction of autolysed yeast, valuable both as a rich source of the B vitamins and for its strong savoury flavour. Yeast (commercially brewers' yeast) is allowed to autolyse, extracted with hot water and concentrated by evaporation.

Commercial preparations are Marmite and Yeastrel, which see.

**yeast fermentation, bottom**   Fermentation during the manufacture of beer with a yeast that sinks to the bottom of the tank. Most beers are produced this way; ale, porter and stout being the principal beers produced by top fermentation.

**yeast filtrate factor**   Obsolete name for pantothenic acid.

**Yeastrel**   Trade name (Brewers Foods Supply Co.) for a yeast extract; contains 4.2 mg vitamin $B_2$ and 40 mg nicotinic acid per 100 g.

**yeasts**   Grouped with the fungi although they are unicellular. Various types are of major importance in the food industry. *Saccharomyces cerevisiae* is used in brewing, wine-making and baking. Varieties such as *Candida utilis* (formerly *Torula utilis*) are grown on carbohydrate or hydrocarbon media as animal feed and potential human food, since they contain about 50% protein (dry weight) and are very rich in B vitamins.

**Yeatex**   Trade name (English Grains Ltd) for yeast extract – autolysed brewers' yeast – used as a flavouring ingredient.
Analysis per 100 g; 41 g protein, 10 g carbohydrate, 1 mg thiamin, 2 mg riboflavin, 40 mg nicotinic acid, 5 mg pantothenic acid, 2.5 mg pyridoxine, 1 mg folic acid.

**yellow colours**   Oil yellow GG – mixture of 4-phenylazoresorcinol and 4,6-di(phenylazo) resorcinol.
Yellow 2G – disodium salt of 1-(2,5-dichloro-4-sulphophenyl)-5-hydroxy-3-methyl-4-*p*-sulphophenylazo-pyrazole.
Yellow RFS – disodium salt of 4-sulpho-4-(sulphomethylamino)-azobenzene.
Yellow RY – disodium salt of 6-*p*-sulphophenylazoresorcinol-4-sulphonic acid.
Sunset yellow FCF – disodium salt of 1-*p*-sulphophenylazo-2-naphthol-6-sulphonic acid; yellow-orange colour used to simulate the colour of eggs or orange; called Yellow No. 6 in the USA.
Oil yellow XP – 3-methyl-1-phenyl-4-(2,4-xylylazo)-5-pyrazolone.
Naphthol yellow S – disodium or potassium salt of 2,4-dinitro-1-naphthol-7-sulphonic acid.

**yellow enzyme**   See *Warburg's yellow enzyme*.

**yellow fats**   See *fats, yellow*.

**yerba maté**   See *maté*.

**Yestamin**   Trade name (English Grains Ltd) for a variety of preparations of dried *Saccharomyces* yeast (debittered brewers' yeast) used to enrich foods.
Analysis per 100 g: 45 g protein, 1–2 g fat, 36 g carbohydrate, 4.5–27 mg thiamin, 3–6.5 mg riboflavin, 20–60 mg nicotinic acid, 1.8–6 mg pantothenic acid, 2–3 mg pyridoxine, 2 mg folic acid.

**yin**   See *macrobiotic diet*.

**yoghurt**   See *milks, fermented*.

**yolk index**   Index of freshness of an egg; ratio between height and diameter of yolk under defined conditions. As the egg deteriorates, the yolk index decreases.

**Yuksov disease**   Another name for Haff disease, which see.

**Yusho disease**   Caused by leakage of polychlorinated biphenyls which contaminated edible oil on the island of Kyushu Japan, 1968.

# Z

**zeaxanthin**   One of the carotenoid pigments in maize, egg yolk and *Physalis* (Chinese lantern); has no vitamin A activity; used as a colouring.

**zearalenone**   See *mycotoxins*.

**zedoary root**   Of *Curcuma zedoaria*, an Indian plant of the ginger family. Used in the manufacture of flavours and bitters.

**zein**   Protein obtained from maize (*Zea mays*), soluble in alcohol but not water or dilute alkali. Of poor nutritive value, as it completely lacks lysine and is poor in tryptophan.

**Z-enzyme**   Enzyme found associated with amylases, that attacks the few 1,3-beta-links present in amylose. Pure, crystalline beta-amylase will convert only 70% of amylose to maltose; it requires the presence of the Z-enzyme for complete conversion.

**zest**   Outer skin of citrus fruits. See *flavedo*.

**zinc**   A dietary essential that is part of the structure of about 20 enzymes, including carbonic anhydrase, alcohol dehydrogenase and superoxide dismutase.

   Deficiency gives rise to hypogonadism, small stature and mild anaemia, and has been found in middle eastern countries and elsewhere. Found in meat (3–5 mg/100 g), whole grains and legumes (2–3 mg).

**zitoni**   See *alimentary pastes*.

**zizanie**   See *rice, wild*.

**zomotherapy**   Treatment of convalescents with raw meat or meat juice – long since discontinued.

**zoopherin**   Vitamin $B_{12}$.

**zooplankton**   Wide variety of very small crustaceans and other invertebrates, mixed with the young of larger fish, which live upon the phytoplankton (although some are carnivorous) and serve, in turn, as a food supply of small fish and other marine life.

**Zucker rat**   A genetically obese strain of rat used in research.

**z-value**   See *decimal reduction time*.

**zwieback** German term for twice-baked bread. Ordinary dough plus eggs and butter, baked, sliced, baked again to a rusk and sometimes sugar coated.

**zymase** Name given to the mixture of enzymes in yeast which is responsible for fermentation.

**zymogens** The inactive form in which some enzymes exist before being liberated by the action of a kinase. For example, trypsinogen and pepsinogen are secreted in the intestine and converted into their active forms, trypsin and pepsin.

**zymotachygraph** An instrument that measures the gas produced in a fermenting dough and the amount escaping from the dough.

# Bibliography

## ADDITIVES AND INGREDIENTS

*Carbohydrate Sweeteners in Foods and Nutrition*, ed. P. Koivis-
toinen and L. Hyvonen. Academic Press (1980)
*CRC Handbook of Food Additives*, 2nd edn, ed. T.E. Furia. CRC
Press (1972)
*Encyclopaedia of Common Natural Ingredients Used in Food and
Drugs and Cosmetics*, A.Y. Leung. Wiley (1980)
*Fenaroli's Handbook of Flavour Ingredients*, 2nd edn, T.E. Furia
and N. Bellanca. CRC Press (1975)
*Food Additives*, ed. A.L. Branen, P.M. Davidson and Seppo
Salminen. Marcel Dekker (1989)
*Food Additives Tables*, ed. M. Fondu, H. Van Gindertael-Zegers
de Beyl, G. Bronkers, A. Stein and P. Carton. Elsevier. Part I:
Classes I–IV (1980), Part II: V–VIII (1982), Part III: Classes
IX–XIII (1984)
*Plant Pigments, Flavors and Textures: The Chemistry and
Biochemistry of Selected Compounds*, N.A.M. Eskin. Academic
Press (1979)

## ANALYSIS AND FOOD COMPOSITION

*Analysis of Food Carbohydrate*, ed. G.G. Birch. Elsevier (1985)
*Analysis of Food Contaminants*, ed. J. Gilbert. Elsevier (1984)
*The Analysis of Nutrients in Food*, D.R. Osborne and P. Voogt.
Academic Press (1978)
*Composition of Foods*, No. 8, B.K. Watt and A.L. Merrill. US
Department of Agriculture Handbook
*CRC Handbook of Nutritive Value of Processed Food*, ed. M.
Rechcigl. CRC Press (1981)
*Developments in Food Analysis Techniques*, ed. R.D. King.
Applied Science Publishers (1978)
*Fat-Soluble Vitamin Assays in Food Analysis*, G.F.M. Ball.
Elsevier (1988)

*Food Composition Data,* ed. William M. Rand, Carol T. Windham, Bonita W. Wyse and Vernon R. Young. United Nations University (1987)

*HPLC in Food Analysis,* ed. R. Macrae. Academic Press (1988)

*Immunoassays for Veterinary and Food Analysis,* ed. B.A. Morris, M.N. Clifford and R. Jackman. Elsevier (1988)

*McCance and Widdowson's The Composition of Foods,* A.A. Paul and D.A.T. Southgate (1978) 1st suppl. *Amino Acids and Fatty Acids* (1979); 2nd suppl. *Immigrant Foods* (1985); 3rd suppl. *Cereals and Cereal Products* (1988); 4th suppl. *Milk Products and Eggs* (1989). Royal Society of Chemistry

*Methods for the Determination of Vitamins in Foods,* ed. G. Brubacher, W. Muller-Mulot and D.A.T. Southgate. Elsevier (1985)

*Nutrients in Processed Foods,* 3 vols, ed. P.L. White and D.C. Fletcher. American Medical Association (1974–75)

*Pearson's Chemical Analysis of Foods,* 8th edn, H. Egan, R.S. Kirk and R. Sawyer. Churchill Livingstone (1981)

*Qualitative Analysis of Flavor and Fragrance Volatiles by Glass Capillary Gas Chromatography,* W. Jennings and T. Shibamoto. Academic Press (1980)

## COGNATE SCIENCES

*Amino Acid Metabolism,* 2nd edn, D.A. Bender. Wiley (1985)

*Basic Biochemistry,* J. Edelman and J.M. Chapman. Heinemann (1978)

*Basic Biotechnology,* ed. P. Prave, U. Faust, W. Sittig and D.A. Sukatsch. VCH (1987)

*Biochemistry,* 2nd edn, A.H. Lehninger. Worth (1975)

*Carbohydrate Chemistry, Monosaccharides and their Oligomers,* Hassan S. El Khadem. Academic Press (1988)

*A Companion to Medical Studies,* Vol. 2, *Anatomy, Biochemistry, Physiology and Related Subjects,* 2nd edn, R. Passmore and J.S. Robson. Blackwell (1976)

*CRC Handbook of Laboratory Animal Science,* 3 vols, ed. E.C. Melby and N.H. Altman. CRC Press (1974–1976)

*Culture Media for Cells, Organs and Embryos,* ed. M. Rechcigl. CRC Press (1977)

*Culture Media for Microorganisms and Plants,* ed. M. Rechcigl CRC Press (1977)

*Dairy Chemistry and Physics,* P. Walstra and R. Jenness. Wiley (1984)

*Durum Chemistry and Technology,* ed. G. Fabriani and C. Lintas. American Association of Cereal Chemists (1988)

312

*Environmental Health Reference Book,* M.H. Jackson, G.P. Morris, P.G. Smith and J.F. Crawford. Butterworths (1988)

*Food, Beverage and Mycology,* ed. Larry Beuchat. AVI (1987)

*Food Biochemistry and Nutritional Value,* D.S. Robinson. Longman (1987)

*Food Biotechnology,* (1 and 2), ed. R.D. King and P.S.J. Cheetham. Elsevier (1988)

*Food: the Chemistry of its Components.* Royal Society of Chemistry (1988)

*Food Engineering Data Handbook,* G.D. Hayes. Longman (1988)

*Food Engineering Fundamentals,* J.C. Batty and S.L. Folkman. Wiley (1983)

*Food Microscopy,* ed. J.C. Vaughan. Academic Press (1979)

*Fundamentals of Biotechnology,* ed. P. Prave, U. Faust, U. Sittig and D.A. Sukatsch. VCH (1987)

*The Human Digestive System, its Functions and Disorders,* ed. L. Van der Reis and H.P. Lazar. Karger (1972)

*Human Growth and its Disorders,* W.A. Marshall. Academic Press (1977)

*Immunology,* ed. A. Baumgarten and F.R. Richards. CRC Press (Vol. I, Pt. I, 1978; Vol. I, Pt. II, 1979)

*Introduction to Biotechnology,* C.M. Brown, I. Campbell, and F.G. Priest. Blackwell (1987)

*An Introduction to Plant Breeding,* K. Moore and G.E. Russell. Blackwell (1982)

*Introduction to the Principles and Practice of Soil Science,* R.E. White. Blackwell (1979)

*Modern Carbohydrate Chemistry,* R. Brinkley. Marcel Dekker (1988)

*Principles of Immunology,* 2nd edn, ed. N.R. Rose and F. Milgrom. Macmillan (1979)

*Principles and Practice of Human Physiology,* ed. O.G. Edholm and J.S. Weiner. Academic Press (1981)

*Process Engineering in the Food Industry – Development and Opportunities,* ed. R.W. Field and J.A. Howell. Elsevier (1990)

*Review of Medical Physiology,* W.F. Ganong. Lange Medical Publication (1979)

*Statistical Procedures in Food Research,* ed. J.R. Piggott. Elsevier (1987)

*Textbook of Physiology and Biochemistry,* 8th edn, G.H. Bell, J.N. Davidson and D. Emslie-Smith. Churchill Livingstone (1972)

*The Theory of Plant Breeding,* H. Mayo. Oxford University Press (1980)

## COMMODITIES AND MATERIALS

*Bailey's Industrial Oil and Fat Products*, 4th edn, ed. D. Swern. Wiley (1979)

*Biscuits, Cookies and Crackers, The Principles of the Craft*, P. Wade. Elsevier (1988)

*Biscuits, Cookies and Crackers*, Vol. 2, N. Almond. Elsevier (1990)

*Brewing Science*, (Volumes 1–3), ed. J.R.A. Pollock. Academic Press (1979–1987)

*Butchering, Processing and the Preservation of Meat*, F. Ashbrook. VNR (1983)

*Cereal Production*, ed. E.J. Gallagher. Butterworths (1984)

*Cheese: Chemistry, Physics and Microbiology*, ed. P.F. Fox. Elsevier (1987)

*Cheese and Fermented Milk Foods*, 2nd edn, F. Kosikowski. Edwards Bros. (1977)

*The Chemistry and Technology of Edible Oils and Fats and their High Fat Products*, G. Hoffman. Academic Press (1989)

*Chemistry of Wine Making*, A.D. Webb. Advances in Chemistry Series No. 137, American Chemical Society (1974)

*Chocolate, Cocoa and Confectionery*, Bernard W.E. Minifie. VNR (1988)

*Citrus Nutrition and Quality*. American Chemical Society. Division of Agriculture and Food Chemistry Symposium (1980)

*Coffee*, 6 Vols, ed. R.J. Clarke and R. Macrae. Elsevier (1985–1988)

*Commercial Vegetable Processing*, ed. B.S. Luh and J.G. Woodroof. AVI (1988)

*Connective Tissue in Meat and Meat Products*, ed. A.J. Bailey and N.D. Light. Elsevier (1990)

*Developments in Food Carbohydrate*, ed. G.G. Birch and R.S. Shallenberger. Applied Science Publishers (1977)

*Developments in Meat Science*, ed. R.A. Lawrie. Applied Science Publishers (1980)

*Developments in Soft Drinks Technology*, ed. L.F. Green. Applied Science Publishers (1978)

*Egg and Poultry-Meat Processing*, W.J. Stadelman, V.M. Olson, G.A. Shemwell and S. Pasch. VCH Publishers (1988)

*Fats for the Future*, ed. R.C. Cambie. Ellis Horwood (1989)

*Fish Smoking and Drying*, ed. J.R. Burt. Elsevier (1988)

*Food Legumes*, ed. D.E. Kay. Tropical Institute, London (1979)

*An Introduction to Animal Husbandry*, J.O.L. King. Blackwell (1978)

*Meat Freezing*, ed. G. Charalambous. Elsevier (1990)

*Meat, Poultry and Seafood Technology*, R.L. Henrickson. Prentice-Hall (1978)

*Meat Science*, R.A. Lawrie. Pergamon Press (1977)

*Meat Technology*, F. Gerrard. Northwood Publications (1977)

*Micronutrients in Milk and Milk-Based Food Products*, ed. E. Renner. Elsevier (1990)

*Milk Production from Pasture*, C.W. Holmes *et al*. Butterworths, New Zealand (1987)

*Modern Cereal Science and Technology*, Y. Pomeranz. VCH (1987)

*Muscle and Meat Biochemistry*, A.M. Pearson and R.B. Young. Academic Press (1989)

*New Crops for Food Industry*, ed. Gerald Wickens, Nazmul Haq and Peter Day. Chapman and Hall (1988)

*Post-Harvest Physiology of Vegetables*, ed. J. Weichmann. Marcel Dekker (1987)

*Potato Processing*, W.F. Talburt and O. Smith. AVI (1987)

*Potato Science and Technology*, ed. G. Lisinska and W. Leszeynski. Elsevier (1990)

*Poultry, Meat and Egg Production*, Carmen R. Parkhurst and G.J. Mountney. AVI (1988)

*Processed Meats*, A.M. Pearson and F.W. Tauber. VNR (1984)

*Protein Resources and Technology*, M. Milner, N.S. Scrimshaw and D.I.C. Wang. Avi (1978)

*Recent Advances in Chemistry and Technology of Fats and Oils*, ed. R.J. Hamilton and A. Bhati. Elsevier (1987)

*Seafoods and Fish Oils in Human Health and Disease*, J.E. Kinsella. Marcel Dekker (1987)

*Seaweeds and their Uses*, V. J. Chapman. Chapman and Hall (1980)

*Seeds and their Uses*, C. Duffus and C. Slaughter. Wiley (1980)

*Technology of Cereals*, N.L. Kent. Pergamon Press (1978)

*Vegetable Production*, I.L. Nonnecke. AVI (1988)

*Water and Food Quality*, ed. T.M. Hardman. Elsevier (1990)

*West African Crops*, ed. F. Irwine. Oxford University Press (1974)

*World Vegetables: Principles, Production and Nutritive Values*, M. Yamaguchi. AVI (1983)

## FOOD PREPARATION AND GASTRONOMY

*Advances in Catering Technology*, ed. G. Glew. Applied Science Publishers (1980)

*The Chef's Guide to Practical Restaurant Cookery*, W. Emery. VNR (1988)

*The Complete Cookbook of American Fish and Shellfish*, J.F. Nicolas. VNR (1984)

*Cook-Freeze Catering Systems*, B. Boltman. Applied Science (1978)

*Food Portion Sizes*, Helen Crawley. HMSO (1988)

*A Dictionary of Gastronomy*, A.L. Simon and R. Howe. Nelson (1970)

*The Food of the Western World (An Encyclopedia of Food from Europe and North America)*, T. Fitzgibbon. Hutchinson (1976)

*Guidelines on Pre-cooked Chilled Foods.* UK Department of Health and Social Security. Committee on Medical Aspects of Food Policy (1980)

*The Hotel and Restaurant Business*, D.E. Lundberg. VNR (1988)

*Large Quantities Recipes*, Margaret E. Terrell and Dorothea V. Headlund. VNR (1988)

*Management for Productivity in the Hospitality Industry*, R.C. Mill. VNR (1989)

*Professional Guide to Alcoholic Beverages*, Kathy and Robert Lipinski. VNR (1988)

## FOOD SCIENCE

*Food Science*, 3rd edn, G.G. Birch, A.G. Cameron and M. Spencer. Pergamon Press (1986)

*Food Science*, 4th edn, N.N. Potter. AVI (1986)

*Food Structure and Behaviour*, J.M.V. Blanshard and P. Lillford. Academic Press (1987)

*Food Structure its Creation and Evaluation*, ed. J.R. Mitchell and J.M.V. Blanshard. Butterworths (1988)

*Food Theory and Applications*, ed. P.C. Paul and H.H. Palmer. Wiley (1972)

*Foundations of Food Science*, J. Hawthorn. Freeman (1981)

*Functional Properties of Food Components*, Yeshajahu Pomeranz. Academic Press (1985)

*Fundamentals of Food Chemistry*, W. Heimann. Translated, C. Morton. Ellis Horwood, AVI (1980)

*Introduction to Food Science and Technology*, G.F. Stewart and M.A. Amerine. Academic Press (1973)

*Principles of Food Science*, Part. I, *Food Chemistry*, ed. O.R. Fennema; Pt. II, *Physical Principles of Food Preservation*, ed. M. Karel, O.R. Fennema and D.B. Lund. Marcel Dekker (1979)

*The Science of Food. An Introduction to Food Science, Nutrition and Microbiology*, 2nd edn, P.M. Gaman and K.B. Sherrington. Pergamon Press (1981)

*Science of Food,* M. Bennion. Wiley (1980)

*Water Activity: Influences on Food Quality,* ed. L.B. Rockland and G.F. Stewart. Academic Press (1981)

*Water Activity: Theory and Applications to Food,* ed. L.B. Rockland and L.R. Beuchat. Marcel Dekker (1987)

*Water Relations of Foods,* ed. R.B. Duckworth. Academic Press (1976)

## GENERAL BOOKS

*Chemical Manipulation of Crop Growth and Development,* ed. J.S. McLaren. Butterworths (1982)

*A Colour Atlas of Food Quality Control,* Jane P. Sutherland and Alan V. Varnam. Wolfe Publishing (1986)

*CRC Handbook of Agricultural Productivity,* ed. M. Rechcigl. CRC Press (1981)

*CRC Handbook of Energy Utilization in Agriculture,* ed. D. Pimentel. CRC Press (1980)

*CRC Handbook of Pest Management in Agriculture,* ed. D. Pimentel. CRC Press (1981)

*CRC Handbook of Transportation and Marketing in Agriculture*: Vol. I, *Food Commodities*; Vol. II, *Field Crops,* ed. E.E. Finney. CRC Press (1981)

*Data for Biochemical Research,* ed. R.M.C. Dawson, D.C. Elliot, W.H. Elliot and K.M. Jones. Oxford University Press (1969)

*Dictionary of Microbiology and Molecular Biology,* P. Singleton and D. Sainsbury. Wiley (1987)

*Energy and Agriculture: Their Interacting Futures,* ed. Maurice Levy and John L. Robinson. Harwood Academic Publishers (1984)

*Fermented Foods of the World,* G. Campbell-Platt. Butterworths (1987)

*Food in Antiquity,* D. Brothwell and P. Brothwell. Thames and Hudson (1969)

*Food Cultism and Nutrition Quackery,* ed. G. Blix. Almqvist and Wiksell (1970)

*Food and Drink Manufacture – Good Manufacturing Practice.* Institute of Food Science and Technology (1987)

*Food Factories,* ed. A. Bartholomai. VCH (1986)

*Foods and Food Production Encyclopedia,* ed. Douglas M. Considine, P.E. and Glenn D. Considine. VNR (1982)

*Food, the Gift of Osiris,* W.J. Derby, P. Ghalioungui and L. Grivetti. Academic Press (1977)

*Food, Health and the Consumer,* T.R. Gormely, G. Downey and D. O'Beirne. Elsevier (1987)

*Food Industries Manual*, 22nd edn, ed. M.D. Ranken. Blackie (1988)

*Food Quality Control*, J.P. Sutherland and A.H. Varman. CRC Press (1985)

*Fundamentals of New Food Product Development*, R.C. Baker, P. Wong Hahn and K.R. Robbins. Elsevier (1988)

*Health or Hoax? The Truth about Health Food and Diets*, A.E. Bender. Elvendon Press (1985)

*Interfaces Between Agriculture, Nutrition and Food Science*, ed. K.T. Achaya. United Nations University (1984)

*An Introduction to Marine Ecology*, R.S.K. Barnes and R.N. Hughes. Blackwell (1982)

*The Merck Index. An Encyclopedia of Chemicals and Drugs*. Merck and Co. Inc., Rahway, N.J.

*Micro-organisms in the Production of Food*, ed. M.R. Adams. Elsevier (1986)

*Organic Chemicals from Biomass*, ed. I.S. Goldstein. CRC Press (1981)

*The Oxford Book of Food Plants*, G.B. Masefield, M. Wallis, S.G. Harrison and B.E. Nicholson. Oxford University Press (1969)

*Pigments in Fruits*, J. Gross. Academic Press (1987)

*Plant Pests and their Control*, P.G. Fenemore. Butterworths (1983)

*Quality Control in the Food Industry*, (Volumes 1–4, Second Edn), ed. S.M. Herschdoerfer. Academic Press (1985–1987)

*The Quality of Foods and Beverages: Chemistry and Technology*, 2 vols, ed. G. Charalabous and G. Inglett. Academic Press (1981)

*The Role of Food Safety in Health and Development*. WHO (1985)

*Safety and Quality in Food*, ed. DSA. Elsevier (1984)

*Soils and Agriculture*, P.B. Tinker. Blackwell (1981)

*Upgrading Wastes for Feeds and Food*, ed. D.A. Ledward, R.A. Lawrie and A.J. Taylor. Butterworths (1983)

*The Utilization and Recycle of Agricultural Wastes and Residues*, ed. M.L. Shuler. CRC Press (1980)

*World Food Marketing Systems*, ed. Erdener Kaynak. Butterworths (1986)


## HYGIENE AND MICROBIOLOGY

*CRC Handbook of Microbiology*, 4 vols, ed. A.I. Laskin and H. Lechevalier. CRC Press (1977–1981)

*Developments in Food Microbiology*, (1–4), ed. R.K. Robinson. Elsevier (1988)

*Factors Affecting Life and Death of Microorganisms*, ed. J.H.

Silliker, R.P. Elliott, A.C. Baird-Parker, F.L. Bryan, J.H.B. Christian, D.S. Clark, J.C. Olson and T.A. Roberts. Vol. I, The International Commission on Microbiological Specifications for Food (1980)

*Food Microbiology and Hygiene*, P.R. Hayes. Elsevier (1985)

*Foodborne Microorganisms and their Toxins*, ed. Merle D. Pierson and N.J. Stern. Marcel Dekker (1986)

*Food Processing and Food Hygiene*, B.C. Hobbs and R.J. Gilbert. Edward Arnold (1978)

*Fungi and Food Spoilage*, J.I. Pitt and Ailsa D. Hocking. Aademic Press (1985)

*Hygiene in Practice*, J.A. Murphy. Gill and Macmillan (1985)

*Introduction to Food Microbiology*, Vol. 8 of *Basic Microbiology*, R.G. Board. Blackwell (1982)

*An Introduction to Microbiology*, ed. J.F. Wilkinson, I.R. Booth, C.W. Gooday, J.I. Prosser, N.A.R. Gow and W.A. Hamilton. Blackwell (1986)

*Laboratory Methods in Food and Dairy Microbiology*, W.F. Harrigan and M.E. McCance. Academic Press (1976)

*Microbial Ecology of Foods*, ed. J.H. Silliker, R.P. Elliott, A.C. Baird-Parker, F.L. Bryan, J.H.B. Christian, D.S. Clark, J.C. Olson and T.A. Roberts. Vol. II, The International Commission on Microbiological Specifications for Food (1980)

*Microbiological Methods*, 6th edn, C.H. Collins and Patricia M. Lyne. Butterworths (1989)

*Microbiology*, ed. A. von Graevenitz: Vol. I, *General Topics*; Vol. II, *Fungi: Medical Mycological Methods*. CRC Press (1977)

*Microbiology of Food*. D.A. Mossel. University of Utrecht (1977)

*Microorganisms in Action: Concepts and Applications in Microbial Ecology*, ed. J.M. Lynch and J.E. Hobbie. Blackwell (1988)

*Practical Food Microbiology and Technology*, G.J. Mountney and W.A. Gould. AVI (1988)

## NUTRITION AND DIETETICS

*Animal Nutrition*, 7th edn, L.A. Maynard and J.K. Loosli. M-H series in Agricultural Sciences, University of Florida (1979)

*Artificial Feeds for the Young Infant*. HMSO (1982)

*Beef Cattle Feeding and Nutrition*, T.W. Perry. Academic Press (1980)

*Bogert's Nutrition and Physical Fitness*, 10th edn, G.M. Briggs and D.H. Calloway. Saunders (1979)

*Clinical Nutrition for the Health Scientist*, D.A. Roe. CRC Press (1981)

*Clinical Nutrition in Hospital Practice*, D.B.A. Silk. Blackwell (1981)

*A Colour Atlas of Nutritional Disorders*, D.S. McLaren. Wolfe Medical (1981)

*CRC Handbook of Nutritional Requirements in a Functional Context*, ed. M. Rechcigl. CRC Press (1981)

*Diets for Mammals*, ed. M. Rechcigl. CRC Press (1977)

*Diets for Sick Children*, D.E.M. Francis. Blackwell (1974)

*Elemental Diets*, ed. R.I. Russell. CRC Press (1981)

*The Facts of Food*, A.E. Bender. Oxford University Press (1975)

*Fats in Animal Nutrition*, ed. J. Wiseman. Butterworths (1984)

*Food Acceptance and Nutrition*, ed. J. Solms, D. Booth, R. Pangborn and O. Raunhardt. Academic Press (987)

*Food, Nutrition and Diet Therapy*, 6th edn, M.V. Krause and L.K. Mahan. Saunders (1979)

*Food Processing and Nutrition*, A.E. Bender. Academic Press (1978)

*Food Science, Nutrition and Health*, B.A. Fox and A.G. Cameron. Edward Arnold (1989)

*Growth of Farm Animals*, T.L.J. Lawrence and V.R. Fowler. Butterworths (1988)

*Handbook of Clinical Dietetics*, American Dietetic Association. Yale University Press (1981)

*Handbook of Enteral and Parenteral Nutrition*, ed. A.M. Grant and E. Todd. Blackwell (1981)

*Handbook of Human Nutritional Requirements*. FAO (1980)

*Handbook of Vitamins*, ed. L.J. Machlin. Marcel Dekker (1984)

*Handbook of Normal and Therapeutic Nutrition*, Eagles and Randall. Raven Press (1980)

*Human Nutrition and Dietetics*, R. Passmore and M.A. Eastwood. Churchill-Livingstone (1986)

*Interfaces between Agriculture, Nutrition and Food Science*, ed. J.S. Kanwar. UNU (1985)

*International Perspectives in Food, Diet and Health*, ed. M.L. Wahlqvist, R.W.F. King, J.J. McNeil and R. Sewell. John Libby (1987)

*Iron Fortification of Foods*, ed. Fergus M. Clydesdale and Kathryn L. Wiemer. Academic Press (1985)

*Laboratory Tests for Assessment of Nutritional Status*, H.E. Sauberlich and J.H. Skala. CRC Press (1981)

*Mineral Nutrition of Animals*, V.I. Georgievski, B.N. Annenkov and V.T. Samokhin. Butterworths (1982)

*Mowry's Basic Nutrition and Diet Therapy*, 6th edn, S.R. Williams. Mosby (1980)

320

*New Protein Foods*, ed. A.A. Altschul. *Technology* 1A 1974; *Technology* 2B 1976. Pergamon Press

*Nutrient Requirements of Poultry*, ed. C. Fisher and K.N. Boorman. Butterworths (1986)

*Nutritional Enhancement of Food (Benefits, Hazards and Technical Problems)*. Institute of Food Science and Technology (1989)

*Nutritional Disorders*: Vol. I, *Effect of Nutrient Excesses and Toxicities*; Vol. II, *Effect of Nutrient Deficiencies in Animals*; Vol. III, *Effect of Nutrient Deficiencies in Man*, M. Rechcigl. CRC Press (1978)

*Nutritional Evaluation of Food Processing*, ed. E. Karmas and R.S. Harris. VNR (1988)

*Nutritional Evaluation of Protein Foods*, ed. Peter L. Pellett and Vernon R. Young. United Nations University (1980)

*Nutritional Requirements*, ed. M. Rechcigl. CRC Press (1977)

*Nutrition in Health and Disease*, ed. R.J. Jarrett. Croom Helm (1979)

*Nutrition in Health and Disease*, M. Winick. Wiley (1980)

*Nutrition for Medical Students*, A.E. Bender and D.A. Bender. Wiley (1982)

*Nutrition, Physiology and Obesity*, ed. R. Schemmel. CRC Press (1980)

*Patient Problems in Clinical Nutrition: A Manual*, ed. M.L. Wahlqvist and J.S. Vobecky. John Libby (1986)

*Protein-Energy Requirement Studies in Developing Countries*, ed. William M. Rand, Ricardo Uauy and Nevin S. Scrimshaw. United Nations University (1984)

*Recent Developments in Pig Nutrition*, ed. C. Fisher and K.N. Boorman. Butterworths (1986)

*The Role of Fats in Human Nutrition*, ed. A.J. Vergroesen and M. Crawford. Academic Press (1989)

*Textbook of Paediatric Nutrition*, ed. D.S. McLaren and D. Burman. Churchill-Livingstone (1982)

*Trace Elements in Human and Animal Nutrition*, 4th edn, E.J. Underwood. Academic Press (1977)

*Trace Metals in Health and Disease*, ed. N. Kharasch. Raven Press (1979)

*The Value of Food*, P. Fisher and A.E. Bender. Oxford University Press (1979)

*The Vitamins*, 6 vols, W.N. Pearson, W.H. Sebrell and R.S. Harris. Academic Press (1967–1972)

*Vitamins in Human Biology and Medicine*, ed. M.H. Briggs. CRC Press (1981)

*Vitamins in Medicine*, 4th edn, ed. B.M. Barker and D.A. Bender. Heinemann Medical (Vol. 1, 1980; Vol. 2, 1982)

# PROCESSING METHODS

*Canned Foods. Thermal Processing and Microbiology*, 7th edn, A.C. Hersom and E.D. Hulland. Churchill Livingstone (1980)

*The Canning of Low Acid Foods*. UK Department of Health and Social Security, and others. Food Hygiene Codes of Practice, 10 (1981)

*Chemical Engineering and the Environment*, Vol. III, *Critical Reports on Applied Chemistry*, ed. A.S. Teja. Blackwell (1981)

*Cook-Freeze Catering Systems*. B. Boltman. Applied Science Publishers (1978)

*CRC Handbook of Tables of Commercial Thermal Processes for Low-acid Canned Foods*, ed. C.R. Stumbo, K.S. Purohit, T.V. Ramakrishnan, D.A. Evans and F.J. Francis. CRC Press (1981)

*Effects of Heating on Foodstuffs*, ed. R.J. Priestley. Applied Science Publishers (1979)

*Energy in Food Processing*, ed. A. Spicer. Elsevier (1986)

*Enzymes in Food Processing*, G. Reed. Academic Press (1975)

*Extrusion of Foods*, J.M. Harper. CRC Press (1981)

*Food Engineering Operations*, J.G. Brennan, J.R. Butters, N.D. Cowell and A.E.V. Lilly. Applied Science Publishers (1976)

*Food Factories, Processes, Equipment, Costs*, A. Bartholomai. VCH Publishers (1987)

*Food Irradiation*, W.M. Urbain. Academic Press (1986)

*Food Processing Technology, Principles and Practice*, P. Fellows. VCH Publishers (1988)

*Food Quality and Nutrition – Research Priorities for Thermal Processing*, ed. W.K. Downey. Applied Science Publishers (1978)

*Food Engineering, Principles and Selected Applications*, M. Loncin and R.L. Merson. Academic Press (1979)

*Food Process Engineering*, 2 vols, ed. P. Link, Y. Malkki, J. Olkku and J. Larenkari. Applied Science Publishers (1980)

*Freeze Drying and Advanced Food Technology*, ed. S.A. Goldblith, L. Rey and W.W. Rothmayr. Academic Press (1975)

*Frying of Food. Principles, Changes, New Approaches*, ed. G. Varela, A.E. Bender and I.D. Morton. VCH-Ellis Horwood (1988)

*Guide Lines for the Preparation and Handling of Chilled Foods*. Institute of Food Science and Technology (1990)

*Heat Transfer and Food Products*, B. Hallstrom, G. Skjoldebrand and G. Tragardh. Elsevier (1988)

*Immobilized Enzymes for Food Processing*. W.H. Pitcher. CRC Press (1980)

*Industrialization of Indigenous Fermented Foods*, K.H. Steinkraus. Marcel Dekker (1989)

*Intermediate Moisture Foods*, R. Davies, G.G. Birch and K.J. Parker. Applied Science Publishers (1976)

*Irradiation of Dry Food Ingredients*, ed. J. Farkas. CRC Press (1988)

*Microwave Heating*, D.A. Copson (1975)

*Microwave Processing and Engineering*, R.V. Decareau and R.L. Peterson. VCH (1986)

*Microwaves in the Food Processing Industry*, R. V. Decareau. Academic Press (1985)

*Pasta and Extrusion Cooked Foods*, ed. Ch. Mercier and C. Cantarelli. Elsevier (1986)

*Physical, Chemical and Biological Changes in Food Caused by Thermal Processing*, ed. T. Hoyem and O. Kvale. Applied Science Publishers (1977)

*Physical Principles of Food Preservation*, ed. M. Karel, O. Fennema and D.B. Lund. Marcel Dekker (1975)

*Physical Properties of Foods and Food Processing Systems*, M.J. Lewis. VCH Publishers (1987)

*Preservation in the Food, Pharmaceutical and Environmental Industries*, ed. R.G. Board, M.C. Allwood and J.G. Banks. Blackwell (1987)

*Radiation Chemistry of Major Food Components*, ed. P.S. Elias and A.J. Cohen. Elsevier (1977)

*Safety of Irradiated Foods*, J.F. Diehl. Marcel Dekker (1989)

*The Technology of Food Preservation*, N.W. Desrosier and J.N. Desrosier. Avi (1977)

*Ultra High Temperature Sterilisation of Milk and Milk Products*, H. Burton. Elsevier (1988)

*Wholesomeness of Irradiated Food*. United Nations World Health Organization, Technical Report Series, 659 (1981)


## REGULATORY

*Butterworths Law of Food and Drugs*, ed. A.A. Painter, Butterworths (looseleaf work)

*Consumers Protection Legislation and the US Food Industry*, M.J. Hinich and R. Staelin. Pergamon (1980)

*Food Legislation of the UK*, 2nd edn, D.J. Jukes. Butterworths (1987)

*The Food Legislative System in the UK*, S. Fallows and J.V. Wheelock. Butterworths (1988)

*International Food Regulation Handbook,* ed. R.D. Middlekauff and P. Shubik. Marcel Dekker (1989)

*International Regulatory Aspects for Pesticide Chemicals,* G. Vettorazzi, CRC Press (1981)

*Meat Inspection,* J. Infante Gil. CRC Press (1989)

*OECD Directory of Food Policy Institutes,* compiled by D. Miller and M. Soranna. OECD (1982)

*The Regulatory Status of Direct Food Additives,* ed. T.E. Furia. CRC Press (1980)

*United States Food Laws, Regulations and Standards,* Y.H. Hui. Wiley (1986)

*Use and Regulation of Vitamin and Mineral Supplements,* A. Bruce, E. Helsing and G. Dukes. WHO (1987)

## SENSORY PROPERTIES

*Applied Sensory Analysis of Foods,* Vols. 1 and 2, ed. H. Moskowitz. CRC Press (1988)

*Biochemistry of Taste and Olfaction,* ed. R.H. Cagan and M.R. Kare. Academic Press (1981)

*Developments in Food Colours,* ed. J. Walford. Applied Science Publishers (1980)

*Flavor of Foods and Beverages: Chemistry and Technology.* American Chemical Society. Division of Agriculture and Food Chemistry Symposium (1978)

*Flavour Science and Technology,* ed. M. Martens, G.A. Dalen and H. Russwurm. Wiley (1987)

*Food Emulsifiers,* ed. G. Charalambous and G. Doxastakis. Elsevier (1989)

*Food Flavours,* ed. I.D. Morton and A.J. MacLeod. Elsevier (1990)

*Food Texture: Instrumental and Sensory Measurement,* ed. H.R. Moskowitz. Marcel Dekker (1987)

*Principles of Sensory Evaluation of Food,* M.A. Amerine, E.B. Pangborn and E.B. Roesler. Academic Press (1966)

*Progress in Flavour Research,* ed. D.G. Land and H.E. Nursten. Applied Science Publishers (1979)

*Sensory Evaluation of Food,* G. Jellinek. VCH (1985)

*Sensory Evaluation Practices,* H. Stone and J.L. Sidel. Academic Press (1985)

*Sensory Properties of Foods,* ed. G.G. Birch, J.G. Brennan and K.J. Parker. Applied Science Publishers (1977)

*Sweetness,* J. Dobbing. Springer-Verlag (1986)

# TOXICOLOGY

*Antinutrients and Natural Toxicants in Foods*, R.L. Ory. Food and Nutrition Press (1981)

*Food Toxicology*, S.L. Taylor and R.A. Scanlan. Marcel Dekker (1989)

*Food Toxicology – Real or Imaginary Problems?* ed. G.G. Gibson and R. Walker. Taylor and Francis (1985)

*Introduction to Biochemical Toxicology*, E. Hodgson and F.E. Guthrie. Blackwell (1980)

*Introduction to Environmental Toxicology*, F.E. Guthrie and J.J. Perry. Blackwell (1980)

*Moulds, Toxins and Foods*, C. Moreau. Wiley (1979)

*Mycotoxins in Food*, Palle Krogh. Academic Press (1987)

*Natural Toxicants in Food*, ed. D.H. Watson. VCH (1987)

*Nutritional Toxicology*, ed. J.N. Hathcock. Academic Press, Vol. I (1982); Vol II (1987)

*Report on the Working Party on Pesticide Residues 1982–1985.* MAFF (1986)

*Toxicity of Pure Foods*, E.M. Boyd. CRC Press (1973)

*Toxic Constituents of Animal Foodstuffs*, I.E. Liener. Academic Press (1974)

*Toxic Constituents of Plant Foodstuffs*, ed. I.E. Liener. Academic Press (1980)

*Toxicological Aspects of Food*, ed. Klara Miller. Elsevier (1987)

*Toxicology*, ed. I. Sunshine. CRC Press (1978)

# Appendix

**Table 1 Prefixes and symbols for decimal multiples and submultiples of units**

| | | |
|---|---|---|
| tera | T | $10^{12}$ |
| giga | G | $10^{9}$ |
| mega | M | $10^{6}$ |
| kilo | k | $10^{3}$ |
| hecto | h | $10^{2}$ |
| deca (deka) | da | $10^{1}$ |
| deci | d | $10^{-1}$ |
| centi | c | $10^{-2}$ |
| milli | m | $10^{-3}$ |
| micro | μ | $10^{-6}$ |
| nano | n | $10^{-9}$ |
| pico | p | $10^{-12}$ |
| femto | f | $10^{-15}$ |
| atto | a | $10^{-18}$ |

**Table 2 European Community proposals for directives on nutrition labelling, vitamins and minerals which may be declared and their recommended daily allowances**

| | |
|---|---|
| Vitamin A (μg) | 1000 |
| Vitamin D (μg) | 5 |
| Vitamin E (mg) | 10 |
| Vitamin C (mg) | 60 |
| Thiamin (mg) | 1.4 |
| Riboflavin (mg) | 1.6 |
| Niacin (mg) | 18 |
| Vitamin $B_6$ (mg) | 2 |
| Folacin (μg) | 400 |
| Vitamin $B_{12}$ (μg) | 3 |
| Biotin (mg) | 0.15 |
| Pantothenic acid (mg) | 6 |
| Calcium (mg) | 800 |
| Phosphorus (mg) | 800 |
| Iron (mg) | 12 |
| Magnesium (mg) | 300 |
| Zinc (mg) | 15 |
| Iodine (μg) | 150 |

**Table 3 Recommended intakes – Food and Agriculture Organisation**

| Subject | Age (years) | kcal | MJ | Protein (g/kg) | Calcium (g) |
|---|---|---|---|---|---|
| Children | 0–1 | 110 per kg | 0.47 | 1–3 | 0.5–0.6 |
| | 1–3 | 1360 | 5.7 | 1.19 | 0.4–0.5 |
| | 4–6 | 1830 | 7.6 | 1.01 | 0.4–0.5 |
| | 7–9 | 2190 | 9.2 | 0.88 | 0.4–0.5 |
| Boys | 10–12 | 2600 | 10.9 | 0.81 | 0.6–0.7 |
| | 13–15 | 2900 | 12.1 | 0.72 | 0.6–0.7 |
| | 16–19 | 3100 | 13.0 | 0.60 | 0.5–0.6 |
| Adults | | 3000 | 12.6 | 0.57 | 0.4–0.5 |
| Girls | 10–12 | 2350 | 9.8 | 0.76 | 0.6–0.7 |
| | 13–15 | 2500 | 10.5 | 0.63 | 0.6–0.7 |
| | 16–19 | 2300 | 9.6 | 0.55 | 0.5–0.6 |
| Adults | | 2200 | 9.2 | 0.52 | 0.4–0.5 |
| Pregnancy | | +350 | +1.5 | +9 | 1.0–1.2 |
| Lactation | | +550 | +2.3 | +17 | 1.0–1.2 |

| Subject | Age (years) | Vitamin C (mg) | Vitamin D (µg) | Vitamin $B_{12}$ (µg) | Folate (µg) |
|---|---|---|---|---|---|
| Children | 0–1 | 20 | 10 | 0.3 | 50 |
| | 1–3 | 20 | 10 | 0.9 | 100 |
| | 4–6 | 20 | 10 | 1.5 | 100 |
| | 7–9 | 20 | 2.5 | 1.5 | 100 |
| Boys | 10–12 | 20 | 2.5 | 2.0 | 100 |
| | 13–15 | 30 | 2.5 | 2.0 | 200 |
| | 16–19 | 30 | 2.5 | 2.0 | 200 |
| Adults | | 30 | 2.5 | 2.0 | 200 |
| Girls | 10–12 | 20 | 2.5 | 2.0 | 100 |
| | 13–15 | 30 | 2.5 | 2.0 | 200 |
| | 16–19 | 30 | 2.5 | 2.0 | 200 |
| Adults | | 30 | 2.5 | 2.0 | 200 |
| Pregnancy | | 50 | 10 | 3.0 | 400 |
| Lactation | | 50 | 10 | 2.5 | 300 |

* If animal foods, comprise 10–25% of energy intake.

From *Requirements of Vitamin A, Thiamin, Riboflavin and Niacin*, WHO Rpt. No. 362 (1967), *Energy and Protein Requirements*, WHO Rpt. No. 522 (1973) and *Requirements of Ascorbic Acid, Vitamin D, Vitamin $B_{12}$, Folate and Iron*, WHO Rpt. No. 452 (1970).

**Table 3** (*continued*)

| Iron (mg) | Vitamin A (i.u.) | (μg) | Thiamin (mg) | Riboflavin (mg) | Niacin (mg) |
|---|---|---|---|---|---|
| 7 | 100 | 300 | 0.4 | 0.6 | 6.6 |
| 7 | 800 | 240 | 0.5 | 0.7 | 8.6 |
| 7 | 1000 | 300 | 0.7 | 0.9 | 11.2 |
| 7 | 1300 | 390 | 0.8 | 1.2 | 13.9 |
| 7 | 1900 | 570 | 1.0 | 1.4 | 16.5 |
| 12 | 2400 | 720 | 1.2 | 1.7 | 20.4 |
| 6 | 1500 | 750 | 1.4 | 2.0 | 23.8 |
| 6 | 2500 | 750 | 1.3 | 1.8 | 21.1 |
| 18 | 2400 | 720 | 1.0 | 1.4 | 17.2 |
| 18 | 2400 | 720 | 1.0 | 1.4 | 17.2 |
| 19 | 2500 | 750 | 1.0 | 1.3 | 15.8 |
| 19 | 2500 | 750 | 0.9 | 1.3 | 15.2 |
| 19 | 2500 | 750 | 0.4/1000 kcal | 0.55/1000 kcal | 6.6/1000 kcal |
| 19 | 4000 | 1200 | 0.4/1000 kcal | 0.55/1000 kcal | 6.6/1000 kcal |

**Table 4 Recommended intakes of nutrients for the UK (1979\*)**

| Age range | Occupational category | Body weight (kg) | Energy (kcal) | (MJ) | Protein (g) |
|---|---|---|---|---|---|
| **BOYS AND GIRLS** | | | | | |
| 0 up to 1 year | | 7.3 | 800 | 3.3 | 20 |
| 1 up to 2 years | | 11.5 | 1200 | 5.0 | 30 |
| 2 up to 3 years | | 13.5 | 1400 | 5.9 | 35 |
| 3 up to 5 years | | 16.5 | 1600 | 6.7 | 40 |
| 5 up to 7 years | | 20.5 | 1800 | 7.5 | 45 |
| 7 up to 9 years | | 25.1 | 2100 | 8.8 | 53 |
| **BOYS** | | | | | |
| 9 up to 12 years | | 31.9 | 2500 | 10.5 | 63 |
| 12 up to 15 years | | 45.5 | 2800 | 11.7 | 70 |
| 15 up to 18 years | | 61.0 | 3000 | 12.6 | 75 |
| **GIRLS** | | | | | |
| 9 up to 12 years | | 33.0 | 2300 | 9.6 | 58 |
| 12 up to 15 years | | 48.6 | 2300 | 9.6 | 58 |
| 15 up to 18 years | | 56.1 | 2300 | 9.6 | 58 |
| **MEN** | | | | | |
| 18 up to 55 years | Sedentary | 65 | 2700 | 11.3 | 68 |
| | Moderately active | | 3000 | 12.6 | 75 |
| | Very active | | 3600 | 15.1 | 90 |
| 35 up to 65 years | Sedentary | 65 | 2600 | 10.9 | 65 |
| | Moderately active | | 2900 | 12.1 | 73 |
| | Very active | | 3600 | 15.1 | 90 |
| 65 up to 75 years | Assuming a | 63 | 2350 | 9.8 | 59 |
| 75 and over | sedentary life | 63 | 2100 | 8.8 | 53 |
| **WOMEN** | | | | | |
| 18 up to 55 years | Most occupations | 55 | 2200 | 9.2 | 55 |
| | Very active | | 2500 | 10.5 | 63 |
| 55 up to 75 years | Assuming a | 53 | 2050 | 8.6 | 51 |
| 75 and over | sedentary life | 53 | 1900 | 8.0 | 48 |
| Pregnancy, 2nd and 3rd trimester | | | 2400 | 10.0 | 60 |
| Lactation | | | 2700 | 11.3 | 68 |

\* Revised figures will be published in 1991.

**Table 4** (*continued*)

| Thiamin | Ribo-flavin | Nicotinic acid | Ascorbic acid | Vitamin A | Vitamin D | Calcium | Iron |
|---|---|---|---|---|---|---|---|
| (mg) | (mg) | (mg equivalent) | (mg) | (µg) | (µg chole-calciferol) | (mg) | (mg) |
| 0.3 | 0.4 | 5 | 15 | 450 | 10 | 600 | 6 |
| 0.5 | 0.6 | 7 | 20 | 300 | 10 | 500 | 7 |
| 0.6 | 0.7 | 8 | 20 | 300 | 10 | 500 | 7 |
| 0.6 | 0.8 | 9 | 20 | 300 | 10 | 500 | 8 |
| 0.7 | 0.9 | 10 | 20 | 300 | 2.5 | 500 | 8 |
| 0.8 | 1.0 | 11 | 20 | 400 | 2.5 | 500 | 10 |
| 1.0 | 1.2 | 14 | 25 | 575 | 2.5 | 700 | 13 |
| 1.1 | 1.4 | 16 | 25 | 725 | 2.5 | 700 | 14 |
| 1.2 | 1.7 | 19 | 30 | 750 | 2.5 | 600 | 15 |
| 0.9 | 1.2 | 13 | 25 | 575 | 2.5 | 700 | 13 |
| 0.9 | 1.4 | 16 | 25 | 725 | 2.5 | 700 | 14 |
| 0.9 | 1.4 | 16 | 30 | 750 | 2.5 | 600 | 15 |
| 1.1 | 1.7 | 18 | 30 | 750 | 2.5 | 500 | 10 |
| 1.2 | 1.7 | 18 | 30 | 750 | 2.5 | 500 | 10 |
| 1.4 | 1.7 | 18 | 30 | 750 | 2.5 | 500 | 10 |
| 1.0 | 1.7 | 18 | 30 | 750 | 2.5 | 500 | 10 |
| 1.2 | 1.7 | 18 | 30 | 750 | 2.5 | 500 | 10 |
| 1.4 | 1.7 | 18 | 30 | 750 | 2.5 | 500 | 10 |
| 0.9 | 1.7 | 18 | 30 | 750 | 2.5 | 500 | 10 |
| 0.8 | 1.7 | 18 | 30 | 750 | 2.5 | 500 | 10 |
| 0.9 | 1.3 | 15 | 30 | 750 | 2.5 | 500 | 12 |
| 1.0 | 1.3 | 15 | 30 | 750 | 2.5 | 500 | 12 |
| 0.8 | 1.3 | 15 | 30 | 750 | 2.5 | 500 | 10 |
| 0.7 | 1.3 | 15 | 30 | 750 | 2.5 | 500 | 10 |
| 1.0 | 1.6 | 18 | 60 | 750 | 10 | 1200 | 15 |
| 1.1 | 1.8 | 21 | 60 | 1200 | 10 | 1200 | 15 |

**Table 5 US recommended daily allowances (1989)**

| Category | Age (years) or condition | Weight (kg) | Weight (lb) | Height (cm) | Height (in) | Protein (g) | Fat-soluble vitamins Vit. A (µg RE)* | Vit. D (µg) | Vit. E (mg µ-TE)† | Vit. K (µg) |
|---|---|---|---|---|---|---|---|---|---|---|
| Infants | 0.0–0.5 | 6 | 13 | 60 | 24 | 13 | 375 | 7.5 | 3 | 5 |
|  | 0.5–1.0 | 9 | 20 | 71 | 28 | 14 | 375 | 10 | 4 | 10 |
| Children | 1–3 | 13 | 29 | 90 | 35 | 16 | 400 | 10 | 6 | 15 |
|  | 4–6 | 20 | 44 | 112 | 44 | 24 | 500 | 10 | 7 | 20 |
|  | 7–10 | 28 | 62 | 132 | 52 | 28 | 700 | 10 | 7 | 30 |
| Males | 11–14 | 45 | 99 | 157 | 62 | 45 | 1000 | 10 | 10 | 45 |
|  | 15–18 | 66 | 145 | 176 | 69 | 59 | 1000 | 10 | 10 | 65 |
|  | 19–24 | 72 | 160 | 177 | 70 | 58 | 1000 | 10 | 10 | 70 |
|  | 25–50 | 79 | 174 | 176 | 70 | 63 | 1000 | 5 | 10 | 80 |
|  | 51+ | 77 | 170 | 173 | 68 | 63 | 1000 | 5 | 10 | 80 |
| Females | 11–14 | 46 | 101 | 157 | 62 | 46 | 800 | 10 | 8 | 45 |
|  | 15–18 | 55 | 120 | 163 | 64 | 44 | 800 | 10 | 8 | 55 |
|  | 19–24 | 58 | 128 | 164 | 65 | 46 | 800 | 10 | 8 | 60 |
|  | 25–50 | 63 | 138 | 163 | 64 | 50 | 800 | 5 | 8 | 65 |
|  | 51+ | 65 | 143 | 160 | 63 | 50 | 800 | 5 | 8 | 65 |
| Pregnant |  |  |  |  |  | 60 | 800 | 10 | 10 | 65 |
| Lactating | 1st 6 months |  |  |  |  | 65 | 1300 | 10 | 12 | 65 |
|  | 2nd 6 months |  |  |  |  | 62 | 1200 | 10 | 11 | 65 |

* RE = retinol equivalents
† α-TE = α-tocopherol equivalents

**Table 5** (continued)

| | Water-soluble vitamins | | | | | | | Minerals | | | | | | |
|---|---|---|---|---|---|---|---|---|---|---|---|---|---|---|
| Vit. C (mg) | Thiamin (mg) | Riboflavin (mg) | Niacin (mg NE)* | Vit. B$_6$ (mg) | Folate (µg) | Vit. B$_{12}$ (µg) | Calcium (mg) | Phosphorus (mg) | Magnesium (mg) | Iron (mg) | Zinc (mg) | Iodine (µg) | Selenium (µg) |
| 30 | 0.3 | 0.4 | 5 | 0.3 | 25 | 0.3 | 400 | 300 | 40 | 6 | 5 | 40 | 10 |
| 35 | 0.4 | 0.5 | 6 | 0.6 | 35 | 0.5 | 600 | 500 | 60 | 10 | 5 | 50 | 15 |
| 40 | 0.7 | 0.8 | 9 | 1.0 | 50 | 0.7 | 800 | 800 | 80 | 10 | 10 | 70 | 20 |
| 45 | 0.9 | 1.1 | 12 | 1.1 | 75 | 1.0 | 800 | 800 | 120 | 10 | 10 | 90 | 20 |
| 45 | 1.0 | 1.2 | 13 | 1.4 | 100 | 1.4 | 800 | 1200 | 170 | 12 | 10 | 120 | 30 |
| 50 | 1.3 | 1.5 | 17 | 1.7 | 150 | 2.0 | 1200 | 1200 | 270 | 12 | 15 | 150 | 40 |
| 60 | 1.5 | 1.8 | 20 | 2.0 | 200 | 2.0 | 1200 | 1200 | 400 | 10 | 15 | 150 | 50 |
| 60 | 1.5 | 1.7 | 19 | 2.0 | 200 | 2.0 | 800 | 800 | 350 | 10 | 15 | 150 | 70 |
| 60 | 1.5 | 1.7 | 15 | 2.0 | 200 | 2.0 | 800 | 800 | 350 | 10 | 15 | 150 | 70 |
| 60 | 1.2 | 1.4 | 15 | 2.0 | 200 | 2.0 | 1200 | 1200 | 350 | 15 | 15 | 150 | 70 |
| 50 | 1.1 | 1.3 | 15 | 1.4 | 150 | 2.0 | 1200 | 1200 | 280 | 15 | 12 | 150 | 45 |
| 60 | 1.1 | 1.3 | 15 | 1.5 | 180 | 2.0 | 1200 | 1200 | 300 | 15 | 12 | 150 | 50 |
| 60 | 1.1 | 1.3 | 15 | 1.6 | 180 | 2.0 | 800 | 800 | 280 | 10 | 12 | 150 | 55 |
| 60 | 1.0 | 1.2 | 13 | 1.6 | 180 | 2.0 | 800 | 800 | 280 | 10 | 12 | 150 | 55 |
| 70 | 1.5 | 1.6 | 17 | 2.2 | 400 | 2.2 | 1200 | 1200 | 320 | 30 | 15 | 175 | 65 |
| 95 | 1.6 | 1.8 | 20 | 2.1 | 280 | 2.6 | 1200 | 1200 | 355 | 15 | 19 | 200 | 75 |
| 90 | 1.6 | 1.7 | 20 | 2.1 | 260 | 2.6 | 1200 | 1200 | 340 | 15 | 16 | 200 | 75 |

* NE = niacin equivalent

There is insufficient information on which to base figures for biotin and pantothenate, so a range of estimated Safe and Adequate Daily Dietary Intakes of these vitamins and the trace elements are stated. (The upper levels for the trace elements should not be habitually exceeded since toxic levels may be only several times usual intakes.)

| Category | Age (years) | Biotin (µg) | Pantothenic acid (mg) |
|---|---|---|---|
| Infants | 0–0.5 | 10 | 2 |
| | 0.5–1 | 15 | 3 |
| Children and adolescents | 1–3 | 20 | 3 |
| | 4–6 | 25 | 3–4 |
| | 7–10 | 30 | 4–5 |
| | 11+ | 30–100 | 4–7 |
| Adults | | 30–100 | 4–7 |

Trace elements

| Category | Age (years) | Copper (mg) | Manganese (mg) | Fluoride (mg) | Chromium (µg) | Molybdenum (µg) |
|---|---|---|---|---|---|---|
| Infants | 0–0.5 | 0.4–0.6 | 0.3–0.6 | 0.1–0.5 | 10–40 | 15–30 |
| | 0.5–1 | 0.6–0.7 | 0.6–1.0 | 0.2–1.0 | 20–60 | 20–40 |
| Children and adolescents | 1–3 | 0.7–1.0 | 1.0–1.5 | 0.5–1.5 | 20–80 | 25–50 |
| | 4–6 | 1.0–1.5 | 1.5–2.0 | 1.0–2.5 | 30–120 | 30–75 |
| | 7–10 | 1.0–2.0 | 2.0–3.0 | 1.5–2.5 | 50–200 | 50–150 |
| | 11+ | 1.5–2.5 | 2.0–5.0 | 1.5–2.5 | 50–200 | 75–250 |
| Adults | | 1.5–3.0 | 2.0–5.0 | 1.5–4.0 | 50–200 | 75–250 |

**Table 6 Average portions of food** (energy and protein content of edible portions)

| Food | Size of average portion (oz) | Energy per average portion (kcal) | (MJ) | Protein (g) |
|------|------|------|------|------|
| Apple | 4 | 50 | 0.21 | 0.4 |
| Apple pudding | 4 | 280 | 1.1 | 3 |
| Bacon, gammon | 2 | 250 | 1.4 | 18 |
| Banana | 4 | 80 | 0.33 | 1 |
| Beans, baked | 4 | 100 | 0.42 | 7 |
| Beans, butter | 2 | 50 | 0.21 | 4 |
| Beans, French | 2 | 4 | 0.02 | 0.4 |
| Beef, lean only | 4 | 250 | 1.04 | 30 |
| Beetroot | 2 | 30 | 0.13 | 1 |
| Blancmange | 2 | 70 | 0.29 | 2 |
| Bread | 3 slices | 280 | 1.17 | 9.6 |
| Bread with butter | | 390 | 1.63 | 9.6 |
| Butter | 1 | 230 | 0.96 | 0 |
| Cabbage | 4 | 10 | 0.04 | 0.8 |
| Cake, cherry | 2 | 260 | 1.09 | 5 |
| Cakes | 2 | 240 | 1.00 | 4 |
| Carrots | 2 | 10 | 0.04 | 0.4 |
| Cauliflower | 2 | 6 | 0.03 | 0.8 |
| Cereal, breakfast | 1 | 100 | 0.42 | 1.9 |
| Cheese | 1 | 120 | 0.50 | 7.2 |
| Chicken, boiled or roast | 4 | 220 | 9.20 | 33 |
| Cod, fried | 6 | 240 | 1.00 | 30 |
| Egg | 2 | 90 | 0.38 | 7 |
| Fish cakes | 4 | 240 | 1.00 | 14 |
| Ham, boiled | 4 | 490 | 2.05 | 18 |
| Jelly | 4 | 90 | 0.38 | 2.4 |
| Kidney, stewed | 4 | 180 | 0.75 | 29 |
| Lettuce, raw | 2 | 5 | 0.02 | 0.6 |
| Luncheon meat, canned | 4 | 380 | 1.6 | 13 |
| Margarine | 1 | 230 | 0.96 | 0 |
| Marrow, boiled | 2 | 4 | 0.02 | 0.2 |
| Milk | 1 glass | 130 | 0.54 | 6.3 |
| Mince-pie | 2 | 220 | 0.92 | 7 |
| Nuts, Brazil, Barcelona | 2 | 360 | 1.50 | 16 |
| Nuts, pea | 2 | 340 | 1.40 | 16 |
| Orange | 4 | 40 | 0.17 | 0.8 |
| Peas, fresh, boiled | 2 | 30 | 0.13 | 3 |
| Pineapple, canned in syrup | 4 | 70 | 0.29 | 0.4 |
| Plaice, fried | 6 | 390 | 1.63 | 30 |
| Plaice, steamed | 6 | 150 | 0.63 | 30 |
| Potatoes, boiled | 6 | 140 | 0.59 | 2.4 |
| Potatoes, chipped | 6 | 410 | 1.71 | 7 |
| Potatoes, roast | 6 | 210 | 0.88 | 5 |
| Salmon | 4 | 160 | 0.67 | 22 |
| Salmon, canned | 6 | 240 | 0.96 | 22 |
| Sardines in oil | 1 | 85 | 0.35 | 6 |

**Table 6** (*continued*)

| Food | Size of average portion (oz) | Energy per average portion (kcal) | (MJ) | Protein (g) |
|---|---|---|---|---|
| Sardines in tomato | 1 | 50 | 0.20 | 6 |
| Sausage roll | 2 | 260 | 1.09 | 4.6 |
| Sausages, fried, pork | 2 | 360 | 1.50 | 13 |
| Spaghetti, macaroni | 4 | 130 | 0.54 | 4 |
| Sprouts | 4 | 20 | 0.08 | 3 |
| Stew, Irish | 4 | 170 | 0.71 | 4.4 |
| Suet pudding | 4 | 420 | 1.69 | 6 |
| Tomato, raw | 2 | 10 | 0.04 | 0.6 |
| Trifle | 4 | 160 | 0.67 | 4 |